Food Allergies

FOR

DUMMIES®

Food Allergies FOR DUMMIES®

by Robert A. Wood, MD, with Joe Kraynak

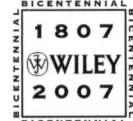

BICENTENNIAL
1807
WILEY
2007
BICENTENNIAL

Wiley Publishing, Inc.

Food Allergies For Dummies®

Published by
Wiley Publishing, Inc.
111 River St.
Hoboken, NJ 07030-5774
www.wiley.com

WILEY

About the Authors

Robert A. Wood, MD, is Professor of Pediatrics and International Health and Chief of Pediatric Allergy and Immunology at the Johns Hopkins University School of Medicine in Baltimore, Maryland. After receiving his medical degree from the University of Rochester School of Medicine, he completed his residency in pediatrics at the Johns Hopkins University, where he also completed an allergy and immunology fellowship. Dr. Wood is an internationally recognized expert in food allergy and childhood asthma and has published over 100 manuscripts in scientific journals, including the New England Journal of Medicine, JAMA, Pediatrics, and the Journal of Allergy and Clinical Immunology, as well as two books and numerous book chapters. He is Deputy Editor of the journal Pediatric Allergy and Immunology, was Associate Editor of the Annals of Allergy, Asthma, and Immunology, and has served on the editorial board of the Journal of Allergy and Clinical Immunology. He is on the Board of Directors of the American Board of Allergy and Immunology. He personally cares for over 4,000 patients with food allergy and has a special interest in this topic as someone with a severe, lifelong peanut allergy.

Joe Kraynak is a freelance author who has written and co-authored dozens of books on topics ranging from slam poetry to computer basics. Joe teamed up with Dr. Candida Fink to write his first book in the *For Dummies* series, *Bipolar Disorder For Dummies*, where he showcased his talent for translating the parlance of psychiatry into plain-spoken practical advice. He then tackled *Flipping Houses For Dummies* with legendary real estate pro Ralph Roberts to produce the ultimate guide for real estate rehabbers. In *Food Allergies For Dummies,* Joe returns to the doctor's office with world-renowned allergist, Robert Wood, MD, to pen the definitive guide to living well with food allergies.

For additional details about the authors, late breaking food allergy research, and more practical information on the diagnosis and treatment of food allergies, visit Dr. Robert Wood's Food Allergy website at www.drrobertwood.com.

Dedication

From Robert Wood: To my wife, Renee Melly Wood, DVM, for her unbelievable patience and support, to my parents, Dr. Bob and Carol Wood, for their consistent support and lifelong example of hard work, integrity, and compassion to all, and to my brother David, for all he taught me about life before his tragic death.

From Joe: In memory of my brother Mitch, a brilliant physician and an outstanding human being who passed away well before his time.

Authors' Acknowledgments

Although we wrote the book, dozens of other talented individuals contributed to its conception, development, and perfection. Special thanks go to acquisitions editor Lindsay Lefevere, who chose us as the authors and guided us through the tough part of getting started. Jennifer Connolly, our project editor, deserves a round of applause for acting as a very patient collaborator and choreographer — shuffling chapters back and forth, shepherding the text and photos through production, and asking a whole lot of questions to ensure that you would have all *your* questions answered. We also tip our hats to the production crew for doing such an outstanding job of transforming a loose collection of text and illustrations into such an attractive bound book.

We owe special thanks to the folks at FAAN (Food Allergy and Anaphylaxis Network), especially FAAN founder Anne Munoz-Furlong, for gathering the recipes for the delectable dishes served up in the appendix and for writing the foreword for our book.

We owe a huge debt of gratitude to a few people who have played a special role in moving the field of food allergy forward. From a scientific standpoint, Drs. Hugh Sampson and Scott Sicherer at Mt. Sinai School of Medicine and Dr. Wesley Burks at Duke University School of Medicine led the way in moving the study of food allergy to the 21st century. From a personal standpoint, we would once again like to acknowledge Anne Munoz-Furlong for what she and FAAN have done to provide the leadership and resources that we all rely on to educate everyone — from patients to schools to doctors — about what it means to live with food allergy.

We owe special thanks to our technical editor, accomplished allergist John M. James, MD, for ferreting out technical errors in the manuscript, helping guide its content, and offering his own advice, guidance, and tips.

Publisher's Acknowledgments

We're proud of this book; please send us your comments through our Dummies online registration form located at www.dummies.com/register/.

Some of the people who helped bring this book to market include the following:

Acquisitions, Editorial, and Media Development

Project Editor: Jennifer Connolly

Acquisitions Editor: Lindsay Lefevere

Copy Editor: Jennifer Connolly

Technical Editor: John M. James, MD

Editorial Manager: Michelle Hacker

Editorial Supervisor: Carmen Krikorian

Editorial Assistants: Erin Calligan, Joe Niesen, LeeAnn Harney, David Lutton

Cover Photo: © Cole Group/Getty Images

Cartoons: Rich Tennant (www.the5thwave.com)

Composition Services

Project Coordinator: Lynsey Osborn

Layout and Graphics: Claudia Bell, Carl Byers, Joyce Haughey, Shane Johnson, Stephanie D. Jumper, Alicia B. South, Julie Trippetti

Proofreaders: Jessica Kramer, Susan Moritz, Sossity R. Smith

Indexer: Aptara

Wiley Bicentennial Logo: Richard J. Pacifico

Publishing and Editorial for Consumer Dummies

Diane Graves Steele, Vice President and Publisher, Consumer Dummies

Joyce Pepple, Acquisitions Director, Consumer Dummies

Kristin A. Cocks, Product Development Director, Consumer Dummies

Michael Spring, Vice President and Publisher, Travel

Kelly Regan, Editorial Director, Travel

Publishing for Technology Dummies

Andy Cummings, Vice President and Publisher, Dummies Technology/General User

Composition Services

Gerry Fahey, Vice President of Production Services

Debbie Stailey, Director of Composition Services

Contents at a Glance

Table of Contents

Part IV: The Part of Tens....................................269

Chapter 16: Teaching Your Child Ten Key Food Allergy Lessons 271

Chapter 17: Packing Ten Key Food Allergy Tips for Camp, College, and Other Outings 279

Foreword

. . . .

*A*s the incidence of food allergy continues to increase in the U.S., particularly in children, the need for an easy-to-read book also has increased. With *Food Allergies For Dummies,* Dr. Wood has provided all of us with a handy reference tool.

As someone who has a peanut allergy, he is in a unique position to write this book. Dr. Wood understands this topic personally and professionally. His easy-to-read writing style and calm demeanor make him a favorite among patients throughout the country and around the world.

The articles he writes for parents are reprinted by organizations around the world. At FAAN's annual meetings, Dr. Wood is a favorite speaker. Families travel thousands of miles to visit his clinic at Johns Hopkins Hospital in Baltimore, Maryland. For those with young children, he helps unravel the mystery and brings a diagnosis and treatment plan that helps the children and their families. Teens, the highest risk group for severe or fatal reactions, visit his office to hear from someone who really does understand the opposing forces of striving for independence while having to be cautious and always ready for the unexpected reaction.

His writing style leaves you feeling like you know him. Most importantly, he touches on all the key topics — including why peanuts cause so many reactions, why food allergy is increasing, and where you are likely to find allergens. Dr. Wood shares his personal experiences with peanut allergy reactions, reminding us all that even one of the world's leading experts sometimes has reactions. He helps us learn from his mistakes and how to assess risks to minimize stress or worry.

If you are looking for a book that you can sit and read quietly, this is it. If you need a book you can use as a reference tool, this one fits that bill too. You won't be disappointed with *Food Allergies For Dummies.* You'll find yourself recommending it to everyone you know, just like the patients who travel long distances just to speak to Dr. Wood.

Anne Munoz-Furlong
Founder and CEO
The Food Allergy & Anaphylaxis Network

Introduction

*W*hen I was about nine months old, my mother gave me a bit of peanut butter on her finger. My face immediately doubled in size. Fortunately, I grew up in a small town and the hospital was only a few minutes away. My mother, who is a pediatric nurse, took me straight to my pediatrician, who also happened to be my father. They quickly treated me and made the diagnosis based on the reaction alone.

When I turned two years old, I had my second reaction. The standard practice at the time was that when you turned two, you would retry any food you had been allergic to as an infant. Bad idea, but at least I got to visit my father at work again.

After that second incident, I led a charmed life. We avoided peanuts and my parents established strict rules around the house. My seven sisters and brothers followed the rules, and I managed to stay safe at home. Away from home, I avoided obvious peanut products but ate everything else — baked goods, desserts, ice cream, candy, you name it. Back then, we had little knowledge of food allergy and certainly no precautionary labels on foods. In retrospect I believe I was just lucky. I was especially lucky because prescribing and carrying epinephrine were not standard practices in those days. I had no real strategy to avoid peanuts, no action plan, no medications. And this was not because proper medical care was unavailable. In fact, I received the best of care and was actually a patient of the world's most renowned pediatric allergist of the 1950s and '60s — Dr. Jerome Glaser.

My charmed existence was rudely interrupted by a tainted brownie in ninth grade. The cafeteria had changed the recipe after receiving a large supply of surplus peanut butter. It really was an awakening for my parents and me. I started paying more attention to what I was eating — as did the cafeteria workers in my school — and was given a vial of epinephrine and a syringe to carry around with me.

A few years later, I experienced another severe reaction when I ate a sugar cookie from a bakery that must have been contaminated. I have since had three more reactions — one to spaghetti when I was in college, one to a piece of coconut cream pie, and a third to another contaminated cookie.

Undoubtedly, my personal experience of living with a severe peanut allergy coupled with the fact that I was raised by medical professionals led me down the path to becoming an allergist specializing in food allergy. Currently, I personally care for over 4,000 patients with food allergies, and I have treated thousands more over the course of my career. I'm also actively and passionately involved in performing cutting-edge research to track down the root cause of food allergies, discover superior preventions and treatment options, and hopefully discover a cure.

In *Food Allergies For Dummies*, I pass along the knowledge and insights I've gathered over my nearly 50 years of living with, studying, researching, and treating food allergies. I present strategies and tips for avoiding exposure and preventing reactions. I reveal medications and treatment options that can quell symptoms ranging from minor to severe. I point out unproven, untested options that simply waste your time and money. I show you exactly what to do in the event of an emergency. And, I offer guidance on how to live well with food allergies at home, school, and work; while dining out; and as you're traveling for business or pleasure.

My capable co-author and I thoroughly enjoyed collaborating on this project to create what we believe is the best food allergy management guide on the planet. We hope that you and your family, friends, teachers, and childcare and healthcare providers enjoy reading this book as much as we enjoyed writing it. We also hope that the information contained in this book protects you from harm and improves your quality of life for years to come.

About This Book

On a daily basis, I see patients who have been undiagnosed, misdiagnosed, and over-diagnosed. Often, they have no idea which foods trigger their symptoms, because they haven't been properly tested and evaluated. In some cases, their doctors subject them to too many tests, misinterpret the test results, and saddle their patients with an overly restrictive diet that not only compromises the patient's quality of life but can actually lead to malnutrition. I've seen young children whose diets are unnecessarily restricted to less than ten foods!

I don't want you or your loved ones to suffer unnecessarily from a bad or nonexistent diagnosis. In *Food Allergies For Dummies*, I arm you with the information and insight you need to assess the care you're receiving and team up with your doctor to identify the foods that ail you, without mistakenly eliminating from your diet foods that are perfectly safe. An accurate diagnosis is key to successful treatment and a fuller culinary and nutritional life.

Food Allergies For Dummies can't and doesn't even attempt to act as a surrogate for skilled and knowledgeable medical care. Your family doctor and allergist play the leading roles in your diagnosis and treatment. This book plays a supporting role, expediting your diagnosis and treatment and enhancing your life by:

- Assisting you in determining if and when you need to seek professional medical advice for diagnosis and treatment based on your symptoms.

✔ Guiding you in selecting the medical professionals who are best qualified to diagnose and treat food allergies (and are covered on your health
insurance policy).

✔ Providing you with the information you need to more effectively team up
with your healthcare providers to arrive at an accurate diagnosis and
obtain the most effective medical treatments, without overly restricting
your diet.

✔ Empowering you to take control of your allergies by presenting practical, plain-English advice, tips, and strategies for living well with food
allergies at home, work, and school, while dining out, and on vacation or
business trips.

✔ Saving your life by showing you how to construct your own food allergy
emergency kit and follow life-saving procedures if you or a loved one
experiences a severe allergic reaction.

Although *Food Allergies For Dummies* is packed from cover to cover with
valuable information, advice, and tips, you don't have to read it from cover to
cover. We broke the information down into easily digestible parts, chapters,
sections, subsections, and even sub-subsections, so you can dip in at any
point in the book and find just the information you need. Of course, I don't
want to discourage you from reading the entire book — if you skip around
too much, you're likely to skip right over some golden nuggets.

Conventions Used in This Book

I don't like to think of *my* book as *conventional,* but I do have some standard
ways of presenting material. For example, whenever I introduce a new, somewhat technical term, such as *anaphylaxis,* I italicize it. A commonly used term
that's not necessarily a technical term, I enclose "in quotes," but for the life of
me, I can't really remember a chapter in which I actually quoted something.
Web site addresses appear in `monofont` and never hyphenated, even if they
run longer than a line of text; simply type the address into your Web browser
exactly as it appears.

In almost every chapter, I include intriguing research on food allergy or stories about people who've walked into my clinic with a suspected food allergy
and emerged after successful diagnosis and treatment feeling a whole lot
better. These stories aren't necessarily about real people — to protect their
privacy, I composed composites of real case studies I've diagnosed and
treated over my many years in practice.

In a few chapters I include fill-in-the-blank forms you can scribble on.
Although you can fill out these forms in the book, you may want to make
copies to write on, especially if you borrowed the book from your library or

plan on re-selling it on eBay when you're done with it. These forms are incredibly valuable at empowering you to take a more pro-active role in your diagnosis and treatment.

Even though you see two author names on the cover of this book — Robert Wood and Joe Kraynak — you see "I" throughout the book when I, Robert (you can call me Dr. Wood or Dr. Bob), am offering expert advice, presenting research data, and describing patients. Joe's the word maestro who fiddled with the language to make it sound just right. Although Joe knows much more about food allergies after having worked with me, he's careful not to hand out medical advice.

What You're Not to Read

The best way to ingest and digest the information in this book is to read every word of it from cover to cover. Joe and I toiled tirelessly to provide you with everything you need to know and do to live well with your food allergy, and I'd hate for you to fast forward through the juicy parts.

You can, however, safely skip anything you see in a gray shaded box. I stuck case studies and technical information you really don't need to know in these boxes, to clue you into the fact that this is optional reading material. I doubt that you'll want to skip the case studies, because they provide real world examples of people who struggle with the same food allergy issues that you and your family now face, and they offer hope for a full, symptom-free life ahead.

Foolish Assumptions

In some books that cover advanced topics, authors must assume that their readers already understand some basic topics or have acquired beginning-level skills. For example, if this were a book about biochemistry, you'd have to know a little about chemistry, first. To read, understand, and apply the information in this book to your life requires no prerequisites. This book, along with expert medical care and a moderate amount of cooperation from those around you, are all you need to start feeling better.

I do, however, make a few foolish assumptions about who *you* are. I figure your situation matches one or more of the following scenarios:

- ✔ You experience unexplained symptoms that seem to arise or worsen after eating.
- ✔ Your doctor has diagnosed you as having a food allergy, but you're still experiencing symptoms.

✔ Your doctor has diagnosed you as having a food allergy and placed you on a severely restricted diet, and you're determined to find ways to introduce more variety into your diet and live a fuller life.

✔ You're a parent or caregiver of someone who has food allergies, and you want to know what you could and should be doing to help.

✔ You're a medical professional who needs or wants to learn more about food allergies in order to diagnose and treat your patients more effectively.

✔ You're a teacher or school administrator who wants some definitive answers about food allergies, so you can more effectively discern real risks from overblown claims and put an effective and reasonable food allergy policy into place.

✔ Your friend has a food allergy, and you want to know what you can do to help.

✔ You're just plain curious.

How This Book Is Organized

I wrote this book so you could approach it in either of two ways. You can read the book from cover-to-cover or pick up the book and flip to any chapter for a quick, stand-alone mini-course on a specific food allergy topic. To help you navigate, I divvied up the 19 chapters that make up the book into five parts. Here, I provide a quick overview of what I cover in each part.

Part I: Feasting on Food Allergy Fundamentals

This part begins with a primer that touches on almost every topic covered in the book, so you can accelerate from 0 to 60 in about 18 pages. I proceed to present you with an explanation of the food-allergy connection, lead you on an exploration of common causes and symptoms, point out the top allergens and their favorite hiding places, and finish up with some practical advice on effectively dealing with the very common, often scary peanut allergy.

Part II: Progressing from Hives to Hope: Diagnosis and Treatment

The key to whipping food allergies is to arrive at an accurate diagnosis, eliminate the problem foods, and treat any lingering symptoms or unexpected reactions with allergy medications. In this part, I show you how to work with your doctor to streamline the diagnostic process, identify the specific foods that are triggering your reactions, and develop an effective treatment plan to keep reactions at bay.

Here you develop skills for deciphering food labels, so you can more effectively avoid the foods that ail you. I reveal the most effective medications for providing symptomatic relief, and I warn you of unproven, often costly, alternative tests and treatments. Finally, I present cutting edge research that may lay the path to an eventual cure.

Part III: Living Well with Your Food Allergies

After you step out of your doctor's office with diagnosis and perhaps prescriptions in hand, you return to your daily life and need to know how to manage your food allergy in your day-to-day activities. The chapters in this part show you how to apply the information your doctor provided to your workaday and play-a-day world, so you can more safely and fully enjoy your life. Here you gain the knowledge and skills required to cope with your food allergies at home, on the road, in daycare, in preschool, and from kindergarten to your senior year in high school.

In this part, I also offer tips that show teens and tweens how to play a more active role in managing their food allergies in the face of sometimes daunting peer pressure. I show you how likely it is (or isn't) that you will eventually outgrow your food allergy, and offer some tips that may assist you in increasing your chances.

Part IV: The Part of Tens

No *For Dummies* book is complete without a Part of Tens. Turn to this part for a list of ten key food allergy lessons to pass along to your children, ten tips to enlighten your child's caregiver at daycare or preschool, ten common dietary substitutions to help out in the kitchen, and the top ten food allergy Web sites where you can gather even more advice and support.

Appendixes: Allergy-Friendly Recipes and Other Treats

Food allergies may reduce your recipe box to a meager collection of index cards for only the blandest of dishes. In this part, you begin to restock your box with several time-tested, patient-recommended recipes that treat the palate, satisfy your appetite, and nourish your body all at the same time.

FAAN (Food Allergy and Anaphylaxis Network) generously provided me access to its vast collection of recipes, and I selected the recipes that my patients most often recommend.

In this part, I also include a collection of food-allergy-related terms and their definitions, making it easy for you to look up a definition as you're reading the book or doing your own extra research.

Icons Used in This Book

Throughout this book, I've sprinkled icons in the margins to cue you in on different types of information that call out for your attention. Here are the icons you'll see and a brief description of each.

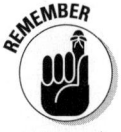

If you remember nothing else in a particular chapter, remember anything that's marked with one of these icons.

Tips provide insider insight from behind the scenes. When you're looking for a better, faster way to do something, check out these tips.

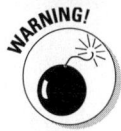

"Whoa!" This icon appears when you need to remain extra vigilant or seek professional medical guidance before moving forward.

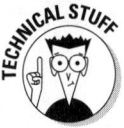

When I drift off and start using more doctor jargon than usual, I warn you by marking the text with this "Technical Stuff" icon. I do, however, try my best to present the more technical material in plain English.

Where to Go from Here

Think of this book as an all-you-can-eat buffet. You can grab a plate, start at the beginning and read one chapter right after another, or you can dip in any chapter and pile your plate high with the information it contains.

If you're looking for a quick overview of food allergies along with their diagnosis and treatment, check out Chapter 1. Chapters 5 and 6 are key, so if you're skipping around, don't miss these essential chapters. They contain everything you need to know to obtain effective medical care and avoid the foods that cause discomfort.

If you're already under the care of a doctor, and you're satisfied with the results, you can safely skip to any of the chapters in Part III to gather tips and strategies for dealing with food allergies in different places and situations.

When you need some quick tips to pass along to your kids or their care-givers, Part IV is the place to go. Here you can also find a list of dietary sub-stitutions and food allergy Web sites.

If you get hungry, head to the appendix at the back of the book, where you can find recipes for breakfast, lunch, dinner, and dessert.

Finally for some quick tips, tricks, and tools, check out the Cheat Sheet pro-vided at the very beginning of this book, just past the front cover. Better yet, tear it out (preferably not in the bookstore or from a library copy), and carry the Cheat Sheet with you for quick reference.

Of course, after reading the book, you're welcome to dip back into it at any time to pick up something you missed or take a brief refresher course.

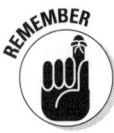

Exposures and reactions are not always preventable, so always carry your medications just in case and be prepared for unexpected reactions.

Part I
Feasting on Food Allergy Fundamentals

The 5th Wave
By Rich Tennant

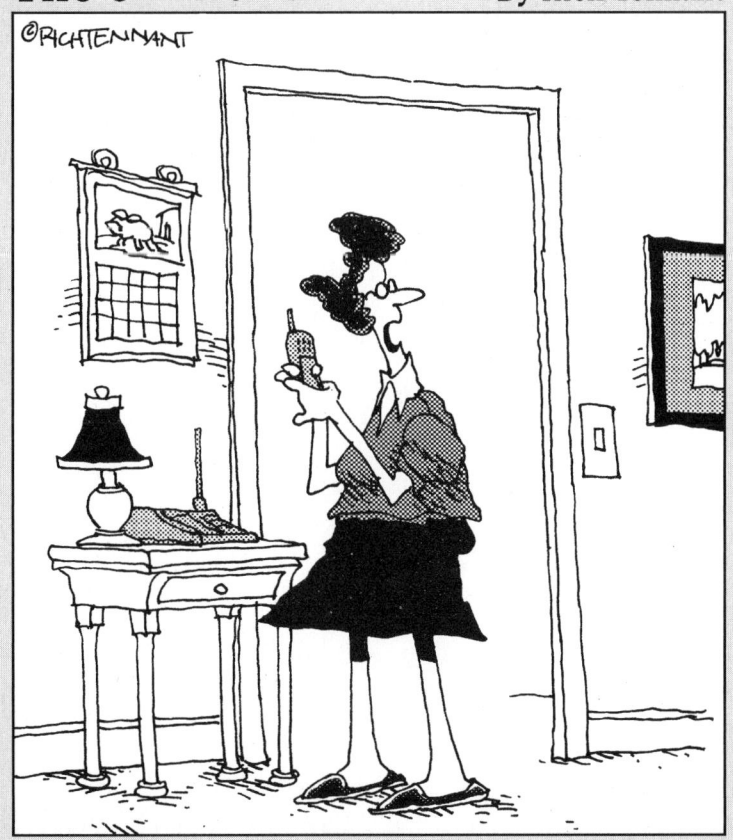

"Beth says she can come to the dinner party, but she's allergic to nuts. Does that mean we can't invite your brother?"

In this part . . .

When your immune system wages war against the very foods that nourish you, your body becomes the battlefield. As your immune system mounts its attack against the invading forces, your body bears the brunt and responds with some form of dis-ease and discomfort — hives, eczema, abdominal cramps, sneezing, wheezing, fainting, or a host of other symptoms . . . perhaps even a potentially deadly case of anaphylaxis.

You don't have to be a casualty of the food allergy war. Armed with the medical intelligence provided in this part, you can gain a deeper understanding of the food–immune system connection and can begin to identify the foods that most commonly confuse the immune system. But first, I provide a quick primer on food allergies to get you up to speed in a hurry and expedite the process of removing offending foods from your diet, pacifying your immune system, and enhancing your postdiagnosis life.

Chapter 1

Breaking Out with Food Allergies

*W*hen you begin to suspect that you or one of your family members has a food allergy, all sorts of questions pop up:

✔ How did I become allergic?

✔ What can I do to stop feeling so miserable?

✔ What should I do if I begin to have a reaction?

✔ Can my doctor cure me?

In this chapter, I get you up to speed in a hurry about food allergies. After pointing out what is an allergy and what's not, I show you how to spot the common signs and symptoms, obtain an accurate diagnosis, avoid the foods that ail you, and relieve your misery with symptomatic treatments. I also reveal what researchers currently believe causes food allergies and some of the possible future cures you have to look forward to.

Pinning Down Food Allergy: What's an Allergy, and What's Not?

Due to a lack of accurate information and an overabundance of misinformation about food allergies, many people have developed misconceptions about what a food allergy really is. Some people think that if you get sick after eating a particular food, you're allergic to that food. Others think that if a food makes you tired, you're allergic to it, or that a craving for a particular food is a sign of allergy, or if your pulse rate rises after eating, you're allergic. The general public often lumps every adverse symptom they have after eating a food as an allergic reaction when this, in fact, is not the case.

In the following sections, I define *food allergy* and then reveal some common conditions that produce similar symptoms to those produced by food allergies but are actually something quite different.

Defining food allergy

Food allergies are sort of like overprotective parents. Trying too hard to do the best for their children, they often cause more harm. In the case of food allergies, an overprotective immune system, attempting to defend you from harmful viruses and bacteria, misidentifies harmless substances in foods as harmful to your health and wages all-out warfare to purge them from your system. This overreaction by the immune system may be enough to kill you.

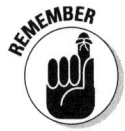

So what exactly is a food allergy? A *food allergy* is an immune system response that creates antibodies to attack substances in a food that your immune system identifies as harmful to you. In the process, the reaction releases huge stores of chemical substances, including histamines, which cause symptoms ranging from a mild case of hives to a potentially life-threatening system shutdown. For a description of exactly what happens during an allergic reaction, refer to Chapter 2.

Identifying imposters

Foods can make you feel sick for a variety of reasons, most of which have nothing to do with food allergies. This leaves the door open to quackologists selling all sorts of ineffective cures and treatments for a host of ailments that they falsely attribute to food allergies. To avoid getting sucked in by misinformation, be aware that the following ailments are rarely, if ever, related to food allergies:

- **Food intolerances:** The inability to digest a particular food, such as milk or wheat, is typically related to a missing enzyme in the digestive system that prevents a person from fully digesting the food.

- **Food poisoning:** Some foods may have toxins or bacteria that make you sick. Just because a food makes you sick one time does not mean you're allergic to it, although you should have your doctor check it out.

- **Histamine poisoning:** When you have an allergic reaction, your body releases histamine into your system, which causes most of the symptoms you experience. Some foods, including strawberries, chocolate, wine, and beer, may contain enough histamine to produce similar reactions, but these are not bona fide allergic reactions.

✔ **Reactions to food additives:** MSG (monosodium glutamate) and sulfites often cause reactions, but in these cases, the body has a chemical reaction, not an allergic reaction, to the additive, not to the food itself.

✔ **Other common ailments:** Food allergy is blamed for everything from migraine headaches to irritable bowel syndrome, but most of these ailments are caused by something other than a food allergy. Don't waste your time chasing the food allergy ghost. Work with your doctor to identify the real cause and obtain more effective treatments.

For additional information on reactions that are often mistaken for food allergy reactions, check out Chapter 2.

Meeting the Many Faces of Food Allergies: Signs and Symptoms

When your immune system flips out and starts dumping histamine into your system, all sorts of nasty stuff can happen. The histamine can attack just about every organ in your body, including your skin, lungs, and gastrointestinal (GI) tract, triggering these common symptoms:

✔ Hives, swelling, or an itchy rash

✔ Itching or swelling of the lips, tongue, or mouth

✔ Tightening of the chest, hoarseness, or coughing

✔ Abdominal cramps, vomiting, diarrhea, or nausea

✔ Fainting or passing out, paleness, blueness, irregular heartbeat

✔ Coughing, wheezing, difficulty breathing

✔ Fear of impending doom, panic, chills, sudden weakness

✔ Death, if effective emergency treatment is not immediately administered

Symptoms can appear within minutes after eating and completely disappear in an hour or two after you eat the problem food, making diagnosis a snap. In many cases, however, symptoms slowly creep up on you over the course of several hours. If you're allergic to a common food, such as wheat or milk, or to several foods, and symptoms arise slowly and take a long time to go away, you may not even suspect food allergy as the cause, and diagnosis can be much more challenging.

An accurate diagnosis is the first step toward obtaining effective treatment. See Chapter 2 for details about symptoms. In Chapter 5, I show you how to team up with your doctor to obtain an accurate diagnosis and identify the food or foods that are causing problems.

Investigating the Conspiracy: Allergens and Other Contributing Factors

When you experience an allergic reaction, your immediate concern is probably not what caused it but how to make it stop. After receiving some relief, however, your curiosity is likely to get the better of you, and you may begin to wonder why you have this condition in the first place.

The following sections explore the two factors that lead to the onset of food allergies and the possible reason why some foods are more likely to trigger allergy onset than others.

Digging up the root cause of food allergy

Research shows that the onset of food allergies is primarily due to a one-two punch of nature and nurture — genetics and environment:

1. You're born genetically susceptible to some sort of allergic condition.

2. Exposure to even a small amount of the food sensitizes your immune system to the food. Your immune system produces antibodies to attack the food next time it enters your system. Upon your first exposure, you may not experience symptoms; your immune system is just gearing up for next time.

3. You consume the problem food again, and your immune system, now sensitized to the allergen, leaps into action to purge the allergen from your system.

Food allergies typically show themselves in the first few months or years of life, and food allergy sufferers often outgrow their allergies by the time they're teenagers. Some food allergies, however, such as allergies to fish and shellfish appear later in life and rarely disappear over time. See Chapter 15 for details about your chances of outgrowing an allergy and for information on the possibility of preventing the onset of food allergies.

Playing the blame game

When people get sick, they naturally try to blame someone or something for their illness. They want to point fingers at the person who "gave me this cold" or blame their chronic headaches on "work-related stress." In the case of food allergies, there's plenty of blame to go around, as I point out in the following sections.

Blaming your parents: Genetic factors

Allergies run in families, but not as you may think. If one family member is allergic to milk, another may be allergic to peanut or develop asthma. If one or both parents have hay fever or asthma, their children may have hay fever, asthma, a food allergy, a combination of the three, or no allergy at all. In short, if any allergic condition is present in a family member, other family members are more susceptible to developing an allergic condition, not necessarily a food allergy.

For details on how genetics and environment co-contribute to the onset of food allergies and to determine the probability that any new addition to your family will develop food allergies, check out Chapter 2. Chapter 15 reveals strategies for possibly preventing the onset of food allergies and the likelihood of outgrowing particular food allergies.

Blaming your foods: Allergens

When you're allergic to a particular food, you may be tempted to blame the food — "I like peanuts, but peanuts don't like me." But the food itself is only partially to blame.

Foods that commonly spark allergic reactions, such as peanuts, eggs, milk, fish, and wheat, have uniquely structured protein molecules in them that make them a more identifiable target for your immune system. How your immune system responds to those proteins determines whether or not you experience an allergic reaction.

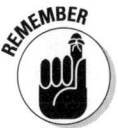

Currently, the most effective treatments for food allergies are to avoid the problem foods (to prevent reactions) and then relieve symptoms when reactions do occur. Researchers are looking for ways to train the immune system not to overreact. See Chapter 9 for details about the most promising research.

Labeling Your Maladies with a Doctor's Diagnosis

The first step in avoiding food allergy reactions and preventing future reactions requires a trip to your doctor, who can record your history, initiate allergy testing, rule out other potential causes, refer you to a qualified allergist, and provide advice and medications to keep you healthy until you can get in to see your allergist.

Then, the real work begins, as your allergist performs a complete food allergy workup to:

- ✔ Pin down food allergy as the cause of your symptoms.
- ✔ Identify the food or foods that trigger symptoms.
- ✔ Rule out foods that are suspected of triggering symptoms but really don't.

In the following sections, I provide a brief overview of the diagnostic process that leads from symptoms to cause. For additional guidance on obtaining the most accurate diagnosis possible, skip to Chapter 5.

Finding a food-allergy savvy allergist

Your family doctor is likely to refer you to an allergist she's worked with in the past. Many allergists, however, are more accustomed to working with hay fever and other environmental allergies and less with food allergies.

Knowing the benefits of a food-allergy savvy allergist

Choosing an allergist who's experienced with food allergies benefits you in four ways:

- ✔ The diagnosis may be quicker and less costly, because the allergist is likely to perform tests that focus on food allergies rather than on a host of other allergies.
- ✔ The allergist may be more aware of the risks of *false positive results* — test results that show you're allergic to something you're not really allergic to. False positives often lead to overly restricted diets that lower your quality of life and may even lead to malnutrition.
- ✔ Because skin tests can cause serious reactions in people with severe food allergies, the allergist is likely to have the necessary emergency medications on hand to properly treat you. (Severe reactions to skin tests are very rare.)
- ✔ The allergist won't order controversial tests that have been used by charlatans or quacks in the past. These tests can be very expensive and have no real bearing on the ultimate diagnosis of food allergy.

Choosing an allergist with the right stuff

If you have input on selecting the allergist, look for a combination of the following qualities:

- ✔ Experience in diagnosing and treating food allergies.
- ✔ Excellent interpersonal skills, so the allergist can effectively work with you to address all your concerns.

- ✔ Covered by your insurance, so you don't have high out-of-pocket expenses.

- ✔ Availability, so you can see the allergist as soon as possible and are likely to have little trouble scheduling follow-up appointments.

For details on selecting a top-notch allergist with the knowledge and experience required to diagnose and treat food allergies effectively, refer to Chapter 5.

Navigating the diagnostic process

A thorough food allergy workup consists of your medical history, a physical exam, and one or more tests to determine if you are, in fact, allergic to certain foods and to identify the problem foods. Your allergist is likely to perform one or more of the following tests:

- ✔ **Skin tests:** Skin tests consist of applying a tiny amount of the suspected allergen below the upper layer of the skin, usually by scratching or pricking the skin. A skilled allergist tests only the foods he suspects may cause reactions, based on the results of your history and physical exam, so no more than a few pokes with a needle are ever required.

- ✔ **Blood tests:** Your allergist may draw a vial of blood and test it for the presence of antibodies that indicate the probability of an allergy to a specific food. These blood tests are commonly referred to as RASTs (short for *radioallergosorbent tests*) but more accurately called *immunoassay for specific IgE*. IgE (or *Immunoglobulin E*) is a type of antibody that your immune system produces to attack a particular allergen. For each allergen, your body produces a different IgE, so if you're allergic to milk, your blood has IgE to attack allergenic substances in milk.

- ✔ **Food challenges:** To confirm a positive test result or gather more diagnostic data, your doctor may perform a controlled food challenge, in which you consume increasing amounts of a suspect food under your doctor's close supervision.

Don't try a food challenge at home. Food challenges carry a risk of serious reactions. Only trained personnel with emergency treatment immediately available should perform the test.

Considering food intolerances

Your body may react to certain foods in ways that can trick you into thinking you have an allergy when you don't. Instead of a food allergy, your body may lack the necessary chemicals to digest a particular food, which is considered an *intolerance,* not an allergy. Lactose intolerance is one such example, in which the body doesn't have the enzyme (lactase) it needs to break down milk sugars.

A lactose intolerant person is likely to experience stomach cramps, nausea, and vomiting — the same symptoms that may afflict someone who has a milk allergy — but the diagnosis and treatments are very different. With lactose intolerance, you can avoid milk or take a lactase supplement to enable you to digest the milk sugars. With a milk allergy, avoiding milk products and treating symptoms in the event of a severe reaction are the primary treatment options.

Battling Back with Medications, Modifications, and Other Therapies

I hate to be the bearer of bad news, but no matter how skilled your allergist is, she can't cure your food allergy at the present time. The best we allergists can do at this point is identify the problem foods, instruct you on how best to avoid them, and treat reactions when avoidance maneuvers fail, as they often do. In some cases, you simply outgrow the allergy, as explained in Chapter 15.

In the following sections, I discuss the three options you have at your disposal — avoidance, symptomatic treatment, and one alternative therapy that shows some promise.

Modifying your diet

The primary defense against future reactions is to stop eating what makes you sick. Yeah, you just shelled out good money for a book that tells you what you already knew. Avoidance, however, is more complicated and challenging than anyone can summarize in a bit of homespun wisdom. Effective avoidance requires vigilance and a coordinated effort to prevent any amount of the allergenic food from entering your system through measures, such as:

- **Meticulously reading labels for hidden ingredients:** I provide several food allergy field guides in Chapter 6 to assist you with this task.

- **Refusing foods from unknown or un-trusted sources:** Even a well-meaning friend can offer you what he considers an allergen-free batch of cookies that has enough of the allergen in it (perhaps from a tainted spoon or spatula) to trigger a reaction. If you're ever unsure about the specific ingredients or cannot confirm the absence of a particular ingredient, don't take chances with the food.

- **Preparing foods properly to avoid cross-contamination:** For example, cross-contamination may occur if you're allergic to milk and the same knife is used to cut a piece of cheese and then slice the meat for your sandwich. Chapter 10 provides guidelines for allergen-free food preparation and cooking.

✔ **Cleaning eating surfaces thoroughly before sitting down to eat:** In a school cafeteria, for example, tables should be thoroughly scrubbed down with a household cleaning solution to remove all remnants of an allergen before an allergic student sits at the table to eat.

✔ **Avoiding situations in which the allergen becomes airborne in high enough concentrations to trigger a reaction:** You may find yourself in this situation if you're allergic to peanuts and dine out at a restaurant where other patrons are cracking open shelled peanuts or you're allergic to fish and are seated at a table close to the kitchen where fish is being fried.

When your immune system is genetically wired to overreact to a food allergen, any amount of the allergen can trigger a reaction and potentially increase the risk of more severe reactions in the future.

In Chapter 6, I provide most of the guidance and information you need to successfully avoid problem foods by carefully reading food labels. Throughout the book, I offer additional tips and strategies to prevent accidental exposure to problem foods.

Muffling your symptoms with meds

You can't pop a pill or take a shot to cure your food allergies, but several medications can help relieve symptoms when avoidance is not 100 percent effective. Consult your allergist and stock your medicine cabinet and your travel bag with medications that can provide symptomatic relief.

Chapter 7 offers detailed information on the most effective food allergy medications and includes a Food Allergy Emergency Action Plan that helps you plan in advance for even the most severe reaction. Here, I provide a brief overview of medications that can assist in relieving your symptoms:

✔ **Epinephrine:** Giving someone who's experiencing a severe allergic reaction a shot of epinephrine (adrenaline) is like throwing a drowning person a life preserver. If your doctor believes that you're at risk for a severe reaction, he can prescribe epinephrine autoinjectors that enable you or someone you're with to give you an immediate injection.

✔ **Antihistamines:** Benadryl (Diphendydramine) and other antihistamines in the category of H1 blockers, given by mouth or by injection, can help symptoms subside. Liquid forms or fast-dissolve pills may offer faster relief, because your system can absorb them more readily.

✔ **H2 blockers:** Zantac (Ranitidine) and Tagamet (cimetidine), which are commonly used to treat ulcers and acid indigestion are often effective, especially when combined with antihistamines in the H1 class.

- **Inhalant medications:** Albuterol and other asthma medications can help if you have difficulty breathing, chest tightness, or coughing.

- **Corticosteroids:** Prednisone and other corticosteroids can help prevent a recurrence in the hours following a severe reaction and prevent late reactions, but they don't work rapidly enough for emergency treatment.

Confronting the alternative (therapy) crowd

Although some alternative therapies may assist by complementing well-established medical treatments, most alternative therapies are useless at best and counterproductive at worst. In addition, they're often costly, your insurance probably won't pay for them, and they siphon off the time, energy, and resources you would be better off investing in a proven medical diagnosis and treatments.

In the following sections, I provide a brief overview of the most useless alternative tests and treatments. In Chapter 8, I do a more thorough job of debunking them and pointing out some therapies that may improve your overall health and well being but have no proven track record of relieving symptoms or curing allergy.

My mind is not completely sealed off to the possibility that more effective treatments and perhaps a cure can come from somewhere other than the established medical community. In fact, in Chapter 9, I shine the spotlight on a Chinese herbal formula that actually holds out some promise for food allergy sufferers. When I pick apart quack tests and treatments, I do it only to show that proponents of these tests and treatments have little, if any, scientific evidence to back up their claims, and I don't want you spending your time and money chasing after a treatment that's certain to be ineffective.

Exposing the most dubious tests

If I were to tell you that I could diagnose your food allergy by watching you swing a rubber chicken over your head, you'd probably question my credentials. Yet, people continue to subject themselves to tests that have no scientifically proven data to back them up. Here are some of the more questionable tests:

- **Cytotoxic testing** douses your skin cells (under a microscope) in a solution that contains the allergen to see if your cells break down or change shape in response to the allergen.

- **ELISA/ACT (Enzyme-Linked Immunosorbent Assay) testing** consists of watching how your white blood cells (lymphocytes) react to particular allergens. Proponents claim that the test can reveal the root cause of 60 percent of all human illnesses.

✔ **NAET (Nambudripad's Allergy Elimination Technique)** requires you to hold a food while stretching your arms out akimbo and having the examiner pull down on your arms to test your muscle strength. Supposedly, you're allergic to a food if the food weakens you, because the food is interfering with your energy pathways. Tests results almost always show the need for acupuncture or acupressure treatments.

✔ **Immune-complex and IgG tests** assess common immune reactions not necessarily related to allergy. IgG tests often identify perfectly harmless foods as allergens, which can lead to poor diet and malnutrition.

✔ **The pulse test** calls for taking your pulse before and after eating a certain food. If your pulse rate increases significantly, supposedly you're either allergic to the food or have an intolerance to it.

What qualifies as scientific proof?

Most of the proof that supports the effectiveness of alternative tests and therapies is in the form of theories or anecdotal evidence rather than scientific evidence. "Theory" is simply another term for "wishful thinking." Anyone can concoct a theory that a certain test, for example, reveals hidden allergens, but if the theory doesn't pan out in clinical practice or a controlled test, it's bunk. With anecdotal evidence, patients simply describe how they felt before and after treatment. This evidence is very open to being influenced by the *placebo effect* — the patient's belief in the treatment is sufficient in making the patient think and report that he feels better.

Scientific proof is gathered only through carefully controlled studies on people who have been accurately diagnosed as having a true food allergy — people who get sick when they eat a particular food and remain symptom-free when they avoid that food. A *controlled study* is one in which a control group — people or other animals who do not receive treatment — is used for comparison purposes.

The accuracy of a study's results vary depending on how the researchers run the study. They may choose from any of the following three testing methods:

✔ **Open:** Researchers and patients all know who's receiving the treatment and who's not. Because everyone is aware of what's going on, results may be influenced by the placebo effect.

✔ **Single-blind:** Researchers know who's receiving treatment and who's not, but the patients don't. Because the researcher may unknowingly communicate, through body language, who's getting treatment and who's not, blind testing may also be influenced by the placebo effect.

✔ **Double-blind:** Neither the researchers nor the patients know who's receiving treatment and who's not until after the study is completed. Results of double-blind testing are the most reliable.

After a particular treatment is proven effective, typically in non-human animals, responsible researchers perform further testing to determine the treatment's effectiveness in humans and its safety. This ensures that mainstream treatments are safe and effective in humans, which you can't always rely on with alternative treatments.

Pulling the plug on unproven treatments

Many alternative medical practitioners want you to believe that your food allergies stem from nothing more than your body having too much or too little of something it needs. They often promise to cure your food allergy and every other illness you have by bringing your system into "proper balance." Following are some of the half-baked schools of thought that drive the development of these unproven treatments:

- **Homeopathy:** A tiny amount of what ails you can supposedly cure you for good.

- **Supplementarians:** Peddling their pet concoctions of vitamins, minerals, and herbs, these folks want you to believe that if your body just had the right chemical balance, you'd never be sick another day in your life.

- **Chelationists:** The theory here is that you've been poisoned by something in the environment, typically a heavy metal like lead or mercury. Leaching the poisons out of your system, through chelation, supposedly will do the trick.

- **Full-body cleansers:** These folks attribute almost every disease to a gummed up colon, liver, kidneys, or gallbladder — nothing a thorough internal scrubbing can't cure!

- **Leaky gutters:** The leaky gutters do have a point. Sometimes your GI tract can let some undigested food particles through its walls (a leaky gut), which may eventually cause a condition called eosinophilic gastrointestinal, which I discuss in Chapter 7. Leaky gut, however, plays no role in food allergies or intolerances.

- **Masseuses, chiropractors, and other body manipulators:** Although a good massage, a chiropractic adjustment, or yoga may make you feel better all around, none of these treatments or practices can cure food allergies.

The National Center for Complementary and Alternative Medicine (NC CAM) Web site at nccam.nih.gov provides some excellent information on alternative tests and therapies. It's not comprehensive (for example, when I searched the site, I found nothing on NAET or ELISA/ACT), but the site does provide some reliable details about specific herbs, supplements, and other alternative and complementary treatments. I recommend that you visit the site before trying any potentially dangerous or utterly useless treatment.

Getting the Lowdown on Potential Futuristic Cures

Although the medical community has no cure for food allergy, researchers are working on it. As I reveal in Chapter 9, we're advancing quickly, and research is accelerating at breakneck speed. I predict that within 20 years, we'll see a cure for food allergy. The following list introduces some of the most promising results of current research:

- **Immunotherapy:** Immunotherapy attempts to desensitize the immune system to a particular allergen over time by subjecting it to increasing doses of the allergen.

- **Ancient Chinese herbal remedy:** An ancient Chinese herbal formula (FAHF-1) has proven effective in virtually curing peanut allergy in mice. Another variant of this herbal brew, fondly referred to as FAHF-2 has proven equally effective in treating mice. For more about FAHF-2, refer to the following sidebar and skip to Chapter 9.

- **Anti-IgE antibody therapy:** Because IgE antibodies are the instigators of most food allergy reactions, scientists are looking for ways to incapacitate these antibodies. Anti-IgE antibody therapy consists of stimulating the body's production of IgG antibodies that bind with the IgE antibodies. IgG renders the IgE powerless and unable to trigger the massive release of histamines, which cause most symptoms.

- **Genetically engineered immunization shots:** Scientists are working on ways to re-train the immune system to function properly by ramping up its response to disease-causing organisms and cranking down its response to harmless substances. Genetically engineered amino acids can often tweak the operation of the immune system to mute its reaction to food allergens.

- **Probiotics:** Beneficial bacteria, such as those found in yogurt, may optimize the functioning of the immune system, improving its ability to defend the body against harmful bacteria and viruses while decreasing its tendency to overreact to food allergens.

Improving the ancient Chinese herbal remedy

The results of an NC CAM–sponsored study sought to test the effectiveness of an ancient Chinese herbal formula known as FAHF-1 in reducing allergic reactions to peanut in mice and possibly preventing the occurrence of life-threatening reactions. The study proved that the formula was effective, but it had some significant drawbacks. FAHF-1 was:

- A complex formula

- Difficult to produce in mass quantities

- Contained two ingredients that were potentially dangerous

The research team removed the two potentially dangerous ingredients, developing a new, improved, and simpler formula called FAHF-2. Test results prove that FAHF-2 is just as effective in treating peanut allergy in mice, and the beneficial effects lasted for up to five weeks after discontinuing treatment.

You can read more about FAHF-2 in Chapter 9.

Living Large with Your Food Allergies

Food allergies limit more than your menu selections. They can place some restaurants off limits, isolate your allergic child in the cafeteria, make you more reluctant to visit family and friends for dinner, and complicate your life with a host of precautionary measures and sometimes paralyzing fear.

Throughout this book, especially in Part III, I attempt to allay any fears and equip you to deal more effectively with food allergies at home (Chapter 10), during your evenings out on the town and wherever you happen to travel (Chapter 11), and at school (Chapters 12 and 13). I reveal common-sense precautions that, once they become habit, enable you to live a full, enjoyable life without becoming paralyzed by undo fears. I equip you with everything you need to decipher labels (Chapter 6), discover tasty alternatives for the foods you love (Chapter 18), and even whip up a few delicious allergen-free meals and desserts in your own kitchen (Appendix).

Avoiding the foods you're allergic to, however, is rarely 100 percent effective in preventing reactions. The trick to dealing with the possibility of a reaction is to be prepared 100 percent of the time. By having the medications you need to immediately respond in the event of an emergency, you can decrease the fear factor by a factor of ten and establish a more relaxed form of vigilance. (For more about medications and preparing from emergencies, check out Chapter 7.)

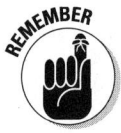

An allergic reaction can be a terrifying experience, but by mastering a few allergen-avoidance techniques and remaining well-prepared to respond immediately in the event of a reaction, you can limit the risk and ease your mind.

Unmasking Common Food Allergy Myths

Before you move on to the next chapter or skip ahead to a chapter you find more fascinating, I'd like to take the opportunity to dispel some of the most common myths about food allergies. By clearing any cloud of misinformation from your brain, I can free up some space for the more accurate and useful information I present later in this book. The following list reveals the most common and tenacious myths:

> ✔ **It's nothing more than a stomachache.** Maybe you're right. Maybe you
> have nothing more than a stomachache, but you should still have it
> checked out, especially if your stomach aches soon after you eat a
> specific food. Without an accurate diagnosis, you're at a higher risk of

experiencing a more severe reaction later and being unprepared to deal with it, if, in fact, it turns out to be allergy related.

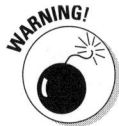

- ✔ **A little taste can't hurt.** To your immune system, even a tiny amount of a problem food is enough to trigger an all-out attack. People with severe allergies can have life-threatening reactions when the same spatula used to serve a cookie containing the allergen is used to serve up their supposedly allergen-free cookie.

- ✔ **A tiny bit may actually help.** Although some food allergy treatments call for exposing the immune system to increasing amounts of a known allergen to desensitize the immune system, trying to do this on your own is very dangerous.

- ✔ **Food allergies make me hyper.** Food allergies are often blamed for psychiatric disorders, such as ADHD (Attention-Deficit/Hyperactivity Disorder). Although food may play a role in the severity of the symptoms, food allergies are not the root cause or even a strong contributor. You're better off seeing a psychiatrist and therapist to receive a proper diagnosis and treatment.

- ✔ **Epinephrine is a dangerous drug.** Some doctors refuse to prescribe epinephrine, particularly for children, because they think it's a dangerous drug. The fact is that epinephrine is a very safe drug, and for a huge majority of food allergy sufferers, the benefits far outweigh the risks. See Chapter 7 for details.

- ✔ **You're allergic to any food that causes problems.** Foods can cause problems for all sorts of reasons, including other ingredients in the food, toxins, high concentrations of histamine, bacteria, and viruses. Don't assume that just because a particular food gives you the collywobbles that you're allergic to that food.

- ✔ **The peanut allergy is the most common.** Peanut may very well be the most common allergy in some populations, but the prevalence of a particular food allergy varies according to age and culture. Kids are more likely to be allergic to peanuts, milk, and eggs, for example, while adults are more prone to seafood allergies. People of Jewish decent have a higher prevalence of allergy to sesame. In Japan and other countries in which fish is a staple, fish allergy is more common.

- ✔ **If you weren't allergic to it before, you can't be allergic to it now.** As explained earlier in this chapter, in the section "Investigating the Conspiracy: Allergens and Other Contributing Factors," the onset of a food allergy is brought on by a genetic susceptibility and exposure to the problem food. The more exposure to the problem food, the higher the risk of developing an allergy to it if you're susceptible. However, some food allergies, including milk and egg allergies, tend to develop earlier in life, whereas seafood allergies tend to appear later in life.

✔ **Bona fide food allergies are rare.** Approximately 7.5 percent of the population of the United States has a bona fide food allergy, and the incidents of food allergies seems to be on the rise.

✔ **I'm allergic to food additives.** Food additives can trigger reactions, even severe reactions, but these are not allergic in nature. Reactions to food additives are chemical reactions that produce symptoms very similar and perhaps even identical to those of allergic reactions.

Chapter 2

Turning Allergies Inside Out: Probable Causes and Common Symptoms

. . . .

In This Chapter

▶ Exploring the food-body connection

▶ Examining your immune system's response to allergens

▶ Investigating the rising prevalence of food allergies

▶ Assessing the risk of your child acquiring a food allergy

▶ Spotting the signs and symptoms of typical and atypical reactions

. . . .

*W*hen you experience an allergic reaction to your food, you may begin to feel as though your food allergy has turned you inside out. You eat a peanut or sample some mayonnaise, and you break out in hives or eczema. What kind of sense does that make? If something you ate made you sick, you'd expect to get queasy or nauseous and feel your stomach doing somersaults, and that's often what occurs, but breaking out in hives? How does that happen?

In this chapter, I get back at food allergies by turning them inside out. I illustrate the main culprits in allergenic foods that trigger allergies and show you how your immune system overreacts when you eat something that you're allergic to. I lead you through some population studies to reveal why you may have developed a food allergy in the first place. Finally, I reveal the symptoms that are commonly attributed to food allergies and symptoms often falsely blamed on food allergies. With this information in hand, you can distinguish fact from fiction when ill-informed practitioners attempt to chalk up all your ills to the foods you eat.

Finding Out What's Wrong with Your Food

When something you eat makes you sick, your natural impulse is to blame the food and never eat it again. With food allergies, however, you can't blame everything on the food. After all, most people can enjoy the same foods that make you sick without experiencing even the slightest reaction.

Food allergy is not solely a problem with a particular food. The problem is your body's response to that food. Some foods clearly are much more prone to inducing allergies than others, but the real problem is with the body's reaction to these foods.

In the following sections, I reveal the stuff (allergens) in foods that trigger reactions and investigate other substances in our food supply that are often mistakenly suspected of triggering reactions or making humans more susceptible to acquiring a food allergy.

Pinpointing problematic proteins

The stuff in some foods that trigger reactions in some people are *proteins* — molecules constructed out of building blocks called *amino acids*. As you know, proteins are essential in building muscle and repairing cells; they also play an important role as hormones, enzymes, and antibodies.

The Brazil nut soybean debacle

In the early days of genetically engineered foods, scientists were looking for a way to make a soy plant more resistant to disease. In doing so, they inserted genetic material from Brazil nuts into these super-duper soy plants. Turns out that the component of Brazil nut that they inserted contained the nut allergen that triggers reactions in people with tree nut allergy. The resulting soybean plant could have resulted in producing several species of soybeans that could be deadly to people with tree nut allergies.

This plant was quickly removed from development, and the government took steps to screen all future genetically engineered foods for their allergic potential. Although these safety measures are not foolproof, they have provided a substantial element of safety.

Every protein has a unique, genetically mapped structure. You probably couldn't discern one protein from another in a police lineup, but your immune system has an eagle eye for identifying proteins. Within seconds after a specific protein enters your system, your immune system identifies it as friend or foe. When your immune system mistakenly identifies a food protein as an enemy invader, it jumps into attack mode and causes all the symptoms that make you miserable — hives, rash, nausea, breathing difficulties, and so on.

What is it about a particular protein that makes it problematic? Researchers continue to study that question, but most suspect that problematic proteins are high-profile molecules that the immune system can easily spot. Problematic proteins commonly exhibit the following traits:

- **Unique shape or folding pattern:** Peanut proteins, for example, are folded with the protein pieces that are responsible for stimulating the immune system exposed rather than concealed inside the molecule.
- **Size:** Protein molecules that trigger allergic reactions tend to be rather large . . . comparatively speaking, of course.
- **Stability:** Allergenic proteins may be more stable, requiring additional time for your system to break them down into innocuous amino acids.

Separating logic from lore

Nature abhors a vacuum, and so does the human mind. When people are unaware of the protein-immune-system connection, they concoct all sorts of theories about what actually causes food allergies. Some of these theories are valid to certain point, others rarely apply, and a few are just plain bunk. In the following sections, I separate logic from lore to paint a clearer picture of what really causes food allergies and reactions and what doesn't.

Fooling Mother Nature (and your immune system) with genetically engineered foods

Can genetically engineered foods trigger allergies? They sure can, although the occurrences are rare. To genetically engineer a food, scientists introduce genetic material from one food into another. If they mistakenly introduce an allergenic protein from one food into another, the receiving food also contains the allergenic protein, which can also trigger a reaction, (see the sidebar, "the Brazil nut–soybean debacle," to find out about a case in which this actually happened).

Putting the heat on histamines

During an allergic reaction, your immune system produces histamines that trigger symptoms, so it stands to reason that consuming histamines would trigger similar symptoms, and consuming histamines sometimes does just that. Several foods contain histamine or histamine-like substances of their own:

- **Scombroid fish:** The Scombridae family of fish, including tunas and mackerels and their close cousins, bluefish and mahi-mahi, contain a toxic histamine generated by bacterial degradation of substances in the muscle protein. This natural spoilage process is thought to release additional by-products that intensify the toxic effect and can cause *scombroid poisoning*.

- **Strawberries:** People who have "allergic reactions" to strawberries are often simply more sensitive to the histamines they contain.

- **Tomatoes:** When tomatoes produce symptoms similar to those of an allergic reaction, histamines may be to blame.

- **Chocolate:** A food allergy to chocolate is rare, but chocolate may contain higher levels of histamines that can trigger allergic-like symptoms.

- **Wine and beer:** Some wines and beers contain elevated levels of histamines. Wine producers have picked up on this and some now offer histamine-low or histamine-free wine. Red wines typically contain more histamines than white wines.

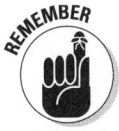

The levels of histamine present in these foods are usually not capable of causing reactions but they can and occasionally do cause allergic-like reactions. Scombroid poisoning can cause severe reactions, but reactions to other foods that contain elevated histamine levels are typically mild, if they even occur.

Accusing food additives

Most processed foods contain additives including dyes, preservatives, and a variety of other chemicals to make foods more stable, prettier, or tastier. If you experience reactions consuming foods that contain a particular additive, the food itself is not at fault, and you're not really experiencing a true food allergy. You're allergic to the stuff in or on the food. Here are the two most common culprits:

- **Sulfites:** Sulfites can cause severe reactions in people who are sensitive to them. Asthma sufferers generally face a higher risk. Food manufacturers often add sulfite to wines, some baked goods, and even on fruits and vegetables to keep them fresh. Strict labeling laws are in place for sulfites, because even low levels can cause severe reactions in some people.

> ✔ **MSG (monosodium glutamate):** MSG is another food additive that occasionally causes adverse reactions. Because Chinese foods commonly contain high levels of MSG, reactions it causes are often referred to as "the Chinese restaurant syndrome." Headache and flushing are the most common symptoms, but sweating, increased heart rate, and anxiety can also occur.

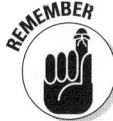

Reactions to other food additives are relatively uncommon. They do occur, especially to food dyes, but a history of such a reaction is usually not borne out by a full evaluation. Many people believe that they have reacted to a dye or preservative, but on closer inspection allergists find that the patient is actually eating the same substance in high concentrations in many other foods without experiencing any reaction. Allergists have no allergy tests for most of these dyes and preservatives. Health history and challenge testing are the best diagnostic tools currently available.

Joe's Alleve and pink champagne story

In 1994, my wife attended the inaugural Brickyard 400 auto race at the Indianapolis Motor Speedway with her sister and brother-in-law. My wife was driving a separate car, and they all planned on meeting at the track. Not a big race fan myself, I volunteered to stay home with the kids. When the race was over, I was pretty worn out and had a terrible headache from a full day with my 8- and 5-year-olds, so I popped an Alleve and washed it down with a couple gulps of pink champagne.

Minutes later, my entire body started to itch, and I had no idea what was happening. My sister-in-law called to say that she and her husband were going to drop by on their way home. Feeling terrible, I told her to just go on — I had had a long day. She said they were coming over anyway.

When they arrived, I was a wreck. My body was covered with hives, my ears had swelled up to the size of oven mitts, and my lips were swollen into a curved smile that made me look like the

Joker on Batman. My sister-in-law called my neighbor, a nurse who lived in the house behind ours. She instructed me to take some Benadryl and sit in a cold bath until she arrived. My poor brother-in-law was assigned the task of keeping my naked body covered with cold, wet towels.

As soon as my neighbor saw my face, she instructed us to head to the hospital. My wife arrived, and then she, my sister-in-law, and my neighbor drove me to the emergency room where the nurse on staff gave me a shot of epinephrine and hooked me up to an IV. I felt immediate relief.

The doctor came in to talk with me a little later. When he saw me with three women and heard my story about the Alleve and the pink champagne, he smirked and asked, "So which one of you is his wife?" After the laughter died down, he followed up with, "And what exactly were you celebrating?"

Investigating other manufactured-chemical troublemakers

Chemical engineers have designed a wide variety of products to improve our lives — everything from pain relievers to zero-calorie artificial sweeteners. But some bodies haven't evolved to assimilate this stuff.

Any of hundreds of manufactured chemicals can trigger allergic-like reactions, but one of the most common classes that cause problems are NSAIDs (Nonsteroidal Anti-Inflammatory Drugs). Pain relievers including aspirin, Motrin, Advil, and Alleve are known as NSAIDs. These pain relievers are great for treating headaches and pain in most people, but they can cause severe reactions in some. My co-author, Joe, experienced a severe reaction to Alleve that he accounts in the preceding sidebar.

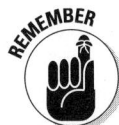

Manufactured chemicals can't be considered foods, so reactions to them are not considered the result of food allergies. The medical community attributes reactions to these substances to *chemical sensitivities*.

Mistaking food intolerances for food allergies

When a food makes you sick, you may be inclined to blame it on a food allergy, but foods can make you ill for other reasons — the most common of which is that you have an intolerance of the food. With a food intolerance, symptoms occur because your body has trouble digesting or breaking down the problem food.

The classic example of a food intolerance is lactose intolerance, in which people experience nausea, vomiting, abdominal pain, or diarrhea because they're unable to break down the milk sugar called *lactose*. Lactose intolerance is completely different from milk allergy in which the immune system has developed a sensitivity to milk protein.

Examining nature's poisons and their purpose

If you try to eat a lion, the lion fights back. Although inanimate edibles can't claw your eyes out, they often contain toxins that protect them from predators or simply exist as part of the plant's chemistry. Almonds, for example, contain cyanide. Fruits commonly have a laxative effect on animals, to enable any seeds that an animal swallows to quickly move through their digestive track, so the seeds are not damaged. Other foods contain chemicals to ward off bacteria and fungus infection.

Some toxins in foods can be quite deadly. Mushroom hunters, for example, have to be able to tell a poisonous mushroom from one that's harmless, because some mushrooms can be deadly. Several varieties of fish also produce their own toxins. One of the most well known is the puffer fish, which can contain a potent toxin.

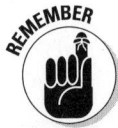

Natural toxins in foods can make you ill, but your illness from those toxins has nothing to do with food allergies.

Paying the price for eating high on the food chain

Some toxins, such as mercury in fish, become more of a problem the higher up you eat on the food chain. Eating lower on the food chain is thought by some to reduce the risk. Eating smaller fish, for example, such as sardines and anchovies (if you can stomach them), rather than larger fish, such as tuna and swordfish, may help you limit your consumption of specific toxins.

But not all toxins move up the food chain, and if you're eating a relatively balanced and varied diet, the amount of toxins you're ingesting is typically not much of a problem, and they're certainly not related to food allergies.

Finding Out What's Wrong with You

A food allergy is not just difficulty digesting a food but rather the immune system's overreaction to a specific food that sparks a reaction. The actual reaction that produces symptoms involves a complex sequence of events that I describe in the following sections.

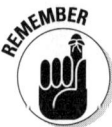

Although food allergies can arise at any stage in life, the vast majority have their onset in childhood, particularly in the first one to two years.

Going wild: Immune systems gone wild

A virgin immune system has no reason to launch an all-out attack on a harmless food. It has to be properly sensitized to the food first (through an initial exposure). *Sensitization* is the process by which the immune system starts producing antibodies to a food that causes the immune system to overreact the next time it's exposed to that food.

The mechanics of exactly what happens to trigger the first reaction can be somewhat complicated. In the following sections, I provide a brief overview of how sensitization leads to future reactions and how the resulting antibodies react when a problem food is reintroduced.

From sensitization to all-out mayhem

A food allergy is an immune system response to a food that the body mistakenly believes is harmful. Here's a blow-by-blow description of what occurs during a typical reaction:

1. Once the immune system decides that a particular food is harmful, it creates specific *IgE (Immunoglobulin E)* antibodies to it. The following section introduces you to IgE.

2. The next time the individual eats that food, the immune system releases massive amounts of chemicals, including histamine, as shown in Figure 2-1.

3. These chemicals trigger a cascade of allergic symptoms that can affect the respiratory system, gastrointestinal tract, skin, or cardiovascular system.

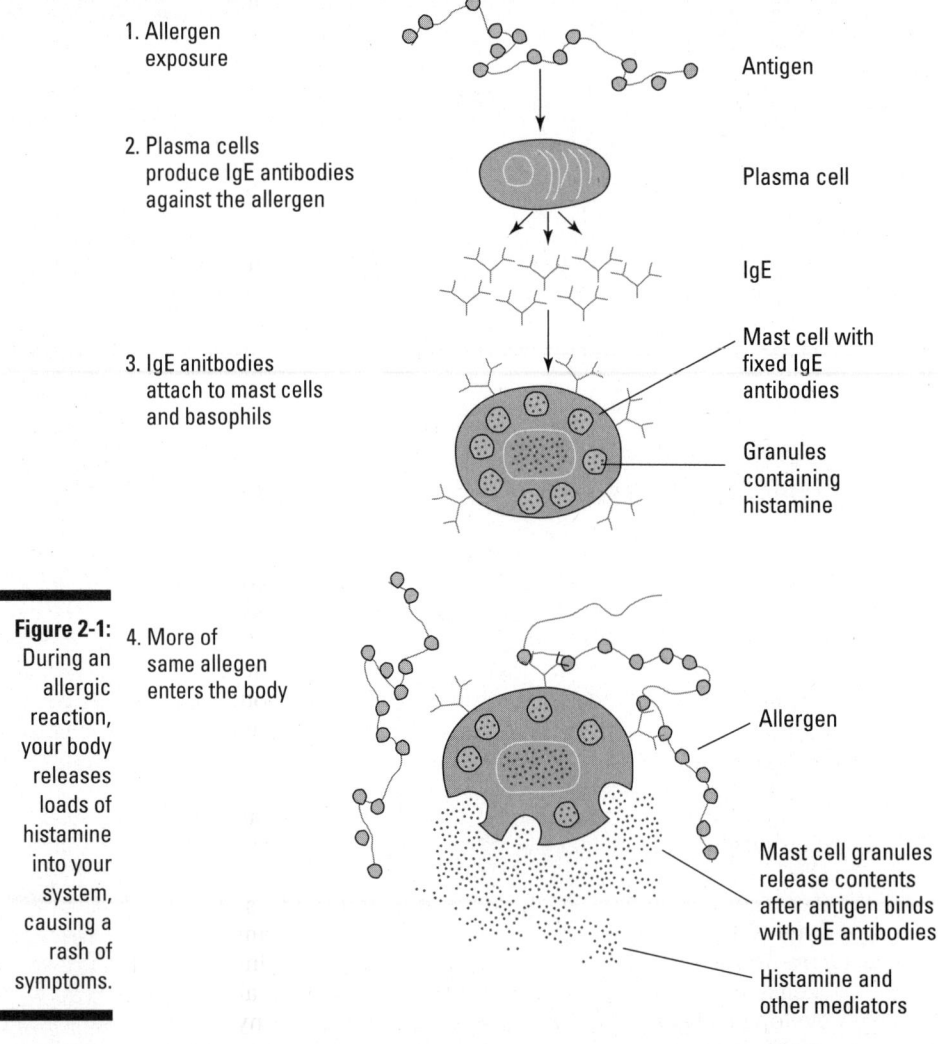

1. Allergen exposure

Antigen

2. Plasma cells produce IgE antibodies against the allergen

Plasma cell

IgE

3. IgE anitbodies attach to mast cells and basophils

Mast cell with fixed IgE antibodies

Granules containing histamine

Figure 2-1: During an allergic reaction, your body releases loads of histamine into your system, causing a rash of symptoms.

4. More of same allegen enters the body

Allergen

Mast cell granules release contents after antigen binds with IgE antibodies

Histamine and other mediators

Although most food allergies are caused by these IgE antibodies, some do not involve IgE but rather other parts of the immune system. These are particularly common with some of the food allergies that affect the gastrointestinal tract and are referred to as *non-IgE-mediated food allergies*.

IgE antibodies and the foods they hate

Your immune system produces four main classes of antibodies — IgG, IgA, IgM, and IgE. The first three types serve to fight infection and are critical to our health. The purpose of IgE is to fight infection, specifically parasitic infections. These IgE antibodies, however, also cause allergic reactions. As parasitic infections have become less common in the developed world, IgE can devote more and more of its energy toward allergy. Here's a quick overview of how IgE comes into play:

1. Once IgE is produced, it sits on the surface of the main allergy cells of the body called the *mast cells* and *basophils*.

2. The IgE that your body produces is specific for one allergen or another, and when that specific allergen reenters the body, it finds the IgE sitting on the surface of the cells.

3. Once the allergen finds the IgE, the immune system triggers the release of histamine and other chemicals that cause allergic symptoms.

The same process occurs with environmental allergens that cause hay fever and other conditions.

Debating the nature or nurture question

What causes you to develop an allergy in the first place? Is it your genetic makeup? Something in our food supply? Something you ate too much of as a kid? A great deal of research has been devoted to answering these questions, and the best answer that researchers have developed so far is that food allergies are caused by a combination of nature (your genes) and nurture (what you eat). The best evidence available for a genetic connection comes from studies of peanut allergy in twins (see the sidebar "Discovering the genetic connection through peanut studies on twins").

The medical community knows that allergies run in families, so the genetic link is well established, but we also know that children in the same families — even twins — do not always share the same allergies. This has led researchers to suspect that genes account only for a susceptibility to food allergies. If parents have hay fever or asthma, for example, their children are more prone to developing an allergic disease, including hay fever, asthma, eczema, or food allergy. One child may develop food allergy, another may develop hay fever, and a third may be allergy-free. Why this happens is still largely a mystery.

Discovering the genetic connection through peanut studies on twins

Studies of peanut allergy in twins have provided the strongest proof that genes play a role in developing food allergy but are not exclusively responsible. An important study shows that an identical twin has a 64 percent chance of sharing a peanut allergy with the twin sibling who is allergic to peanut. With nonidentical twins the risk drops to a mere 7 percent.

The study clearly demonstrates a strong genetic link to peanut allergy but also proves that food allergy is not purely a genetic disease. What leads one of the identical twins to develop the allergy and spares the second is unknown. Allergy specialists believe that exposure plays a role in developing a food allergy, but determining exactly what each twin is exposed to in the uncontrolled testing environment of daily living is nearly impossible.

Triggering allergies through exposure

A genetic predisposition to a food allergy is like a genetic predisposition to bruising. Even if you bruise easily, you won't get a bruise unless you get whacked with something. With food allergy, you're highly unlikely to develop an allergy unless you're predisposed to react to a particular allergen and then exposed to that allergen. This sensitizes your immune system to the allergen, making you susceptible to future reactions.

The formula that causes the onset of a food allergy is well known:

Genetic Predisposition + Exposure = Sensitization

After your immune system is sensitized to a particular allergen, exposure to that allergen potentially leads to symptoms, as shown in Figure 2-2.

The exposure piece of the equation gets pretty complicated. For those who are predisposed to developing a food allergy, the type of exposure may influence the likelihood that the exposure triggers onset, as the following general tendencies reveal:

- **Repeated low-dose exposure to an allergen early in life is most likely to sensitize you to a specific allergen.** In other words, you're more likely to develop a food allergy to an allergen that repeatedly enters your system in small amounts, such as in breast feeding, trace amounts in foods, or even incidental contact.

✔ **Large-dose exposures early in life may make you less likely to develop a food allergy.** Odd, but true — increased exposure to an allergen may actually make you less sensitive to that food. Hold on. Don't start feeing your baby peanut-based formula or advising nursing mothers to gobble up more peanuts. At this point, doctors have no reliable way to implement this observation in a preventive treatment plan. Based on the best information currently available, the recommendation is still to *avoid peanut and other common allergens early in life.*

✔ **Avoidance diets may or may not help ward off the development of a food allergy.** Although my colleagues and I recommend that parents limit exposure to common food allergens early in their children's lives, research results waffle on the conclusion. While some studies show that avoidance diets early in life ward off the onset of food allergies, others have failed to uphold these results. We commonly see children who are born into allergic families where exposure has been virtually or completely eliminated develop the allergy. The mother may never have eaten peanut during pregnancy or breast feeding, all peanut has been banned from the premises, and incidental contact is highly unlikely, but the child still develops a peanut allergy. My belief is that these children are so genetically prone to developing the allergy that even inhaling a few errant molecules of peanut protein in the grocery store or shopping mall may be enough to trigger the sensitization process.

Figure 2-2: A genetic predisposition combined with exposure leads to sensitization, which produces symptoms when the offending food is re-introduced.

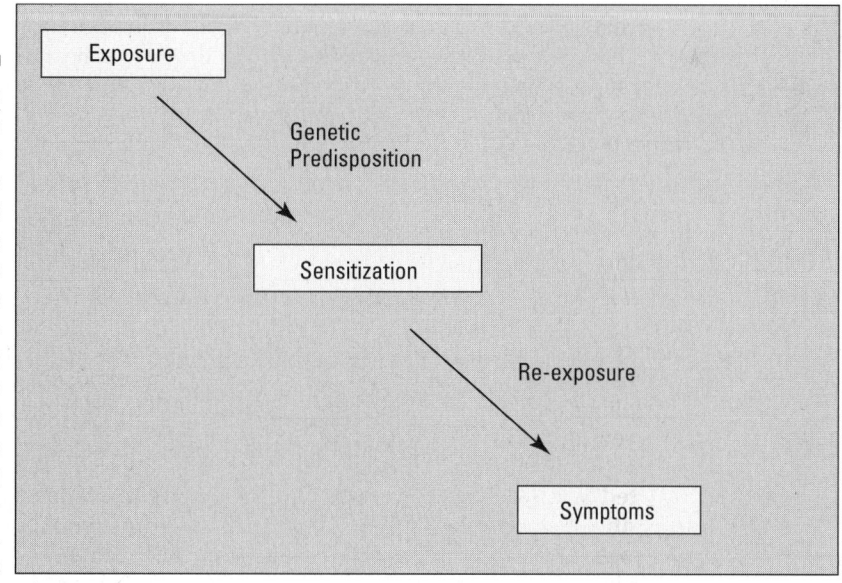

Exploring the Sudden Rise in Food Allergies

If you grew up in the '60s or '70s, you may never have heard the term "food allergy." Your classmates and playmates probably were able to eat whatever they wanted free from the fear of a reaction. Perhaps your entire school had only one or two kids with food allergies if your school even had a kid with food allergies.

Over the last 20 years, however, the prevalence of food allergy appears to have risen sharply. Researchers can't pin an absolute number on the increase, because no reliable comparative data over the 20-year period is available — studies being performed today follow different procedures from those performed 20 years ago, so you can't really compare the numbers. Allergists do, however, have plenty of evidence that points to a dramatic increase in food allergy:

- ✔ Evidence gathered over the last 10 years using the same methods show that the prevalence of peanut allergy has doubled in the last 5–10 years.

- ✔ Anecdotal and clinical evidence shows a significant increase in food allergy. Pediatricians tell me that they see far more food allergy than ever before. School nurses report that while a decade ago they had one or two children in the school with epinephrine prescriptions, they now have 20 or 30. Some of this could be due to what we refer to as a *detection bias*; that is, increasing awareness about a problem leads to its being diagnosed more efficiently. However, most experts believe that the increase is real and not simply the result of increased awareness.

- ✔ Reliable asthma studies show at least a 100 percent increase in the prevalence of asthma (an allergy-related disease) over the last 30 years. The rise in asthma appears to have preceded the rise in food allergy (which is a source of confusion) although experts believe that similar mechanisms likely underlie the dramatic increases in all allergic diseases.

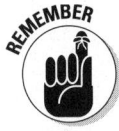

The jump in all allergic diseases across the board suggests that a collection of contributing factors not present 20 or 30 years ago is responsible. Researchers have presented many theories to explain the increase, but the only clear conclusion is that no one, single cause can explain it.

Examining the hygiene hypothesis

When you're growing up, adults, whom you assume know what's good for you tell you to practice proper hygiene. By the time you're six years old, the phrases "Wash your hands," "Brush your teeth," "Don't let the dog lick your face," and "Stay out of the mud," play like Zen mantras in your head.

Perhaps our obsession with cleanliness is at the root of the increase in allergies. This theory, referred to as the *hygiene hypothesis*, is the most popular explanation for the rise in allergies. Simply stated, the hygiene hypothesis proposes that the less the immune system is exposed to germs and bacterial by-products the more energy it has to unleash on allergens. If this sounds kooky to you, examine the evidence before dismissing this theory:

- Allergies are much more common in developed countries, and the prevalence in allergies rises pretty much in direct proportion to the rise in development.

- Allergies are less common in children who grow up on farms, who attend daycare in early life, and who have multiple older siblings.

- Allergies may be less common in families that have pets, perhaps because pets increase exposure to bacteria and bacterial by-products.

Before you move out to the country, surround your family with livestock, and start rolling around in the pig pen, realize that the hygiene hypothesis has some holes in it, suggesting that other factors may play a role. The inner-city environment, for example, defies the hygiene hypothesis. Children growing up in the inner-city should reap all the benefits of poor hygiene in warding off the onset of allergies, but inner-city kids have some of the highest rates of asthma and allergy anywhere. This suggests that other factors, such as air pollution or environmental allergen exposure, may trump the hygiene hypothesis.

Investigating other possible suspects

When you consider all the new developments in foods, medications, and other substances introduced into our lives over the past 30 years, you can easily become suspicious of numerous items that may have influenced the rise in food allergies. In the following list, I name several of the top suspects and provide my professional opinion on just how likely they contribute to the upward trend:

- **Vitamins:** One study suggests that vitamin supplements may promote allergy. Another study suggests that vitamin deficiency, especially vitamin D, may promote allergy. Conclusion? We just don't know yet.

- **Antacids:** Some evidence shows that antacids or other medicines designed to suppress stomach acids may promote allergy. This makes sense, because these products may reduce the breakdown of allergenic proteins in the stomach. The jury's still out on this one.

- **Immunizations or antibiotics:** No evidence at this time provides reliable evidence that immunizations or antibiotics promote allergy development.

✔ **Tobacco smoke:** Of all the studies ever done, the only factor that consistently has been associated with increases in allergy is exposure to tobacco smoke. The first studies in this regard looked at childhood asthma, and nobody was surprised to learn that exposure to tobacco smoke may lead to an increased susceptibility to asthma. This was presumed to be due to tobacco smoke's irritating effects on the airways. Research has now shown that exposure to tobacco smoke actually stimulates the immune system to promote the development of allergy. Other air pollutants may also play a role, although most studies have shown that exposure to air pollution has relatively little effect on the development of allergy.

Gauging Your Child's Risk for Developing a Food Allergy

Families frequently ask my colleagues and me to estimate the risk that their next child will develop food allergy. These are typically families who already have at least one child with food allergy, so the odds may already be tipped against them. Although we're reasonably good at predicting the chance of developing some form of allergic disease, our track record for specifically predicting food allergy is less impressive.

In the following sections I present data that can assist you in guesstimating the odds that your next child will develop some sort of allergic disease — based on family history and gender. I then investigate the role that age plays in the onset of an allergy-related condition.

Following the guidelines

You can use the following guidelines and the graph shown in Figure 2-3 to formulate your own prediction:

✔ If both you and your mate have an allergic disease, your children have a 40–60 percent chance of developing some form of allergic disease, not necessarily food allergy.

✔ If only you *or* your mate has an allergic disease, the likelihood drops to 30–40 percent.

✔ I would estimate that in the most allergic families that already have one or two children with a food allergy, the odds are less than 20–25 percent that the next child will also have food allergy. The next child is almost guaranteed to have some form of allergic disease but not necessarily food allergy.

✔ All allergies, including food allergies are about twice as common in boys as girls. This evens out later in childhood, and then, by adulthood, asthma and allergies are more common in women.

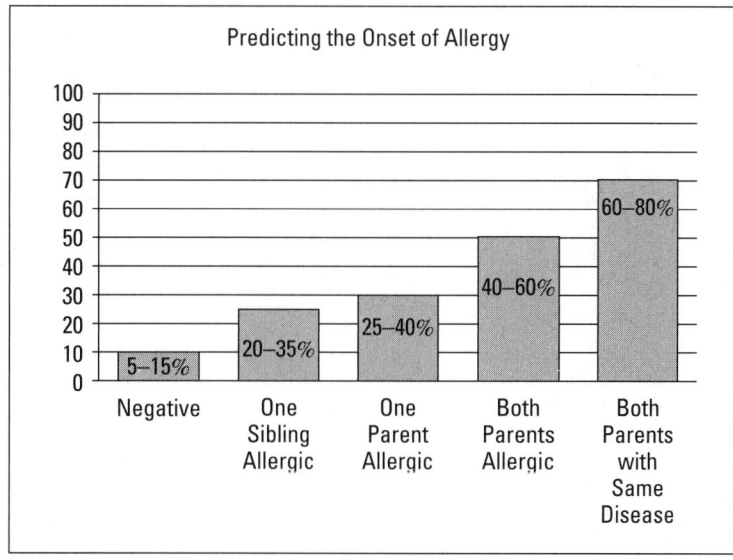

Figure 2-3: Family history can help predict the likelihood that your next child will have some form of allergy, not necessarily food allergy.

See Chapter 1 for details on preventing the onset of food allergies.

In a family with several members who have food allergy, the likelihood of the next child being allergic is highly probable, but whether the allergy takes the form of food allergy is impossible to predict.

Weighing the age factor

The age factor carries a lot of weight in determining the onset of allergies. The vast majority of allergies develop early in life. Food allergy hits its peak prevalence at one year of age, and at least 80 percent of childhood food allergies are likely to develop by the age of one.

Why are young children so much more susceptible to developing a food allergy? Because the intestinal tract of the infant provides a less complete barrier against allergenic proteins, so as proteins escape the intestinal tract, they become high-profile targets for the body's immune system. This barrier slowly closes by about six months of age. The only problem with this theory is that allergies very commonly worsen over the first two to three years of life, even if a child is destined to outgrow them later. A one-year-old who's allergic to milk or egg, for example, is likely to develop a more severe allergy by the time they are two to three, even if they eventually outgrow the allergy.

A few allergies defy this rule and tend to crop up more frequently in later years.

- **Shellfish and fish:** Allergies to shellfish and sometimes fish most often develop later in life.

- **Fruits and vegetables:** Allergies to fruits and vegetables may arise later in life as a secondary allergy related to a pollen allergy that you acquired earlier in your life. Allergies to fruits and vegetables often don't get into full swing until your pollen allergies have become sufficiently strong to spill over and cause a food allergy. Reactions to fruits and vegetables typically result in oral allergy syndrome covered in detail in Chapter 7.

Exploring Common Signs and Symptoms

Food allergy may *present* with a wide array of signs and symptoms. (The term *present* is doctor lingo for how a condition shows up in your body.) Food reactions typically involve the following three major organ systems in your body along with a fourth system that plays a role in severe reactions:

- Skin, such as hives or eczema

- Gastrointestinal tract, including nausea, stomach upset, and diarrhea

- Respiratory tract, including rhinitis (sneezing, runny nose) and difficulty breathing (or asthma)

- Cardiovascular system, sometimes involved in severe reactions (see the section "Uncovering anaphylaxis: The shocking story," later in this chapter for more information)

Some reactions are isolated to a single system, such as hives on the skin, while others may involve multiple systems, as sometimes occurs in an anaphylactic reaction. This myriad of presentations is one of the many reasons why some food allergies are so difficult to diagnose. In the following sections, I bring you up to speed on the most common symptoms, introduce some rare symptoms, and deliver several tips on how to rule out symptoms unrelated to (but often mistaken for) food allergy.

Getting under your skin

A food allergy can literally get under your skin. Skin reactions are the most common manifestations of food allergy. Symptoms, such as hives, may occur very acutely or as a much more chronic, low-grade condition. In the following sections I give you the skinny on the most common *cutaneous* (a fancy doctor term for *skin*) manifestations of food allergy.

Itching with eczema (atopic dermatitis)

Eczema (or *atopic dermatitis*) is a chronic skin condition characterized by extreme dryness and itchiness. It typically begins early in life and hits its peak prevalence at about one year of age. At that point, 15 to 20 percent of all one-year-olds have some degree of eczema, ranging from extremely mild to involving only tiny areas of skin to extremely severe cases involving the entire body.

Tracing eczema back to a food allergy requires some savvy detective work for various reasons.

- ✔ Eczema may not involve food allergy. Your doctor may not even suspect food allergy as the cause. Other factors that can contribute to eczema's onset and severity include
  - Genetic susceptibility
  - Heat
  - Humidity
  - Certain types of clothing
  - Soaps or detergents
- ✔ Food reactions that trigger eczema are typically low-grade and difficult to identify.
- ✔ Reactions may be delayed by several hours.
- ✔ Symptoms can wax and wane over time, due to temperature, humidity, and environmental irritants.
- ✔ Foods that typically trigger eczema are common foods eaten on a very regular basis. If you drink milk or eat wheat several times a day, detecting any clear connection between a specific food and your eczema symptoms can be nearly impossible.

Based on a large number of studies, we know that food allergy is at the root of about 40 percent of all cases of children with moderate to severe eczema. This means that at least 50 percent of children with eczema, including some with severe eczema, do not have food allergy. For the remainder, however, identifying the underlying food allergy and restricting the allergenic foods often leads to a marked improvement in symptoms. And given that eczema is an extraordinarily uncomfortable condition due to the severe itching that it creates, anything that makes you more comfortable is of extreme value.

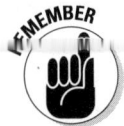

When food allergy is involved in eczema, the five most common food allergens are the prime suspects — egg, milk, peanut, soy, and wheat. Other foods can certainly be involved, but these top five are the most important to remember. In fact, if a child with eczema tests negative to these five foods by either skin testing or blood testing, the likelihood of any food allergy is extremely low.

Once you and your doctor have accomplished the daunting task of tracing your eczema to a food allergy, you can find symptomatic relief in Chapter 7.

Scratching the surface with hives

Hives (also known as *urticaria*) are itchy, raised splotches on the surface of your skin. About 20 times itchier than a mosquito bite, hives make you want to tear off your clothes and then your skin. When most folks have their first encounter with hives, they assume the condition is caused by something they ate. In most cases, however, hives are the result of other conditions:

- ✔ **Viral illness:** In many cases, a viral illness can trigger an outbreak of hives.
- ✔ **Anxiety:** When some people get real nervous, they get hives. This condition is called *cholinergic urticaria.*
- ✔ **Heat or Cold:** Cholinergic urticaria can also result from an increase in a person's core body temperature or other temperature extremes. Some people can't even perform their normal exercise routine without breaking out in hives.
- ✔ **Vibration:** Any vibration against the surface of the skin, even from clothing rubbing against it, can trigger a bout of hives in those prone to cholinergic urticaria. This is rare, indeed. In fact, I've never seen a case of vibratory urticaria.
- ✔ **Chemical reaction:** A reaction to penicillin or other medications can cause hives.

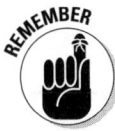

If you haven't eaten anything remotely suspicious in the few hours before experiencing hives, you can safely assume that your hives have nothing to do with a food allergy. Determining the cause of a random outbreak is usually impossible.

If, however, hives occur shortly after eating a new food, food allergy could certainly be the cause, especially if you just ate one of the more highly allergenic foods. A typical scenario is a baby who develops hives after his first taste of yogurt or scrambled eggs or peanut butter. When hives are due to food allergy they typically occur almost immediately (within 30 minutes) after eating the food and rarely beyond four hours after eating a suspicious food. If you ate shrimp on Saturday and got hives on Monday, it's not the shrimp.

A case of hives is not, in itself, serious, but it may be a sign of something more serious now or in the future. Keep the following important points in mind:

- ✔ Hives accompanied by other symptoms including vomiting or restricted breathing may be a sign of the onset of a severe allergic reaction. The more different parts of your body that are involved in a food reaction, the more dangerous it may be.

- ✔ A mild outbreak of hives can indicate the possibility of more severe allergic reactions in the future. This doesn't guarantee that your next reaction will be worse, but you should certainly be prepared for that possibility. When I teach doctors about food allergy, I always tell them that just because that first reaction caused only hives, you have no guarantee that a future reaction will not be more severe.

If you're experiencing repeated bouts of hives and are unsure of the reason, try keeping a food diary for a week or two to see if you can trace your recurring hives to a specific food. While you're logging your encounters with hives, consult your doctor and draw up an emergency plan just in case your next reaction is more severe.

Digging deeper with angioedema

Angioedema means swelling. Although it may occur alone, it most often accompanies hives. In fact, many doctors think of angioedema as hives to the nth degree, although hives tend to be more localized. During a reaction, angioedema can produce a wide range of symptoms:

- ✔ Welts, particularly on the face and around the eyes.

- ✔ Swollen lips.

- ✔ Intestinal swelling, often resulting in painful stomachache.

- ✔ Restricted or obstructed breathing, due to swelling of the airway. This is the most serious manifestation of angioedema, because the swelling can completely block the airway. Keep in mind that your windpipe is less than an inch in diameter and considerably narrower in children — a little swelling can easily pinch it shut. Angioedema's ability to obstruct breathing is the most common cause of life-threatening and fatal food reactions.

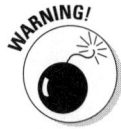

Patients often wonder if having angioedema externally, such as a swollen eye, indicates some internal swelling that they can't observe. External swelling can occur without internal swelling, but even so, when you observe significant external swelling, you need to be concerned about the possibility of swelling in the airway.

Taking a breather: Respiratory reactions

Food reactions can involve the airway anywhere from the tip of the nose to the bottom of the lungs, resulting in any or all the following symptoms:

- Nasal congestion or runny nose.

- Swelling of the throat or airway, as described in the previous section.

- Swelling of the bronchial tubes and even smaller airways in the lungs. When this occurs, the asthma-like symptoms occur as a result of a combination of airway swelling, muscle constriction, and mucus production. Asthmatic patients are much more likely to have these lower respiratory difficulties as part of a food reaction. In fact, patients with asthma are at far greater risk of having life-threatening or fatal allergic reactions because of this lower airway component.

When the lower airway — the throat and lungs — is involved in an allergic reaction, immediate administration of epinephrine is critical. Antihistamines have virtually no effect on these reactions. Asthma medications may be effective or completely useless, so don't rely on them. Epinephrine is king. See Chapter 7 to find out more about medications and emergency procedures.

Although acute food reactions often involve the respiratory tract, chronic congestion and other chronic respiratory conditions, such as asthma, are rarely the work of a food allergy. So, if you have chronic nasal congestion or asthma, without other food allergy symptoms, such as hives, eczema, or intestinal problems, your doctor is unlikely to suspect or test for food allergy as a cause. Environmental allergies become the prime suspect in these cases. Check out *Asthma For Dummies* (Wiley) for more information on asthma.

Having a gut reaction . . . literally

The most obvious victim of a food reaction is your gastrointestinal (GI) track — your digestive system, which starts in your mouth and ends in the waste canal. Because this system processes everything you eat and drink, you'd suspect it to suffer during a food allergy reaction, and it often suffers plenty.

Like skin reactions, GI reactions may range from very acute to very chronic, as the following sections describe. For details on treating specific gastrointestinal disorders, check out Chapter 7.

Observing acute gastrointestinal symptoms

Acute food reactions that attack the GI tract typically occur within moments after eating the offending food, and often produce the following symptoms:

- ✔ Itching in the mouth
- ✔ Swelling of the tongue
- ✔ Nausea
- ✔ Vomiting
- ✔ Abdominal pain
- ✔ Diarrhea (sometimes)

Although these symptoms can occur alone, they're often accompanied by other symptoms, such as hives and angioedema.

Taking note of more chronic gastrointestinal symptoms

Chronic gastrointestinal symptoms behave much more like eczema — these symptoms indicate a more delayed and lower-grade reaction than in acute cases. Symptoms include the following:

- ✔ **Gastroesophageal reflux.** In infants with reflux, food allergy plays a role in up to one-third of cases and may be the sole cause of the reflux. In infants who can't seem to hold down their food, doctors should at least consider the possibility of food allergy. Food allergy is less likely in older children, adolescents, or adults with reflux, although it certainly occurs occasionally and should not be overlooked.

- ✔ **Persistent abdominal pain.** A chronic stomachache can be the sign of a food allergy. Of course, it can also be a sign of eating too much junk food. Have it checked out.

- ✔ **Weight-loss and poor growth in children.** These are usually related conditions that arise as a result of chronic gastrointestinal reactions, because patients may be eating less and be unable to fully absorb nutrients due to chronic gastrointestinal inflammation.

- ✔ **Constipation.** Although food allergy can cause constipation, it's not common. If you have a difficult case of constipation that doesn't respond to other treatments or your constipation is accompanied by other food allergy symptoms, such as hives or eczema, you may want to be tested for food allergy. Otherwise, the cause is probably something else.

Uncovering anaphylaxis: The shocking story

Anaphylaxis (often called *anaphylactic shock*, but I'll get to that later) is an allergic reaction that involves multiple organ systems. If you experience symptoms in any two or more of the following organ systems, you're experiencing anaphylaxis:

✔ **Skin:** The most common symptoms of anaphylaxis are urticaria (hives) and angioedema (swelling of the tissues under the skin), but these symptoms are absent in up to 20 percent of anaphylactic reactions.

✔ **Respiratory tract:** Respiratory symptoms occur in about 50 percent of people who have anaphylaxis and are especially common in people who also have asthma. Low blood pressure can cause lightheadedness, dizziness, tunnel vision, and loss of consciousness (passing out).

✔ **Gastrointestinal tract:** Gastrointestinal symptoms occur in 30 percent of people.

✔ **Cardiovascular system:** Anaphylactic shock (extremely low blood pressure) occurs less commonly but may be increasingly common with age, occurring in up to 30 percent of adults who have a reaction. (See "Taking the pulse of cardiovascular symptoms," later in this chapter for details on cardiovascular symptoms.)

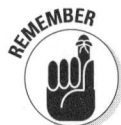

Anaphylaxis isn't always anaphylactic shock. In medical circles, *shock* refers to a drop in blood pressure to a dangerously low level. You can experience anaphylaxis with or without the shock (the dangerous drop in blood pressure).

In the following sections, I reveal the various ways that anaphylaxis attacks, explore the potentially dangerous cardiovascular symptoms that may be present, and describe the factors that increase a person's odds of experiencing anaphylaxis.

Exploring how anaphylaxis attacks

Anaphylaxis typically unfolds according to one of the following three scenarios:

✔ **Uniphasic:** A single wave of symptoms.

✔ **Biphasic:** In about a third of the cases, the reaction appears to resolve but recurs one to eight hours later.

✔ **Protracted:** Rarely, a pattern referred to as *protracted anaphylaxis* occurs, with signs and symptoms persisting for up to 48 hours despite treatment.

Thankfully, not all anaphylaxis is severe and life-threatening. Some reactions even resolve on their own without treatment, but that's impossible to predict, so you must treat all anaphylactic reactions promptly with epinephrine. See Chapter 7 for a comprehensive approach for treating anaphylaxis.

Taking the pulse of cardiovascular symptoms

Whenever the core of your being — your heart and all the pipelines through which it pumps your blood — is involved in a reaction, all sorts of really bad stuff can happen, and it can happen in a hurry:

 ✔ **Hypotension:** *Hypotension* (a drop in blood pressure) is the most common symptom. When your blood pressure drops, you often get dizzy, feel lightheaded, and sometimes pass out. An extreme drop in blood pressure results in anaphylactic shock.

 ✔ **Heart arrhythmia:** A *heart arrhythmia* is a variation in the beating of your heart — beating too fast, too slow, or irregularly.

 ✔ **Heart attack:** A severe food allergy reaction can give you a heart attack.

In children and young adults, anaphylactic shock is relatively uncommon even with the most severe reactions, because their cardiovascular system is so resilient. This does not mean, however, that younger people are immune to severe anaphylaxis. Anaphylaxis in younger people typically results in breathing difficulty — a constricted or blocked airway that causes the fatal and near fatal reaction. In a fatal reaction, the heart stops only because the body eventually runs out of oxygen.

Exploring the risk factors

Anyone who has food allergies should remain on the lookout for the signs and symptoms that presage a severe reaction, but some people may need to remain more vigilant than others. The following factors contribute to increasing your risk for experiencing a severe or fatal anaphylactic reaction.

 ✔ **Naming the high-risk foods:** While any food allergen can cause anaphylaxis, a few are particularly skilled at doing so. The most sinister of the bunch are peanuts, tree nuts, sesame, and shellfish. Peanuts and tree nuts alone are responsible for 80–90 percent of all fatal reactions. Other foods, including milk, egg, and wheat can cause severe reactions, as well. In fact, I see many patients with reactions to these foods that are just as severe as the worst peanut reactions. The reality though is that while most people with peanut and tree nut allergy are at risk for severe reactions, a far lesser proportion of people allergic to most other foods share the same risk.

 ✔ **Increasing the severity with asthma:** People with asthma are more likely to experience anaphylaxis and to have more severe respiratory problems during anaphylaxis. The combination of food allergy (especially to peanuts and tree nuts) and asthma seems to put people at risk for dangerous attacks.

 ✔ **Repeating bouts of anaphylaxis:** People who've had an anaphylactic reaction in the past are at increased risk of future anaphylactic reactions. However, everyone with anaphylaxis has had their first reaction once, so just because a food allergy has not previously caused anaphylaxis does not place you in the low-risk category.

Taking the focus off of food allergy

No doubt about it — food allergies can cause a wide variety of symptoms ranging from a mild tummy ache to a major system shutdown, but food allergy can't be blamed for every medical condition known to humankind. Unfortunately, people commonly suspect food allergy as the root cause of a host of maladies. In the following sections, I encourage you and your doctor to consider more obvious causes and cures before pointing the finger at a food allergy.

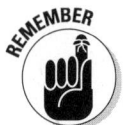

The risk involved in mistakenly suspecting food allergy as the cause of other medical and behavioral issues is that the time, energy, and resources you spend in pursuing an unlikely cause is wasted. You're better off seeking help from specialists who treat these conditions.

Meeting the rare breed of symptoms

Medical wisdom advises doctors that "When you hear hoof beats think of a horse rather than a zebra." In other words, suspect the most common causes first before testing for causes that are less likely.

Food allergies, for example, can cause other conditions — arthritis, inflammatory bowel disease, migraine headaches, or recurrent ear infections, but when these conditions arise, you need to investigate their more common causes first before suspecting food allergies. Only after ruling out more likely causes (or if these conditions are accompanied by other symptoms that can be more readily attributed to food allergy) should you suspect food allergy as the cause.

Keeping food allergies out of the psychiatrist's office

Some people want to blame everything on a food allergy, including psychiatric and behavioral disorders, such as attention deficit disorder, hyperactivity, and depression. As I write these words, a quick search on the Internet revealed over four million Web pages dealing with the relationship of attention deficit disorder and hyperactivity with food allergy. These conditions, however, are rarely, if ever, due to a true food allergy.

In caring for patients with food allergy, I've learned to never say "never," so I'm not claiming that behavioral disorders and other conditions can't possibly be related to food allergy, but the likelihood is extremely low.

I see many families who are hoping to find an easy and quick fix to significant behavioral issues by first exploring the possibility of a food allergy. In doing so, their children might be missing out on some wonderful therapies that are available elsewhere.

Chapter 3

Spotting the Usual Suspects: Wherefore Art Thou, Allergen?

In This Chapter

▶ Spotting the foods that most commonly trigger reactions

▶ Comparing ingestion, contact, and inhalation reactions

▶ Gauging how much of an allergen can cause a reaction

▶ Predicting the severity of subsequent reactions

*I*gnorance may be bliss when knowledge causes undue anxiety, but with food allergies, ignorance can be deadly and may amplify your anxiety. Not knowing which foods trigger your reactions, how much of a particular food is problematic, and the various ways the allergen can and cannot enter your system, is like jumping into the boxing ring wearing a blindfold. You don't know when your opponent is going to hit you, where you're going to get hit, how much it will hurt, or what you can possibly do to fend off the blows. You don't even know if your opponent is in the ring!

This chapter strips away the blindfold and empowers you with the knowledge you need to identify the most common allergenic foods and orient yourself to the three ways that the allergens in these foods can enter your system — by ingestion, contact, or inhalation. I attempt to assuage your fears of incidental contact allergies by revealing the real level of risk. And I place inhalation allergies in their proper perspective, so you won't freak out at the sight of a peanut butter and jelly sandwich.

By the end of this chapter, you'll be well prepared to identify the most common allergenic foods and establish a healthy vigilance without becoming unduly anxious.

In this chapter, I also answer the two questions that most of my patients ask:

✔ How much of an allergen does it take to trigger a reaction?

✔ How serious will my next reaction be?

Naming the Common Culprits

When you begin to explore the wide variety of foods that people consume all around the globe, you're likely to be surprised at the number of foods that don't cause allergic reactions in most people. Only a handful of edibles are predominantly responsible for causing the most problems. In fact, I can count the number of common suspects on my fingers and still have one finger left. In the United States, the following foods cause the most problems:

- Cow's milk
- Hen's eggs
- Peanuts
- Soy beans
- Wheat
- Tree nuts
- Fish
- Shellfish
- Sesame seed, sunflower seed, and other seeds

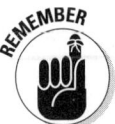

Because allergies are caused by a genetic disposition combined with exposure, common allergic foods vary by geographical location and culture. Populations that consume more fish, for example, have a higher incidence of fish allergies.

In the following sections, I introduce you to the nine foods that are responsible for the lion's share of food allergies and present a character sketch of each suspect.

Condemning cow's milk

Milk is often touted as "the perfect food." One distraught lactose-intolerant patient amended that claim by stating, "Milk is the perfect food . . . for cows." Around the world, cow's milk is the most common cause of food allergy, especially in children, because they drink the most milk at an age when allergies are most likely to develop.

The amount of milk protein that triggers a reaction and the severity of the reaction vary tremendously from one person to another. An extremely sensitive person can have a severe reaction to a small amount of milk protein hiding in a candy bar, while another person who's allergic to milk may be able to drink a half glass of milk and have little or no reaction to it. If you have milk allergy, consult your allergist to determine just how sensitive you are.

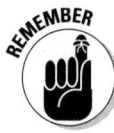

Don't confuse milk allergy with lactose intolerance:

- ✔ Milk allergy is an allergic reaction to one or more of the major milk proteins, the most important of which are *casein, whey,* and *lactoglobulin.* When you're allergic to milk, your doctor is likely to recommend that you avoid all forms of milk protein.

- ✔ Lactose intolerance has nothing to do with milk proteins, but with the sugar in milk. People who are lactose intolerant don't have the enzyme required to break down the sugar in milk.

Avoiding all forms of milk sounds bad enough. No milk? No cheese? No butter? *No ice cream?!* But the reality is even worse. Milk is an ingredient in a multitude of foods, from baby foods to breads to baked goods and milk chocolate, as well as all kinds of processed foods, so avoiding milk typically involves scratching about half of the most common foods off your grocery list. The good news is that the food industry offers plenty of milk, cheese, butter, ice cream, and yogurt substitutes, as described in Chapter 18.

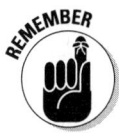

Children often outgrow a milk allergy later in childhood. In Chapter 15, I explain the likelihood of growing out of various food allergies and show you how to safely introduce foods later in life with your doctor's supervision.

Cracking open the mystery of hen's eggs

Eggs are a great source of protein for some and an equally great source of distress for people who are allergic to them. As with milk, several egg proteins can cause allergic reactions, the most common of which is called *ovalbumin.* Although you can't miss the eggs in your grocery store's dairy section, you really have to look hard to spot them out in the real world. Here are some tips to guide you in finding hidden eggs and avoiding them:

- ✔ Read labels carefully, because eggs hide in many food products. Chapter 6 offers an egg identification key that can assist you in deciphering labels.

- ✔ Most egg substitutes contain eggs or egg proteins, but in Chapter 18, I name one egg substitute that's completely safe.

- ✔ While the egg white is much more allergenic than egg yolk, most people with egg allergy need to avoid all forms of egg. Why? Two reasons. First, because the egg yolk contains allergenic proteins. Second, because no one can separate an egg any better than you can — all egg yolks also contain egg white allergens.

- ✔ Some vaccines, especially the common flu shot, contain egg protein.

Pointing the finger at peanuts

Peanut allergy ranks about third on most top-food-allergy lists, but this ranking is misleading. Peanut allergy occurs in less than 1 percent of young children, but then becomes more common than milk and egg allergy as people outgrow those allergies. (You're less likely to outgrow peanut allergy than you are to outgrow milk or egg allergy.) The medical community doesn't have the statistics to know for sure, but more Americans may be allergic to peanut than to any other food.

Peanut allergy also earns a top spot on the common-food-allergy charts, due to the potential severity of its reactions. While milk and egg allergies can and do cause very serious reactions in some people, most people with peanut allergy are at risk of severe reactions.

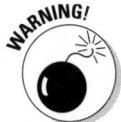

Peanuts commonly cause reactions with very small exposures, so even a contaminated product, such as a sugar cookie that shared a spatula with a peanut cookie, is capable of causing a severe reaction.

Researches have thoroughly characterized the specific peanut proteins that commonly cause allergic reactions, and have observed unique aspects to the way these proteins are constructed that make them such potent allergens. Skip to Chapter 4 to find out more about what makes peanut proteins so sinisterly special and gather tips on how to survive and thrive with a peanut allergy.

Censoring soy

Soy, short for *soybean*, is a member of the legume family, and as such, it's in the same family as the peanut. Of course, the peanut is the black sheep of the legume family due to its notoriety for causing the most severe allergic reactions, but soy has its own nefarious reputation because soy is *everywhere*. And since exposure is a key component to the acquisition of a food allergy, soy's widespread use makes soy a very common problem food. In fact, one of the first major uses of soy was as a substitute for milk protein in infant formulas, where it was introduced largely because the medical community in the 1950s and '60s thought it to be much less allergenic than milk.

Because of the widespread use of soy, avoiding soy is a monumental challenge. Food manufacturers commonly use soy flour in breads and other bakery items, and soy makes its way into a number of food substitutes, especially substitutes designed for those with peanut, milk, and egg allergies. Because soy is high in protein, it helps boost the protein content of many foodstuffs. Skip to Chapter 6 for guidance on how to spot soy on ingredient labels and identify common foods that contain soy.

Blaming the bakery: Wheat

Western diets are chock full of wheat. It's the main ingredient in most breads, cereals, pastas, and almost all baked goods. It also finds its way into numerous crackers and a host of popular snacks and finger foods. When you realize just how ingrained wheat is in the Western diet, when you look out over the aisles at your local grocery store, you may begin to envision amber waves of grain.

As with the other entries on our list of common allergenic foods, wheat's proteins instigate the trouble, and separating the protein from the grain is nearly impossible. If you have wheat allergy, read food labels carefully and remain aware of the foods that most commonly contain wheat, as explained in Chapter 15. For assistance in finding wheat substitutes, including replacements for bread and cereal, check out Chapter 22.

Wheat commonly sneaks its way into soups and sauces as a thickening agent, so don't let your guard down by thinking that you're safe ordering the soup without the French bread. Find out what's in the soup, too.

Shaking the tree for tree nut allergies

Most people don't know or care where their nuts come from, but people who have tree nut allergies sure need to know. While peanuts, which aren't really nuts, grow below the soil, almonds, Brazil nuts, cashews, hazelnuts, macadamias, pecans, pistachios, and walnuts hang out in trees. Like peanuts, however, these tree nuts have a nasty habit of causing severe reactions through even the smallest exposure.

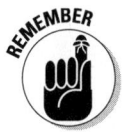

Technically, tree nuts have no family ties with peanuts, but their allergens share structural characteristics, which may explain why they are so potent and why 30 to 40 percent of the people who have peanut allergy also have tree nut allergies. If you're allergic to one tree nut, chances are pretty good that you're allergic to at least one or two other members of the tree nut family, so you're best bet is to avoid the entire family.

For a tree-nut allergen identification chart and instructions on how to pick the tree nuts out of a food label, refer to Chapter 6. Finding a suitable substitute for tree nuts can be quite a challenge. If you're not allergic to seeds, sunflower seeds may be nutty enough to satisfy your cravings.

Fishing for allergens in fish

For those with a genetic predisposition to allergies, the more fish they eat, the more likely they are to develop a fish allergy. Consequently, if you troll the globe and compare the prevalence of fish allergies in various countries, you find that countries that consume a lot of fish have a higher incidence of fish allergies than countries that consume less fish. Fish allergy is far more common, for example, in Japan and Scandinavian countries than it is in the United States.

As with the tree nut family, when you're allergic to one fish you're usually allergic to others, and your doctor is likely to recommend that you shun every member of the fish family.

Prying into shellfish allergies

Although shellfish allergy ranks eighth on our list of common food allergies, it's the number one most common food allergy in adults. Consider it a late bloomer, developing later in a person's life, commonly in young adults. A recent study shows that more than 2 percent of adults have shellfish allergy.

When you're dealing with a shellfish allergy, you may be tempted to lump all shellfish together, but they're actually divided into two major groups:

- ✔ Crustacea, including shrimp, crab, and lobster
- ✔ Mollusks, including clams, scallops, oysters, and mussels

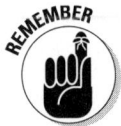

Complete shellfish avoidance is usually the rule once a shellfish allergy develops, although many people with a crustacea allergy may be able to tolerate mollusks, and vice versa. Discuss this with your allergist before indulging.

Suspecting sesame, sunflower, and other seedy culprits

Batting clean-up on the food allergy roster is sesame seed and other seed allergies, but in at least one country, Israel, sesame allergy is number one. If you hung with me through the previous sections, you can probably guess why that is — the Israeli diet includes a lot of sesame seeds and oil.

In the United States, the medical community has witnessed a surge in sesame allergy over the past 10 to 20 years, and some allergists estimate that sesame may well now be in the top five bracket. One reason for this dramatic increase may be due at least in part to the introduction of more sesame in our diets. With restaurants offering sesame seed buns and bread sticks and the increased use of sesame oil in dressings and other food products, exposure is on the rise.

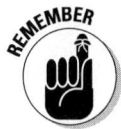

Other seed allergies, such as allergies to sunflower seeds, poppy seeds, and pumpkin seeds, do occur but are much less common, and most people with one seed allergy do not need to avoid all seeds.

Ingesting Allergens with Your Food

One of the main characteristics that distinguishes food allergens from other allergens, such as pollen, is that you generally eat food allergens. As I explain later in this chapter, allergens can also enter your system through physical contact and via the air you breath, in the case of airborne allergens, but most food reactions occur as the result of eating an allergen.

The fact that eating an allergen triggers most reactions inspires two of the most common questions I field on a daily basis:

- ✔ How much of an allergen does it take to cause a reaction?
- ✔ How severe will my next reaction be?

Unfortunately, the answers to those two questions vary from one individual to another and can even vary for one individual over time. In the following two sections, I reveal why the answers to those questions are so tentative and provide guidance on how to work with your doctor to discover answers that more specifically address your food sensitivity.

Gauging how much it takes to trigger a reaction

When someone asks me the amount of food required to trigger an allergy, I ask them to rephrase that question. A better question is "How much of a particular food is required to trigger *my* allergy?" The point here is that everyone's different. Each person who has a food allergy has a specific *threshold* — a specific dose of the food that sets the allergic reaction in motion. For some people that dose is incredibly small, for example 1/1000 of a peanut, but below that amount no reaction may occur. For others the threshold dose is quite large, for example five or six whole peanuts.

Several factors further complicate the process of coming up with a concrete answer that covers all cases:

- ✔ **The dose that causes a reaction may change over time.** In other words, you may be more or less sensitive to a food a couple months or years down the road. If you're lucky, your sensitivity tapers off completely and you outgrow your allergy, as explained in Chapter 15. If you're not so lucky, your sensitivity can increase over time (unfortunately a common occurrence with some allergies), and then you may react to lower and lower doses and your reactions may increase in severity.

✓ **You may be more sensitive when your immune system is revved up.** A recent food reaction or a bad pollen season, for example, can lower your threshold.

✓ **Your tolerance level can fluctuate.** You may be able to tolerate a given amount of food very intermittently, but as you expose yourself to it more regularly, you begin to react to it.

✓ **Some evidence suggests that in some people, exposure to even a small amount of food, even though the exposure doesn't cause an obvious reaction, makes it harder to outgrow the allergy.** The idea here is that these small exposures rev up the immune system and prolong the allergy, sometimes even making the allergy stronger and more dangerous.

Patients who can tolerate small amounts of a known allergen on an occasional basis may benefit from a *rotation diet,* as discussed in Chapter 6. For example, if you have milk allergy and the bread you enjoy contains tiny amounts of milk, you may be okay eating that bread once a week. Don't try this on your own; consult your doctor first. Exposing yourself to even a small amount of the offending food could result in a severe reaction, and even if it doesn't, the exposure could compromise your chances of outgrowing your allergy.

Predicting the severity of an ingestion reaction

Once you've experienced an allergic reaction, the first question is often "How bad will the next one be?"

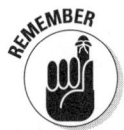

The rule of thumb for predicting the severity of your next reaction is that the higher your sensitivity and the more allergen you ingest above and beyond your threshold the worse the reaction. In other words, if you eat an oatmeal cookie that shared a spatula with a peanut butter cookie and you have a mild reaction, you can very likely expect a much more severe reaction if you gobble up a cookie with five peanuts in it.

Like most rules of thumb, this one begins to break down upon closer examination. Allergies tend to defy rules and common logic and toss in variables that call predictions into question:

✔ **Your threshold can change.** Say you eat 25/1000 of a peanut on a day when your threshold is 1/1000 of a peanut. On another day, you eat 40/1000 of a peanut when your threshold is 35/1000 of a peanut. You can expect a more severe reaction in the first case, even though you consume much more peanut in the second case.

✔ **Your reactivity can change.** If you've had a recent reaction or you're in the midst of a bad pollen season, you may react more strongly than normal.

✔ **Having asthma can increase the severity of reactions, especially reactions that cause breathing problems.** In general, the worse the asthma, the more severe the reaction. In other words, you can expect less severe reactions on days when your asthma is under control. (Asthma and food allergies commonly occur in the same people.)

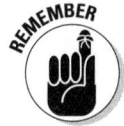

People (including many doctors) often say that severity increases with each subsequent reaction. However, while this may occur, allergies follow no predictable pattern. You really can't predict the severity of your next reaction. The best approach is to play it safe and team up with your doctor to track your allergy's ups and downs. Most importantly, always assume that a worse reaction may occur and be prepared to treat it, as I point out in Chapter 7.

Calming the Fears of Contact Reactions

When AIDS first captured the headlines, mobs of the irrational and uninformed gave their fears free reign. They imagined the worst possible scenarios — their children catching AIDS by sharing a desk with a fellow student who had AIDS, the possibility of passing AIDS through a handshake or a hug, mosquitoes carrying the AIDS virus over the neighbor's fence. None of that happened, but the fears whipped many people and even entire communities into a frenzy.

Although everybody knows that you can't catch an allergy from someone else, uninformed food allergy sufferers and uninformed parents of children who have food allergies occasionally develop similar overblown fears, often quite justifiably. They may read an article written by an ill-informed writer, hear a rumor, or let their imaginations run wild because they know first hand how serious a reaction can be.

In any event, most of the fears and concerns over contact reactions are overblown. In the following sections, I attempt to calm any lingering fears you may have.

Contact reactions occur when a problem food touches the skin. Common examples of this include having milk spilled on you, being touched by someone who has peanut butter on his hands, or being kissed by someone who has just eaten eggs (something that's not all that pleasant even if you don't have an egg allergy).

Predicting the severity of a contact reaction

Although contact reactions are very common, they're generally much less severe than reactions you experience when you eat an offending food. Contact reactions are also typically localized to the site of the contact; that is, the allergen doesn't get into your system and trigger a full-body response.

Contact reactions, however, can be more serious, depending on the amount of contact and on the location of contact — the body part that comes in contact with the allergen. Following are descriptions of three scenarios in which the contact reaction may be more severe:

- ✔ **Significant exposure:** Having a few drops of milk splashed on you typically results in mild reaction, if any. If you (or some clumsy ox) spills a glass of milk on you, that may cause a more severe reaction.

- ✔ **Contact with the eyes:** Your eyes are more than a gateway to your soul. They can be a gateway to allergens, as well. Your eyes are one of your most sensitive body parts, and even a little allergen can cause major swelling. Your eyes can even absorb allergens, which is almost like eating the food, because the allergen can travel *systemically* (throughout your entire body).

- ✔ **Hand contact to mouth ingestion:** If your hands come in contact with an allergen and then you put your hands to your mouth or touch some non-allergenic food you're eating, the contact reaction can turn into an ingestion reaction. This scenario causes additional concern in relation to young children who may be less aware of their surroundings and more prone to putting their hands in their mouths.

- ✔ **Mouth to mouth ingestion:** Kissing someone who has recently eaten a food you're allergic to can cause a reaction, sometimes severe. By following a few simple precautions, you can virtually eliminate this risk. In Chapter 14, I provide some safe-kissing tips for teenagers.

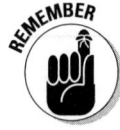

Thankfully, although these three scenarios engender tons of worry, none of them are at all common.

Washing peanut worries away

Concerned patients and caregivers and the always curious press call into our office daily to ask about the risk of contact reactions. To more accurately answer these questions, we did a study published in 1994 called the "Distribution of Peanut Protein in the Environment." The purpose of this study was to look for peanut allergen under various conditions and examine the effectiveness of cleaning agents for allergen removal. We went into schools and looked for peanut contamination on cafeteria tables and other surfaces and measured the presence of residual peanut protein after using various cleaning products on hands and tabletops.

We found that after hand washing with liquid soap, bar soap, or commercial wipes, peanut protein was undetectable. Plain water and antibacterial hand sanitizer left detectable peanut on 3 of 12 and 6 of 12 hands, respectively. Common household cleaning agents removed peanut allergen from tabletops, except dishwashing liquid, which left the protein on 4 of 12 tables. We evaluated 6 preschools and schools and found peanut protein on 1 of 13 water fountains, 0 of 22 desks, and 0 of 36 cafeteria tables. We concluded from these investigations that peanut allergen is relatively easy to clean from hands and tabletops with common cleaning agents and does not appear to be widely distributed in preschools and schools. Antibacterial gels, however, were very ineffective in removing the allergen, and we don't recommend them for this purpose.

Revealing the low risk of hidden dangers: From library books to monkey bars

If we let our imaginations run wild, we can think of innumerable ways in which contact reactions might occur. Just think of a day at school and imagine that a few children walk into school with peanut butter all over their hands. As the pass through the school, they might leave a deadly trail of peanut on door knobs, drinking fountains, library books, art supplies, computer keyboards, basketballs . . . even the monkey bars!

What, though, is the real risk? The answer is that the likelihood of these incidental contact exposures actually leading to a reaction is extremely small. I care for thousands of patients with food allergy and have dealt with tens of thousands of reactions. Of all the reactions I've witnessed, I can count on one hand the number that we could trace back to this sort of hidden, unsuspected exposure.

Refusing to let your allergies control your life

I've cared for many families who ultimately decided to home school their children specifically over fear of potential contact reactions. I have seen children become so paranoid that they won't hold hands with another child or even touch a door knob. While sensible precautions are warranted, remain rational and keep your imagination in check, for your own good as well as the good of those under your care. Follow these sensible precautions to allay your concerns:

- ✔ **Remain aware of your environment and of any potential hazards without becoming obsessed over them.**
- ✔ **Pay attention to major exposures, and let the little stuff go.**
- ✔ **Keep your hands clean and out of your mouth.**
- ✔ **Be careful kissing.** A peck on the cheek is fine, but kissing on the lips is riskier. See Chapter 14 for safe-kissing tips.
- ✔ **Wipe down tables before meals.** My colleagues and I have shown in our research that peanut protein can be cleaned from hands and tables with soap and water, as well as most types of wipes. (See the sidebar, "Washing peanut worries away," to find out about a study that shows just how easy it is to remove peanut remnants from hands and eating surfaces.)

Don't let the myriad of possible contact exposures run (and ruin) your life or foster irrational fears in a child.

Clearing the Air About the Risks of Airborne Allergens

Can peanut dust make you sick? If someone's eating a peanut butter sandwich next to you in the cafeteria, can that make you sick? What about airborne particles from other foods . . . do they pose a danger?

The short answer to these questions is yes, airborne allergens can affect people who are sensitive to those allergens. In some, relatively rare cases, airborne allergens can induce severe reactions. The level of risk, however, requires a somewhat longer answer, as I serve up in the following sections.

Dr. Bob weighs in on airborne peanut risks

I have a severe peanut allergy. A number of years ago I hired a new nurse to work in my food allergy clinic. We worked in different offices in the morning and afternoon and we would often share a ride between offices. For the first week she ate a peanut butter sandwich in my car every day for lunch. The smell was so offensive that I could barely eat my lunch, but I had no allergic reactions.

My nurse soon learned from one of our patients that I had a severe peanut allergy and she was absolutely mortified. I told her it was the best example I could ever give her of just how low the risk is to be around peanut butter. In spite of the smell, no peanut protein was shooting out of her sandwich, and I was really at no risk.

A few months later, we went to a meeting where for some inconceivable reason they were serving peanuts in the meeting room. Peanut shells carpeted the floor, and we were in very cramped quarters. I promptly excused myself because this situation really did put me at risk. The sponsor of the meeting, who had selected the peanuts as entertainment before the lecture, was less than pleased since they lost their speaker for the evening!

Recognizing the risk: When allergens take to the air

Whenever someone cracks open a peanut, tears open a package of powered milk, kneads bread dough, or fries a fish, allergens can take to the air and travel across a room where unsuspecting food allergy sufferers can inhale them. Although these situations commonly occur, serious reactions from airborne exposure are not terribly common, though they can and do happen. The trick to dealing with such situations is to acquire the skills for differentiating between situations that pose a real risk and those that pose little or no risk.

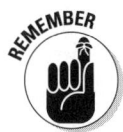

The risk of experiencing an airborne reaction varies greatly depending on the concentration of food protein in the air. And this hinges on how the food is handled, how close you are to the food being handled, and how confined a space you're in. With peanuts, for example, you face four levels of risk, as explained in the following sections.

Assessing level-one risks

Level-one risks arise when someone is eating a food next to you that contains the allergen as part of its ingredient; for example, a peanut butter or grilled cheese sandwich. In this instance, the risk that food protein becomes airborne and causes a reaction, especially a severe reaction, is extremely low. Even though you can smell the peanut or cheese, the scent arises from aromatic oils and has nothing to do with the protein that triggers a reaction. Not enough peanut or milk protein emanates from that sandwich to put you at any real risk, and reactions with this type of exposure are rare, even if you are in close proximity to the sandwich eater. (For a first-hand look at the comparative dangers of inhalation risks from peanut, check out the sidebar, "Dr. Bob weighs in on airborne peanut risks, earlier in this chapter.")

Assessing level-two risks

One step up from level one are level-two risks; for example, you're on an airplane where your fellow passengers are tearing into their tiny bags of peanuts. In this case, small amounts of peanut dust, which does contain the protein, may become airborne, especially since the bags of peanuts are being opened in the negative-pressure environment of the airplane cabin. The risk may further increase because you're in close proximity to the peanuts, you're in very confined space, and the air's re-circulating, potentially making matters worse.

Severe reactions have occurred on airplanes that appeared to be due to this airborne exposure, but you have to put the risk in perspective:

- ✔ Tens of millions of people with peanut allergy have flown with peanuts being served on board, yet only a very small number of people have reported reactions.
- ✔ If the risk were high and planes were routinely making emergency landings due to allergic reactions, they would have stopped serving peanuts a long time ago.
- ✔ As someone with a serious peanut allergy, I have flown thousands of times with no reactions.

Several major airlines have stopped serving peanuts to address the concerns of their passengers who have peanut allergy. The decision to go peanut-free is more for public relations reasons than to reduce the true allergy risk.

I tell my patients to arrange for peanut-free flights, at least for their peace of mind, but personally, I don't spend a lot of time looking for peanut-free flights when I travel. Skip to Chapter 11 for more travel tips.

Assessing level-three and -four risks

Risk levels three and four occur when people are shelling peanuts around you. This clearly causes more disturbance and a greater likelihood that peanut protein can become airborne, especially when the peanut shells cover the floor around you and people are walking on them, kicking up more dust. The key features that differentiate risk levels three and four are the proximity to the peanuts and, more importantly, how confined the space is, as demonstrated in the following two examples:

✔ **Level-three risk:** In an outdoor environment — for example, a baseball game — reactions are very uncommon because the allergen is swept away very readily by the open air.

✔ **Level-four risk:** In an indoor space, especially a small space like the waiting area of a restaurant, the risk of reactions rises dramatically.

Assessing the risks of airborne allergens in cooking

When you're cooking at home, you have control over what you cook and how you cook it. By following the precautions in Chapter 10, you're safe in your own home. When you go out to eat or drop in at your local coffee shop, however, the risks of experiencing an airborne reaction increase. Food allergists commonly see reactions triggered by the cooking of eggs, fish, and shellfish, especially on an open stove.

To reduce the risk, take the following precautions:

✔ **Steer clear of the cooking area.** If you're eating dinner at someone's house, stay in another room while your host prepares the meal. If you're in a restaurant with an open kitchen, sit at the table farthest from the open area.

✔ **Run an efficient ventilation fan.** Of course, you don't have any control over this at a restaurant, but if you're at someone else's house, you can ask them to turn on the exhaust fan.

✔ **Tell people about your food allergies.** When eating at someone else's house, let them know what you're allergic to. Most friends and family members are willing to adjust the menu if they know what to do.

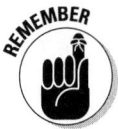

Remain vigilant of possible exposures from cooking and food preparation. In one week alone, I saw two patients who experienced airborne reactions at restaurants. One patient reacted in a restaurant with an open kitchen (the server unfortunately seated the family right next to the kitchen). Another patient, a curious two-year-old with milk allergy was allowed to sit on the counter at a coffee house and watch them froth the milk for his mother's latte. A few minutes later, hives erupted on his face, presumably appearing where microscopic droplets of milk landed on his skin.

Predicting the severity of an inhalant reaction

As with contact reactions, inhalant reactions typically are not severe. They most often begin with a rash or hives on the face, itchy eyes, or a runny nose — places where the airborne food comes in contact with the body. In most instances, you can quickly recognize the early symptoms and flee the scene (or at least move away from the cooking area) to halt the progression of symptoms.

The severity of a reaction is usually in direct proportion to the level of exposure. Severe airborne reactions primarily occur in the following situations:

- ✔ **You get a huge dose all at once.** For example, if you have a severe wheat allergy and walk into a bakery where hundreds of loaves of bread are being made, this huge single dose of allergen may trigger a severe reaction even if you immediately exit.

- ✔ **You can't leave.** If you're on an airplane, you can't just get up and walk off the plane.

- ✔ **You won't leave.** Sometimes people are too stubborn or embarrassed to leave. I've seen a patient with a fish allergy take a new job as a dishwasher in a seafood restaurant. I've also seen a number of teenagers who knew they were beginning to react but didn't leave the party where their friends were eating mass quantities of peanuts.

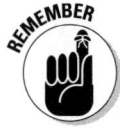

Be sensible about the risks, remain aware of your surroundings, and be prepared to take action when you observe serious risks, but don't let your food allergy run (and ruin) your life.

Chapter 4

Picking On Peanuts: A Potentially Deadly Foe

In This Chapter

▶ Identifying the stuff in peanuts that causes problems

▶ Recognizing the seriousness of the risk

▶ Uncovering the peanut's favorite hiding places

▶ Dining out on the peanut-free fare

*P*eanuts are the bad boys of allergenic foods. They're tasty, tempting, and pervasive, showing up in all sorts of foods where you'd never expect to see them. They can cause extreme, life-threatening allergic reactions, even airborne reactions. That's why I devote an entire chapter to the curse of the peanut.

In this chapter, I reveal the sometimes sinister nature of peanuts, uncover many of their favorite hangouts, separate fact from fiction concerning airborne peanut allergens, and show you how to avoid peanuts in the real world without being overly concerned.

Investigating the Allergic Nature of Peanuts

Although "peanut allergy" isn't exactly synonymous with "food allergy," peanut allergy exemplifies the food allergy phenomenon in a nutshell. It functions as a key to understanding just how common food allergy is, how the prevalence of food allergy has risen, and just how deadly a food allergy can be.

Because peanut allergy typifies food allergy, researchers have focused a great deal of research on it over the past 20 years, seeking answers to these most fundamental questions:

- ✔ Why are peanut reactions so serious?
- ✔ Why do you get peanut allergy?
- ✔ Why is peanut allergy becoming more common?
- ✔ What can be done to prevent peanut allergy?
- ✔ Can doctors treat peanut allergy?

The whole purpose of this book is to address these questions for any food allergy you have and express the answers in a way that assists you in living well with your food allergies on a daily basis. With peanuts, however, the third question, "Why are peanut reactions so serious?" earns additional attention, provided in the following sections.

Probing the peanut protein connection

As I explain in Chapter 2, a handful of proteins are primarily responsible for triggering allergic reactions, because your immune system sees them as the bad guys. Peanut proteins — specifically the three proteins fondly referred to as Ara h 1, Ara h 2, and Ara h 3 — look more like the bad guys than most other food allergens. (A *protein* is made up of a long string of building blocks called *amino acids*, which are folded into all sorts of shapes and sizes. No two proteins look exactly alike.)

Without becoming too technical, what makes peanut proteins so capable of stimulating an allergic reaction is the way in which they're folded. (Molecular size and stability may also be contributing factors.) Peanut proteins are folded in such a way that the protein pieces responsible for stimulating the immune system are very much exposed, rather than concealed inside the molecule. This gives the molecule a high profile that's easy for your immune system to recognize.

Although peanut proteins are easy for your immune system to recognize, researchers still do not know why some people's immune systems react to them so strongly. Do they look like something more sinister? Hopefully, future research can provide the answer.

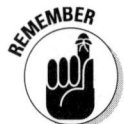

Most people with peanut allergy have IgE antibodies against all three high-profile peanut proteins — Ara h 1, Ara h 2, and Ara h 3, so when you eat a peanut, you're often getting a triple dose of allergen.

Acknowledging the deadly risk

Not all people with peanut allergy have life-threatening reactions to it, but this lowly legume, more than any other food allergen, is capable of causing severe and sometimes fatal reactions. Moreover, peanut can trigger these reactions with exquisitely small exposures. In studies of fatal food reactions, peanut and tree nuts are responsible for the vast majority of all such reactions.

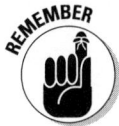

If you have peanut allergy, remain on the lookout for even trace amounts of peanut, which unfortunately shows up in a wide variety of foods. In the following sections I guide you on your quest to stay peanut free.

Playing Find-the-Peanut on Your Plate

Because of this risk of severe reactions with even minute peanut exposures, people with peanut allergy must play a never-ending game of hide and seek with the elusive peanut. Peanuts veil their presence in a surprising number of foods and travel incognito under a host of food label pseudonyms, so you can't assume that just because a particular dish or food sounds safe, it really is safe.

In the following sections, I point out the foods that pose the highest risk and show you specifically how to avoid peanut when dining out.

Uncovering peanut's favorite hideouts

The brilliant inventor George Washington Carver discovered 300 uses for the peanut. Food manufacturers and cooks have discovered infinitely more uses for peanut, many of which make the peanut nearly impossible to detect. Fortunately, food labeling is conservative, typically warning consumers even if the food "may contain peanuts." Unlabeled and prepared foods are responsible for a high majority of reactions. These foods generally fit in one of the two following categories:

- Foods in which you would least expect peanut, such as in sauces and salad dressings, that contain peanut as an ingredient.
- Foods that do not contain peanut as an ingredient but have been contaminated by peanut during production or preparation.

In the following sections, I point out the most suspect foods.

The greatest risk for peanut contaminated foods occurs when other products that do contain peanut are processed or prepared in close proximity to or using the same equipment as the food that you assume is peanut free. This risk is amplified in smaller facilities where the risk of significant cross contamination may be greatest, such as a bakery, restaurant, candy shop, or ice cream parlor.

Deconstructing cookies

Of all foods, cookies may well be responsible for the greatest number of accidental peanut exposures. Peanuts pop up in cookies you'd never suspect would contain peanuts, and cookies that are supposedly peanut free often are the victims of cross contamination. Following are some common scenarios that should make you think twice about eating a cookie you haven't baked yourself:

- ✔ **A baker decides that a few ground peanuts, a little peanut butter, or even peanut flour would make this batch really special.** Because the peanut is pulverized and is used in such small quantities, it's completely disguised, making detection by sight, smell, or even taste nearly impossible. Pulverized peanuts also find their way into some pie crusts.

- ✔ **A restaurant serves typically peanut-free chocolate chip cookies.** A new cook is hired who always sticks ground up peanuts in the dough to make the cookies a little crunchy. The server assures you that the restaurant's cookies are peanut free, not knowing that the change of cooks resulted in a change in the recipe.

- ✔ **The server assures you that a particular brownie doesn't have peanut in it, but when she dishes up your dessert, she uses the same spatula she used to serve up a dessert that contains peanuts.** You may think that the amount of peanut residue would be miniscule, and it is, but it's enough to cause a severe reaction in some people. Cross contamination may occur when the baker or server uses the same mixing bowl, cookie sheet, spatula, or tongs.

Digging into other baked goods

While cookies and similar products carry the greatest risk, all baked goods are suspect. Cakes and cupcakes that seem perfectly safe commonly cause peanut reactions. How can this happen? Cross contamination and hidden ingredients are often the root causes:

- ✔ **A dirty spatula or other serving utensil:** A serving utensil used to serve an unsafe food can sometimes transfer enough of that food to a safe food to trigger a reaction.

- ✔ **A contaminated knife:** A knife used to spread peanut butter icing on one cake and then spread peanut-free icing on your cake or cut your cake can spoil your dessert.

- ✔ **A flavoring that seems safe:** You wouldn't suspect that something called "Almond Extract" would trigger a peanut reaction unless you're also allergic to almonds, but I recently saw a girl who had a severe reaction after eating a supposedly safe cupcake a neighbor gave her. It turned out that the particular artificial almond extract the neighbor used was actually made of peanut.

Assuming my way to severe reactions

When I was growing up, my school system baked the best brownies. Even better for me was that they were peanut free. For nine years, I had eaten the brownies without experiencing a single reaction or even a tinge of suspicion. All that changed in my sophomore year of high school. That's when the high school cafeteria modified its age-old brownie recipe to take advantage of a peanut butter surplus. I never thought to ask if the brownie was safe, because I had eaten the "same" brownies for so many years. As soon as I ate that peanut-butter-laced brownie, I started to feel its ill effects, which ultimately led to a severe reaction. From that day forward, I made it a rule to never eat a baked good that I didn't personally prepare myself or that my mom hadn't baked for me. (I've never had a single reaction at home since the time I was diagnosed with a peanut allergy.)

I made an exception to the rule just once, about 15 years ago . . . after I had become an allergist

and had learned a great deal about peanut allergy. We were celebrating the holidays with a number of my co-workers and a colleague of mine — a world-renowned authority in food allergy. My colleague presented me with a gift of beautifully decorated cookies. As he handed them to me, without me even asking, he reassured me — in fact, he promised me — that these cookies were peanut free. Unfortunately, however, he didn't know that his wife had also made peanut butter cookies that morning and that she had used the same spatula between those cookies and mine. The level of contamination was enough to cause a very severe reaction. In fact, this was probably my most severe reaction ever. Over the course of that evening I needed five shots of epinephrine. The doctor, his wife, and I are still very close friends, but I have not broken my "no cookie rule" ever since. And thankfully, I've had no reactions since that time.

Uncovering peanuts in candies

If you're looking for a tough challenge, mosey down the candy aisle at your local grocery store or pharmacy and try to find candies (especially chocolates) that don't contain peanuts. Even candy bars that contain no discernable peanuts may have labels that warn people with peanut allergies to avoid them with messages like "May contain peanuts," "Traces of peanuts," and "Produced in a facility that uses peanuts."

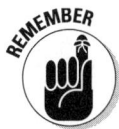

Candies produced by major manufacturers are almost always a safe choice, as long as the label does not list peanut as one of its ingredients. By being a diligent, vigilant label reader, you can consume these candies with a very low risk of reaction. For more about reading labels, see Chapter 6.

The most suspect candies fall into one of the following categories:

- **Candy from smaller manufacturers:** Watch out for smaller manufacturers who don't follow strict labeling guidelines or don't label their candy.

- **Unlabeled candies and other goodies:** For example, you'd have a tough time finding a safe candy in a fudge or candy shop... or in a gift box from a fudge or candy shop.

✔ **Cross contaminated candies and other goodies, especially from candy or fudge shops:** Even if a small candy or fudge shop does not mention peanut on a label, most of these shops have far too much peanut around to successfully prevent cross contamination. I would be very nervous, for example, eating a box of chocolate fudge or chocolate covered cherries, even if the ingredient list contains no hint of peanut.

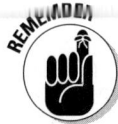

Stick with candies from major manufacturers, and eat those only after carefully studying the label each time you get them. Another alternative is to purchase candy from one of the guaranteed nut-free candy and baked good manufacturers that have popped up in the last few years. Check out:

✔ **Vermont Nut Free Chocolates** (www.vermontnutfree.com)

✔ **Kellie's Candies Nut-Free Confections** (nutfreecandy.com)

✔ **Rebecca's Nut Free** (rebeccasnutfree.com)

✔ **Nothin' Nutty** (nothinnutty.com)

Finding peanuts in ice creams and tasty toppings

The rules I described for cookies and candies in the previous sections apply to ice cream, too:

✔ **Stick with ice cream from major manufacturers and carefully read the labels.** Although ice cream produced in North America is rarely manufactured on dedicated peanut-free lines, I believe that ice cream from major manufacturers is generally safe. However, be careful of the small manufacturers — one study a few years ago of small ice cream manufacturers found that peanut contamination was quite common. Allergic reactions to peanut are rarely traced back to cross-contaminated ice cream from the major companies. You can call a company to learn more about how they handle and clean their equipment.

✔ **Make your own ice cream.** Some patients decide that the only truly safe ice cream comes from their own ice cream maker in their own kitchen.

✔ **Avoid scooped ice cream from parlors.** The ice cream reactions that allergists witness on a regular basis occur with scooped ice cream from ice cream parlors. As with candies and cookies, ice cream from parlors may contain undeclared peanut as an ingredient or, more often, become contaminated from shared ice cream scoops or nearby peanut toppings. At an ice cream shop, the server typically uses the same scoop for all the flavors, merely rinsing (not washing) it between orders. Once the server opens a container of ice cream and dips into it, you're likely to be served a scoop of contaminated ice cream.

✔ **Avoid the soft serve parlor, too.** Soft serve ice cream resolves the problem of the contaminated scoop, but it's not a foolproof solution. Most soft serve shops regularly offer a peanut flavor as the flavor of the day. You may arrive at the shop elated to see that strawberry is today's flavor of the day, but the shop may be dispensing today's strawberry ice cream from yesterday's peanut machine. Soft serve dispensers are extremely difficult to sanitize, and today's ice cream is almost certainly contaminated by yesterday's batch.

✔ **Skip the toppings.** Almost every ice cream parlor on the planet has a can of chopped peanuts on hand. Watch the servers rush through a couple orders, and you quickly notice that the peanut sprinkles often fly into the chocolate syrup, hot fudge, and other toppings. Sometimes, the servers use the same spoon to sprinkle on different toppings. Topping dispensers that haven't been properly cleaned and sanitized between flavor changes can also cause problems.

Some resourceful patients bring their own scoop to the ice cream parlor to reduce the risk of cross contamination. However, unless the person behind the counter opens a new tub of ice cream for you to use with your nice clean scoop, this really is not a safe practice. I do have a few patients with peanut allergy who found local soft serve ice cream parlors where they were comfortable. They know that the chocolate or vanilla machine never handles any other flavor, watch the ice cream come out of the machine and into their cup, and simply avoid toppings altogether.

Discovering peanuts in your chili bowl and other unsuspecting places

Just looking at a bowl of chili, you may never guess that any cook worth his wire whisk would consider sticking peanuts in her chili. Flip through a few gourmet cookbooks, however, and you quickly discover that peanut or peanut butter is a pretty standard ingredient. Cooks may add it to thicken the chili, spice it up with an interesting flavor, or add a little protein in a vegetarian version.

The risk of chili became quite well known a number of years ago when a college student at Brown University died after eating chili in a local restaurant. Hidden peanut can, however, show up in a host of other apparently safe foods, including these:

✔ **Spaghetti sauce:** I had never imagined someone sticking peanut butter in spaghetti sauce until I dined on some spaghetti laced with peanut. To find out what happened, check out the sidebar "Who slipped these peanuts into my spaghetti sauce?!"

✔ **Chicken dishes:** For some cooks, the marriage of chicken and peanuts is a match made in heaven. For those with peanut allergy, any fancy chicken recipe is suspect. I've even seen fried chicken recipes that call for ground peanuts.

✔ **Vegetarian dishes:** Without meat, vegetarians have to hunt for their protein elsewhere, and many of them find it in legumes, including peanuts. Be careful around any vegetarian dishes.

Who slipped these peanuts into my spaghetti sauce?!

Rarely is spaghetti sauce named as a suspect in a peanut allergy incident, but it can (and did) happen, and it demonstrates the need to always consult the cook before placing your order and to always be prepared for a reaction. I learned my lesson the hard way.

When I was in medical school, my future wife and I went out to eat at a health food restaurant. We ordered the spaghetti. After one bite I knew I was in trouble when I developed intense itching in my mouth. We asked the server who said she was sure our food was peanut free. We went straight into the kitchen and asked the chef, who said "Yes." She had tried a new

spaghetti sauce recipe that day that included peanut butter as an added source of protein.

My reaction quickly went from bad to worse, but fortunately, I had an epinephrine autoinjector in my pocket. Otherwise, I may well have not been around to tell this story.

The take-home message here is to always be prepared. When you least expect it, a food that appears completely harmless, a change of cooks, or a change of recipes can expose you to a dangerous amount of allergen. Being properly prepared at all times can literally save your life, as it did mine.

The risk of hidden peanut in chili and other dishes is very real and can be life-threatening, but you can protect yourself by following these tips:

- ✓ **Check with the chef, not only the server.** Ask the chef very direct questions and answer any questions the chef has to ensure that your food is safe. See Chapter 11 for additional tips on working with the restaurant staff to create a safe eating experience.

- ✓ **Always be prepared to deal with a reaction at any time.** Immediate treatment is key to your survival and success. No matter how careful you are, you will get burned at some time. Some creative cook will find a new way to use peanuts where you least expect it.

Deciphering the mysteries of peanut oils

On its surface, my recommendation for peanut oil may sound paradoxically paranoid — most peanut oil is safe, but avoid all peanut oil. Let me clarify that recommendation:

- ✓ **Highly purified peanut oil is safe.** A heat-processed peanut oil is typically completely or nearly completely free of the peanut proteins that trigger reactions. Studies show that these highly purified oils do not cause reactions even in people with severe peanut allergy.

- ✓ **Cold-pressed peanut oil is dangerous.** Because the oil is not heated during processing, it's raw oil that always contains large amounts of peanut protein.

✔ **Almost all peanut oil is suspect, even peanut oil that's advertised as peanut-free.** In your daily life, you can rarely be sure of the purity of a peanut oil used in preparing your food. To be safe, strictly avoid all forms of peanut oil.

If the world were perfect, discerning which peanut oil is safe and which one is not would be a simple matter of reading the label or talking to the cook. The reality though is that when you look at your bag of potato chips, you're likely to see peanut oil listed, void of any useful details concerning the purity of that oil.

A few years ago, I ran into a series of peanut oil induced reactions, when a local restaurant chain started serving potato chips fried in cold-pressed peanut oil. Many of the people who reported reactions knew about the peanut oil but had been reassured by the fact that most peanut oils are indeed safe. They ate the chips thinking that the chips would be okay . . . they weren't. In my patients I see peanut oil related reactions, including scenarios such as this one, at least once a month.

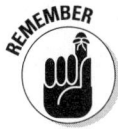

The relative purity of peanut oil makes my rule about avoiding it absolute — avoid all peanut oil. Follow these tips to remain peanut oil free:

✔ **Carefully read labels and avoid any food that contains peanut oil.** Not all peanut oils are created equal.

✔ **Assume that all peanut oil, no matter how it's processed, contains peanut protein.** You just can't tell how peanut-protein-free any peanut oil is.

✔ **Ask the restaurant manager and cook if peanut oil is used.** In most cases, the restaurant manager or cook replies that the restaurant uses "only vegetable oil." Peanut is a vegetable, so find out the specific ingredients in that vegetable oil.

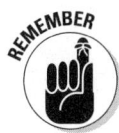

Don't panic unnecessarily if your waiter comes out after you have eaten your French fries and says she made a terrible mistake — your fries were really cooked in peanut oil. The risk of any given peanut oil exposure is truly very low. Discuss with your allergist on what to do if such an incident occurs.

Dining out without peanuts

When you're eating in, you can avoid peanuts by following the precautions I present in Chapters 6 and 10. When dining out, however, you must remain even more careful and vigilant to avoid peanuts by following these four steps:

1. **Choose a restaurant that is less likely to use peanut in their dishes.**

2. **Cross off any menu items that are likely to contain peanut.**

3. **Study the menu carefully to find foods that are more likely to be peanut-free.**

4. **Confirm that the food you are interested in ordering is indeed safe.**

In the following sections, I step you through this four-step process.

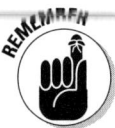

Follow these same steps if you have a tree nut allergy, keeping in mind that peanuts are more common than tree nuts in American cuisine. More and more restaurants, however, are sprinkling tree nuts over salads and adding them to other menu items.

Choosing a peanut-lite restaurant

Vegetarians avoid the local beef house and gravitate toward vegetarian restaurants to take advantage of the expanded selection of vegetarian dishes. Likewise, if you have peanut allergy, you can expand your menu selections by dining at restaurants that offer a wider variety of peanut-free dishes. Focus on the following types of restaurants:

- ✔ **Fast food chains:** A doctor's telling you to eat fast food? Well, not exactly, but most large fast-food chains are relatively safe places to eat for people with peanut allergy. The most common risk with fast foods involves the use of peanut oil, especially in the deep fryer. A number of French fry chains, as well as one national fried chicken chain I can think of, uses peanut oil. Even if you're eating at a relatively safe fast-food joint, don't get lulled into a false sense of security. For example, one of the major chains serves a milkshake made with peanut butter candies.

- ✔ **Steak houses:** Your local steak or beef house may be one of the best places to avoid peanuts altogether. These meat-and-potato restaurants commonly serve up pure beef along with potatoes and salads. You still need to be careful about the chef's secret sauce or barbecue rub and the salad dressings and other items, but a brief conversation with the cook can help you work around these minor complications.

- ✔ **American cuisine:** In the United States, we prefer our peanuts in baked goods and desserts, not in the main course, so restaurants that serve the standard American fare are pretty safe.

- ✔ **Italian (et tu Pizza):** While Italian cuisine may pose an issue for people with tree nut allergy, Italian dishes and pizza are usually safe for those with peanut allergy, although my co-author informs me that he knows of a gourmet pizza joint that serves peanut-butter pizza. As mentioned earlier, make sure the spaghetti sauce is peanut free.

- ✔ **Seafood restaurants:** As long as you don't have a seafood allergy in addition to your peanut allergy, seafood restaurants are about as safe as steak houses.

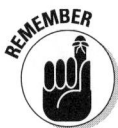

Just because I list a type of restaurant as a safer choice doesn't mean that it's 100 percent safe. You still have to perform your due diligence and talk with the server, cook, or restaurant manager each and every time you dine out.

Some types of restaurants, particularly those that serve up more exotic cuisine, may be places to avoid:

- **Thai:** Thai foods probably pose the greatest risk, because so many of the main courses contain peanut.

- **Chinese:** Chinese foods almost always have at least a few dishes with peanut. Although they're generally safer than Thai restaurants, Chinese restaurants fall into the same high-risk category.

- **Japanese and Korean:** Japanese and Korean dishes typically do not call for peanuts, but the cooks often use imported sauces that may contain peanuts or be contaminated with peanuts. Imported products are not held to the same manufacturing and labeling standards as those produced in the United States. I have some patients who have found Japanese or Korean restaurants where they are completely comfortable eating. However, I personally feel that avoiding these restaurants is the safest option.

- **Indian, Pakistani, Afghani, and Napalese:** Indian foods often contain peanut and pose a huge risk, although some dishes do not commonly use peanuts and therefore may be safe (except for the possibility of cross contamination). Again, I would avoid all Asian restaurants.

- **African, especially Sub-Saharan:** African restaurants often serve up peanut soups and a variety of peanut sauces.

- **Mexican:** While Americanized Mexican food rarely contains peanuts, the same cannot be said for authentic Mexican dishes. Beware of mole sauces, some of which may contain peanut or tree nuts. I do not recommend that you absolutely refrain from Mexican cuisine, but you must certainly approach it with caution.

- **Mediterranean and Middle Eastern countries:** If you're doing the Mediterranean Diet or eating out at a Middle Eastern restaurant, you're generally safe concerning peanuts, but if you're allergic to tree nuts, too, tread carefully in these foreign eateries. Pine nuts are a common ingredient, and these cultures have found a million and one ways to use pistachios and other tree nuts.

- **Health food restaurants:** Health food restaurants may serve up cuisine that's healthier for the general populace, but for those with peanut allergies, these restaurants can pose some hidden risks, especially in vegetarian restaurants, where peanuts are sometimes used to replace meat proteins.

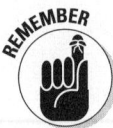

Asian foods are a common source of accidental peanut exposures both because peanut is easily disguised in these dishes and because peanut is used in enough other foods to lead to cross contamination. If the customer before you ordered the Kung Pao chicken, all sorts of peanut remnants can show up in your supposedly peanut-free dish. This is not just a theoretical concern but rather a very common cause of reactions.

I used to eat Asian foods and thought that if I spoke to the chef and ordered carefully I was safe. Luckily, I never had a reaction related to these Asian foods, but the more I get into this field, the more I realize that I was playing a game of Asian roulette.

Crossing off dishes that are likely to contain peanuts

Some types of prepared dishes have "peanut" written all over them. The following list can help you hone your skills for identifying the riskiest selections:

- Foods with sauces or gravies
- The entire dessert menu, including the ice cream

Highlighting dishes that are less likely to contain peanuts

Whether you're dining out at a peanut-safe or a peanut-risky restaurant, examine the menu carefully to separate the low-risk from the high-risk items. Highlight the following types of menu items as less risky:

- Simple, straightforward dishes that you would never dream could contain peanuts
- Grilled foods, including chicken, beef, and fish, served with no fancy sauces or gravies
- Pizza and most Italian foods
- Greek foods
- Fried foods, as long as you know the type of oil being used

Low-risk doesn't mean no-risk. Even if a menu item looks like it can't possibly contain peanut, you can't be sure, and you don't know until you talk with the cook how the item was prepared, as I explain in the following section.

Confirming that a menu item is peanut-free

When the server arrives to take your order, make sure that the server talks to the cook directly, or ask to speak with the cook yourself to ensure that your meal not only does not contain peanut as an ingredient but also that the cook prepares it following a peanut-free protocol. In Chapter 11, I offer guidance on how to communicate with restaurant personnel no matter what food you're allergic to. Chapter 11 also includes a restaurant card that can provide the cook with additional details without having to step out of the kitchen during the dinner rush.

Before placing your order, explain that you have a severe peanut allergy and that even a trace amount could kill you. Then place your order, as in the following examples:

- ✔ "I would like the house salad and the grilled chicken with a baked potato. I need to confirm with the chef that these dishes do not contain any peanut or tree nuts and that contamination with any form of nut cannot occur."

- ✔ "I would like to order a cheeseburger and French fries. I need to know exactly what type of oil is used in your deep fryers." If the server or cook answers, "We use pure vegetable oil." Respond with, "I need to know what type of vegetable oil you're using today."

Ask the server to be sure to wash his hands before serving your food, just in case he handles another plate between orders that contains peanut residue. However, don't rely only on the server's word alone for details about what a particular dish contains. Be sure that the server speaks to the cook about your order and if you have any doubt, speak directly to the cook.

Inhaling Peanut Dust: Airborne Reactions

More fear than actual peanut dust swirls through the air concerning airborne peanut reactions. As I explain in Chapter 3, many people think that just sitting in a chair next to a peanut butter sandwich can cause a severe reaction. Although airborne peanut reactions are possible, the risk is actually lower than you may think. In the following sections, I separate fact from fiction to calm fears and point out the real dangers.

Ruling out airborne reactions in peanut butter and candy bars

Concern over peanut exposure is justified, because peanut is so pervasive, but only by establishing a realistic risk assessment can you identify the true risks and let down your guard in low-risk situations. The truth is that an airborne peanut reaction from peanut butter, candy bars, and even peanut butter crackers is very unlikely. Here's why:

- ✔ Peanut butter and candy bars tend to bind the peanut dust with other stuff like chocolate or caramel, so rarely does a sufficient amount of peanut protein escape into the surrounding air to cause a reaction.

✔ Even though you can smell the peanut from these foods, evidence shows that the odor emanating from peanut butter or candy bars does not contain the protein that could cause a reaction when someone handles or eats these foods.

You could experience an airborne peanut reaction if the peanut eater was in your face, talking and laughing, and essentially spraying small droplets of peanut at you. Aside from this kind of situation, however, the risk is nearly negligible and identifying cases of peanut reactions from this kind of exposure is very difficult.

Designating peanut-free zones

Is your child's lunchroom permeated with peanut? Does your child need to sit at a peanut-free table? Should the entire school ban peanuts of any kind from the premises? These are all valid questions, but you can safely say that we have no universally correct answers to these questions. Parents, students, and school administrators often hold opposing views. Even different doctors can be in total disagreement.

I'm quite certain that prior to 1990, the peanut-free table was unheard of. Considering peanut-free tables since then has often been thought to be borderline un-American. Now peanut-free tables are the norm in most schools, and some schools ban peanut products altogether. So who's right? Following is the approach I recommend:

✔ **Designate peanut-free zones up to the third or fourth grade.** Preschool-age children are much more likely to be tempted to share food, to have lots of peanut on their hands, and have difficulty keeping their hands to themselves. As children grow older, these risks lessen.

✔ **Phase out peanut-free zones in higher grades.** I am not convinced that peanut-free zones provide any additional safety for older students. In fact, I now write many more letters to get kids out of peanut-free tables than I do to get kids seated at peanut-free tables. This typically occurs in older children who have become fed up with being isolated at a peanut-free table and whose parents accept that the risk of eating at regular table is incredibly small.

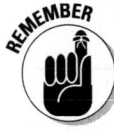

My recommendations may seem too safe for some and too risky for others. You, your child, and your school must work together to establish an acceptable level of safety that keeps kids safe without emotionally isolating them or preventing them from fully experiencing their school years. Chapters 12 and 13 offer additional guidelines on developing allergen-free policies.

Spotting peanuts at bars and restaurants

Among the places where airborne reactions do occur are bars and restaurants where peanuts are being served as a snack. In these settings, peanuts are usually served in the shell, and the process of cracking shells leads to small amounts of protein becoming airborne, sometimes in high enough concentrations to trigger a reaction. This may be further exacerbated when the peanut shells accumulate on the floor and patrons and servers kick up the dust, especially in an enclosed area.

When you're allergic to peanuts, your best bet is to avoid restaurants and bars that serve peanuts in their shells, even if that means leaving your friends behind at the local pub. The worst reactions I've seen in these situations occur when the airborne peanut protein is combined with large doses of alcohol and denial, so that the reaction gets out of hand before the person experiencing the reaction has a chance (or inclination) to leave. Otherwise, simply leaving the area usually leads to a rapid cessation of symptoms, especially when combined with medication.

Mixing peanuts with baseball

What would a baseball game be without shelled peanuts? For someone who suffers from peanut allergy, the game would be a heck of a lot more enjoyable. By the third or fourth inning, the stadium floor is carpeted in peanut shells, and people with peanut allergies often begin to spend more time looking at the exit signs than at the scoreboard.

In the open-air venue of a baseball field, however, the risk of an airborne peanut reaction is relatively low. In fact, most people with peanut allergy experience no symptoms in an outdoor stadium, even when surrounded by a crowd of peanut shelling fans.

So, can you safely take Junior to see his favorite baseball team in action? Well, that depends on whether Junior is old enough to sit in his seat and enjoy the game. Taking young children who are prone to picking up things off the ground, including every peanut shell in sight, is just not worth it.

Steering Clear of the Other Nuts

Unlike peanuts, which are really legumes (in the bean family), tree nuts are really nuts. Tree nuts include almonds, Brazil nuts, cashews, hazel nuts, hickory nuts, macadamia nuts, pecans, pine nuts, pistachios, and walnuts. As opposed to peanuts, which grow in the ground, tree nuts, as their name implies, grow on trees.

In food allergy circles, most people lump together peanuts and tree nuts. Botanically speaking, associating peanuts with tree nuts is absurd. Allergically speaking, however, the association makes a lot of sense. Following is a list of similarities:

- ✔ Like peanuts, tree nuts can cause severe allergic reactions.

- ✔ Tree nuts are capable of causing severe reactions with minute exposures.

- ✔ Peanuts and tree nuts tend to travel in the same circles — baked goods, ethnic foods, candies, and ice creams are the most common causes of accidental tree nut exposures.

- ✔ Tree nut oils and extracts all contain the allergenic proteins, so you must avoid the oils and extracts, too.

In studies of fatal food allergic reactions, tree nuts rank second only to peanuts.

Even though tree nuts and peanuts are botanically unrelated, people with tree nut allergy often have peanut allergy, and vice versa. Several studies show that 30 to 40 percent of people with peanut allergy also develop tree nut allergy. We allergists used to struggle to explain the link between peanut and tree allergy, and we thought it was most likely due to the fact that peanuts and tree nuts are both just very potent allergens. New research, however, has uncovered actual structural similarities between peanut protein and many of the tree nut proteins.

At this point, you're probably wondering, "If I have a peanut allergy, should I avoid tree nuts?" The short answer is "Yes." For a longer answer, discuss with your doctor the pros and cons of avoiding tree nuts. In my clinic, we recommend that patients with peanut allergy avoid tree nuts for the following three reasons:

- ✔ Peanuts and tree nuts are all too often processed together or at least near enough to one another to pose sufficient risk.

- ✔ Manufacturers often use peanuts as a substitute for tree nuts, because peanuts are cheaper.

- ✔ In young children with peanut allergy, staying away from tree nuts may help prevent the child from developing a tree nut allergy.

For those with a tree nut allergy, many forms of peanut can be safe, especially major brand peanut butter and some candies. Be careful though; dry roasted peanuts are often tree-nut contaminated, and a gourmet peanut butter may have shared equipment with almond or cashew butter. In my clinic, we encourage patients with tree nut allergy to avoid peanuts, as well, generally for the same reasons we tell our peanut-allergic patients to avoid tree nuts.

Part II
Progressing from Hives to Hope: Diagnosis and Treatment

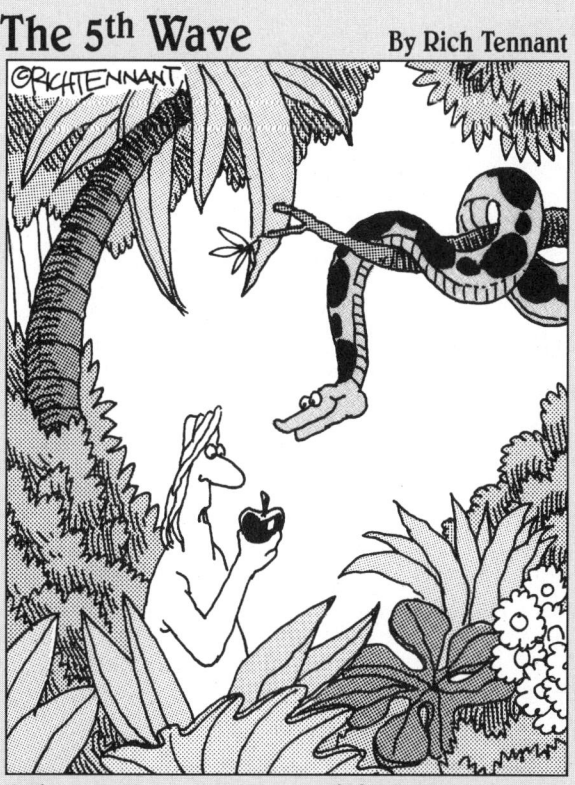

The 5th Wave   By Rich Tennant

"This isn't some sort of fad diet, is it?"

In this part . . .

In this part, I lead you step by step through the diagnostic process and show you how to team up with your allergist to identify your specific problem foods. I guide you on purging the offending foods from your diet without overly restricting your diet, and I provide you with the tools you need to decipher food-label gobbledygook.

To assist you with any lingering symptoms, I present the most effective medications and other symptomatic relief currently available and steer you clear of unproven alternative tests and treatments that can empty your bank account faster than you can say "anaphylaxis."

Finally, I reveal cutting-edge research that may lay the path to an eventual cure. By the end of this part, you and your doctors can form a unified front to accurately diagnose and successfully treat your food allergy and fill you with hopeful expectations for a reaction-free future.

Chapter 5

Labeling Your Ailments with an Accurate Diagnosis

. . . .

In This Chapter

▶ Understanding what to expect

▶ Deciding when you need to see your doctor

▶ Teaming up with your doctors to find the problem food(s)

▶ Picking a food allergist who's best qualified to treat you

▶ Assessing the usefulness of allergy tests and other diagnostic tools

. . . .

*W*hen you can't eat without breaking out in hives, having your ears puff up like muffins, or getting the collywobbles, obtaining an accurate diagnosis can calm your anxieties. I'm not saying that being diagnosed with a food allergy is cause to celebrate, but diagnosis is the first step to relief.

In this chapter, you take the first step on your diagnostic journey by completing a self-screening test. Although this test isn't intended to be a self-diagnosis, it can assist you in deciding whether you need to visit your family physician or an allergist for a more thorough workup. The self-screening test also guides you through the process of logging information that can be very useful in your diagnosis.

With your self-screening test in hand, you and your doctor can then embark on your search for the offending food(s). To assist you, I provide plenty of guidance and tips on how to team up with your family physician (or pediatrician) and allergist to more effectively determine if you do, in fact, have a food allergy, and (if you do) expedite the process of identifying the food(s) that ail you without overly restricting your diet. I also show you the sorts of allergy tests and other diagnostic routines you can expect, so you won't be taken off guard by any of your doctor's recommendations.

In this chapter, I refer to many of the common symptoms of food allergy. For a more complete discussion of symptoms and possible causes, check out Chapter 2.

Taking a Flyover View of the Diagnostic Journey

The path from the point at which you feel ill to the point at which you receive a diagnosis and treatment plan can be a long and winding road. To assist you in navigating that path, check out this eye-in-the-sky overview of the diagnostic process:

1. **Your general practitioner (GP) performs a physical exam and jots down your medical history.** The history is critical in ruling out other possibilities, identifying the likely problem foods, determining which tests are most appropriate, and guiding the interpretation of test results. See "Taking a Trip to Your General Practitioner."

2. **Your GP refers you to an allergist.** An allergist, particularly one with experience in diagnosing and treating food allergies, can perform additional tests and is usually more qualified to interpret the test results. See "Seeking an Allergist's Advice."

3. **Your allergist performs a complete food allergy workup.** Like your GP, your allergist is likely to perform a physical exam and take additional notes about your medical history. Your allergist is likely to perform several tests to identify the problem food(s) and rule out suspects that are not involved:

   - **Skin tests:** Skin testing is used only in the diagnosis of IgE-mediated food allergies — allergies in which your immune system produces IgE antibodies to a specific food. An allergy specialist (rather than your GP) should perform the tests, because of both the risk of anaphylaxis and the skill required to properly interpret the results. A positive skin test to a particular food indicates only the possibility that you're allergic to that food. Your allergist may need to perform additional tests to confirm that eating the food causes you to react. In contrast, a negative skin is about 90 percent accurate in determining that you're not allergic to the tested food. See "Poking around with skin tests," for details.

- **RASTs:** Short for *radioallergosorbent tests*, RASTs look for the presence of food-specific IgE in the blood. These tests are widely available and are unaffected by the presence of medications. In at least one study, RASTs have proven very effective in diagnosing several of the major food allergies in children. RAST results show the concentration of IgE in the blood, and we have established RAST levels that can predict with about 95 percent accuracy whether a child is allergic to egg, milk, peanut, tree nut, or fish. A child with a test result exceeding the established value, in combination with a positive skin test, does not require food challenge for definitive diagnosis. See "Hunting for IgE with RASTs," later in this chapter.

- **Food diary:** Your allergist may ask you to keep a food diary listing the foods you eat and drink and recording any reactions to those foods. A food diary can be useful in identifying overlooked foods, hidden ingredients, and patterns of reactions. See "Preparing to have your history taken," later in this chapter.

- **Diagnostic elimination diet:** Your allergist may order you to stop eating one or more foods to see if symptoms disappear, which would identify the problem foods. The allergist needs to pay careful attention to nutrition whenever removing an essential food from the diet of a growing child. See "Discovering your allergens by avoiding them," later in this chapter.

- **Food challenges:** A food challenge consists of eating the problem food under your allergist's supervision. Results of a food challenge provide the most definitive data for diagnosing a food allergy. Your allergist will select foods for testing based on the history and the results of skin and/or RASTs. Only a qualified allergist who's familiar with food-allergy reactions and is equipped with the necessary emergency medications should perform a food challenge. See "Daring a food to make you react: Food challenges," later in this chapter.

4. **Your GP and allergist may order additional tests if symptoms persist.**
   You may have a non-IgE mediated food allergy, as discussed in "Pursuing the causes of non-IgE mediated allergies," later in this chapter, or you may have a food intolerance (see "Ruling out food intolerances," later in this chapter).

The journey from problem to solution often requires time, patience, and persistence. Don't try to take a shortcut by reaching for untested, unproven alternative tests and treatments. See "Avoiding the untested and unproven," later in this chapter, for details.

Self-Screening for Food Allergies

Funny thing about people in general (specifically men) — they don't like going to the doctor. They often prefer to tough it out, hope it goes away, or convince themselves that the doctor "can't do anything" rather than seek immediate medical care. With food allergies, however, avoiding the doctor can be dangerous, because the longer you tough it out without an accurate diagnosis, the more likely your reactions are going to increase both in frequency and severity.

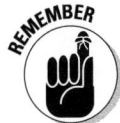

Allergic reactions begin and intensify with increased exposure to allergenic foods. Early diagnosis and an effective treatment plan can not only make you feel better now but also prevent you from feeling much worse down the road.

If you or a loved one is experiencing mysterious symptoms, particularly a couple minutes to a couple hours after consuming food or beverages, you may have a food allergy. Complete the self-screening test, shown in Figure 5.1. This self-screening test serves three very important purposes:

- ✔ Assists you in deciding whether you need to see your doctor or allergist. (If you have any doubt after completing the test, see your doctor anyway.)

- ✔ Provides you with a log of symptoms and other concrete details that you can present to your doctor or allergist, which may be key to an accurate and early diagnosis.

- ✔ Hones your observation and record-keeping skills, which are two of the most valuable skills for any person who has a food allergy or is caring for someone with a food allergy.

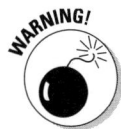

This self-screening test is not a self-diagnosis. Identifying specific allergens is tricky, even for a well-trained and experienced allergist, and you may be allergic to multiple foods. In addition, other conditions can produce symptoms similar to those of allergic reactions. Use the self-screening test only as a tool to facilitate a professional medical diagnosis and treatment.

Food Allergy Pre-Screening Test

Complete the following form to determine whether a visit to a food allergist would be a good idea. Take the form with you to your family doctor or allergist to assist in your diagnosis.

I have the following symptoms a couple minutes to 2 hours after eating or drinking:

Symptom	Food or Beverage	Amount consumed
☐ Tingling or itching in and around the mouth	_____	_____
☐ Swelling of the tongue and throat	_____	_____
☐ Flushing of the face or neck	_____	_____
☐ Rash	_____	_____
☐ Eczema	_____	_____
☐ Hives and swelling	_____	_____
☐ Vomiting	_____	_____
☐ Abdominal cramps	_____	_____
☐ Diarrhea	_____	_____
☐ Wheezing	_____	_____
☐ Difficulty breathing	_____	_____
☐ Drop in blood pressure (feeling faint or weak)	_____	_____
☐ Loss of consciousness	_____	_____

Figure 5-1:
Complete this self-screening test in preparation for your diagnosis.

Symptoms commonly arrise within _____ (minutes/hours) after eating or drinking and last _____ (minutes/hours) after eating or drinking.

I first noticed these symptoms _____ (days/months/years ago)

I have had similar symptoms _____ times in the past.

I have treated my reactions with: _____ , _____ , _____ , with the following results: _____.

Taking a Trip to Your General Practitioner

When you first suspect that you have any health problem, the first doctor you typically go to see is a general practitioner (GP for short) — your family physician, pediatrician, or internist. In the following sections, I reveal how a GP can and cannot help you with food allergies, when and how to request a referral to a food allergist, and how to avoid quacks who promise everything, deliver little or nothing, and often discourage you from seeking effective treatment.

Why see your GP?

In the case of food allergy, seeing your GP first is a good idea for several reasons:

- Your GP possesses a breadth of knowledge and training that's often useful in identifying not only food allergies, but also other conditions that may produce similar symptoms.

- The GP can coordinate the oversight and management of all your health-care needs, not only your concerns about allergies.

- Your GP often has access to your entire health history and may be able to spot patterns in your family history that make certain conditions more likely than others.

- Your health insurance may require you to see your "primary care physi-cian" (your GP) before approving your visit to a specialist.

- Your GP can refer you to a qualified food allergist, often one that's in the same insurance network and perhaps in the same office complex.

Knowing what to expect from your GP

Some GPs know quite a bit about food allergies. Pediatricians may even know a bit more, because food allergy is most common in young children. So what's your GP supposed to do? In the following sections, I describe the standard care you can expect from your GP. If you're not receiving a standard level of care, express your expectations to your GP. If you're still not satisfied, you may need to look for another doctor.

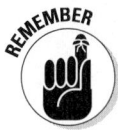

Most patients love their GP's and are satisfied with the general care they provide, but the number one complaint I hear from patients is this: "How could my doctor (pediatricians included) have been so ignorant about food allergy?" Many patients report symptoms of food allergy to their GP's for years before their GP's take the reports seriously. (GP's generally take reports of severe reactions seriously and refer patients to an allergist immediately, but they frequently miss the signs of more subtle reactions.)

Recording your history and equipping you for potential emergencies

The least your GP should do is ask you a lot of questions, record a detailed history of symptoms and what makes them better or worse, and determine the likelihood that you're at risk for severe or life-threatening reactions — that is, whether you may have an IgE-mediated allergy, as described in Chapter 2. If your doctor suspects that you have an IgE-mediated allergy, she will likely take the following steps:

- ✔ Identify suspected food(s) to avoid until you can get in to see the allergist.

- ✔ Refer you to an allergist.

- ✔ Hand you a prescription for autoinjector, such as an EpiPen or Twinject, as a precaution in the event that you experience a future anaphylactic reaction. (See Chapter 10 for details on getting your emergency kit together.)

To err on the side of safety, assume that the next reaction is going to be more severe than the previous reaction and equip yourself to deal with it. Just because a child developed hives only on her face during her first reaction to milk or egg, you can't assume that the next reaction is going to be of a comparable intensity.

Initiating allergy testing

Your GP may or may not decide to initiate allergy testing. Very few GP's have the training or materials to perform skin tests, but any doctor can perform blood testing for allergies (see "Hunting for IgE with RASTs," later in this Chapter). RAST (radioallergosorbent test) results can be very helpful in proving that the suspect food really triggered your reaction. However, searching for culprit foods with extensive panels of tests — that is, by ordering tests for hundreds of foods — is usually a huge waste of time and money and risks returning a number of false positive tests which only complicates the diagnosis.

Tracking down other potential causes

If your doctor doesn't suspect an IgE-mediated allergy, then she should attempt to determine whether the reaction represented some other type of food allergy or a nonallergic food reaction (a *food intolerance*, as explained in

"Ruling out food intolerances," later in this chapter). The diagnosis and management of non-IgE-mediated food allergy often requires the assistance of a gastroenterologist as well as an allergist. In some cases, the history may be insufficient for discerning the cause of a particular reaction. This is most often the case with patients who have isolated gastrointestinal symptoms. In such instances, your GP should arrange for further evaluation and proceed as if the reaction were IgE-mediated, including equipping you with epinephrine if suspicion is sufficiently high.

Advising you until further notice

Based on your history and any test results, your GP should tell you which foods to avoid until further evaluation. Your doctor should carefully interpret the RASTs, since you can often test positive for safe foods, and you don't want to be saddled with an overly restrictive diet. In some cases, a GP orders RASTs but is not fully competent in interpreting the results. Have your RAST results forwarded to the allergist you decide to see.

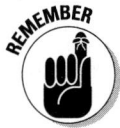

When you're on an extremely restrictive diet, meeting your nutritional needs can be tough, especially for infants and children. If your doctor prescribes extreme restrictions, he's likely to refer you to a nutritionist, as well. If he doesn't refer you, request a referral, as explained in the section, "Navigating the referral process," below.

Navigating the referral process

You visited your GP, she took a detailed history, told you that you probably were suffering from a food allergy, and referred you to an allergist. Good for you. You're now on your way to a more thorough workup and can skip ahead to the section, "Teaming up with your allergist for optimum results." If, on the other hand, your GP offers no reasonable alternative diagnosis or effective treatment and is reluctant to refer you to an allergist, you may have to crank your efforts up a notch:

- ✔ **Ask your GP if she thinks the symptoms could be symptoms of food allergy.** Sometimes, this is enough to lead a GP on the right path.

- ✔ **State the reasons why you suspect food allergy.** Use your powers of persuasion to convince your GP that food allergy is a possibility and that a specialist can help confirm your suspicions or rule them out.

- ✔ **Request a referral.** If your insurance plan requires a written referral from your GP in order to cover your visit to a specialist, your goal is to walk out of your doctor's office with a referral. (See the following sidebar, "Referrals past and present," for details.) Don't be shy, and don't take no for an answer.

✔ **Call your insurance company.** Look on the back of your insurance card for a toll-free number. Following are some guidelines and talking points:

- Always write down the name of the insurance company's representative you talked with, the date and time, and specifically what the person told you.

- Ask if your policy requires referrals (some don't). You may be able to see an allergist without your GP's referral. If your plan doesn't require a referral, the cost of seeing an allergist is typically the same as it would be if you had a referral; you'd have to make a co-pay out of pocket.

- Ask what happens if you see an allergist without a referral or one who's not in the insurance company's network. Your policy may not cover out-of-network doctors or cover a lower percentage of the cost than if you were to see an in-network specialist with a referral from your GP.

✔ **See a food allergist without your doctor's referral or your insurance company's approval.** This is usually the most costly option, because your insurance company may not pay any of the cost.

If you have to pay out of pocket for tests and treatments, mention this to your doctor. Doctors are human beings who are well aware of the high-cost of medical care. They may offer you a discount or be willing to set up a reasonable payment plan and will often be willing to charge you what they would normally get back from the insurance company (an average of a 36 percent discount).

Referrals past and present

In the not-so-good-old days, health insurance companies often set strict limitations on referrals. Sometimes they penalized GPs for sending too many patients to specialists or offered rewards to GPs who issued fewer referrals. (In the real old days, prior to 1990, GP's didn't need to worry about this nonsense.) Fortunately, most insurance companies have ended their Draconian policies and now give their doctors carte blanche to make as many referrals as necessary. Some companies don't even require referrals, so patients are free to see whichever doctor they deem most helpful.

If your GP seems reluctant to refer you to an allergist, don't be quick to blame your insurance company. In most cases, your GP's reluctance is based more on the fact that your GP really does not believe that you have a food allergy. If your doctor is unwilling to assist you in obtaining a referral to an allergist, become more proactive. Contact an allergist yourself, and see if your allergist can obtain the insurance approval you need.

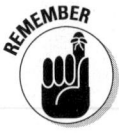

GPs often have the mistaken notion that allergists can't perform allergy tests on children until they're two or three years old. This is clearly wrong. The consensus of food allergists is that the GP should make the referral as soon as possible after concerns of food allergy arise, even in a two- or three-month-old. The medical community has plenty of evidence that early diagnosis and treatment greatly benefit children and their families.

Avoiding quackologists

Alternative therapies for food allergies abound. Chiropractors, nutritionists, acupuncturists, and a variety of other alternative practitioners claim the ability to diagnose and treat food allergies. Some of these healthcare providers may even be quite knowledgeable about food allergies and beneficial in your care. Other practitioners who are more on the fringe or way out there, tout their snake-oils, magic potions, crystals, and other treatments that range from entertaining diversions to dangerous delusions.

Don't fall for pumped-up promises of miracle cures. Seek well-trained, qualified medical practitioners to diagnose and manage your food allergies. If you do decide to pursue alternative routes — a chiropractor with an interest in food allergy, for example — I always advise that you see a traditional allergist as well. For details about the most common quack tests and treatments, skip to Chapter 8.

Seeking an Allergist's Advice

Your doctor decided to call in an allergist, or you decided on your own to pursue this option. Now you're in the market for a top-notch allergist. But what exactly qualifies an allergist as top-notch? Here are the qualities to look for in an allergist:

- ✔ **Training and experience with diagnosing and treating food allergies:** This may seem like a "well, yeah, duh" recommendation, but many allergists are better trained to deal with general allergies, such as allergies to pollen or pets. Not all allergists are up to speed on food allergies, particularly in complicated cases.

- ✔ **Well-honed interpersonal skills:** Some allergists are extremely bright and well-informed but have the interpersonal skills of a manikin or a personality that clashes with yours. They may take your concerns lightly, rush you through your visit without answering your questions, or have some other issues that make for a less than ideal fit.

In the following sections, I show you how to track down an ideal (or at least close-to-ideal) allergist and team up with your allergist to obtain the most accurate diagnosis and most effective treatment plan.

Tracking down a qualified food allergist

Tracking down a local allergist who's best qualified to diagnose and treat food allergies is a four-step process:

1. **Gather recommendations from your doctor, friends, and family.**
2. **Ensure that your insurance policy covers the allergists on your list.**
3. **Verify the allergist's credentials.**
4. **Check the allergist's availability and make an appointment.**

The following sections explain each step in greater detail.

Gathering recommendations

Your first recommendation typically comes from your GP. Your GP should be familiar with the allergists in your area, hopefully knows which allergists have expertise in food allergy, and may even know who would be the best fit from a style and personality standpoint.

If your GP doesn't recommend a suitable allergist or you want additional input, ask everyone you know and trust, especially friends and family members who've already seen an allergist. Ask other doctors if you happen to know any. These people are often even more capable than your GP in helping you find the perfect doctor.

If you're in a food-allergy support group, which isn't likely at this point because you're just getting started, recommendations from fellow members are pure gold. People often change allergists later based on recommendations from other members of the group.

Checking insurance coverage

Now that you have a long list of candidates, you can start paring down your list by crossing off any allergists not covered on your insurance policy. To see if a particular doctor participates in your insurance network, do one of the following:

- ✓ **Call the doctor's office, provide them with your insurance company's name and the network you're in (almost always printed on the health insurance card), and ask if the doctor is in your network.** Most allergists participate with all the larger insurance companies, so your selection shouldn't be overly limited.

- ✓ **Check the approved provider list supplied by your insurance company.** Many insurance companies offer members a book of approved healthcare providers, typically grouping providers by location and specialty. If you don't have such a book, request one. Your insurance company may also have a Web site where you can look up the names and contact information for allergists and other doctors and specialists in the company's approved network.

- ✓ **As a last resort, try calling the company for additional information, especially if you lost or misplaced your approved provider list or it's a couple years old.** A newer list may contain the name of the allergist you want to see.

Verifying the allergists' credentials

When your GP refers you to an allergist, ask about the allergist's credentials and bedside manner to learn as much as possible about his training and experience. If your GP is less than forthcoming or you obtained a recommendation from someone who has little solid information, the following organizations can help you gather information and can even provide you with additional names if you've come up short after talking to your GP, friends, and family:

- ✓ **American Academy of Allergy, Asthma & Immunology** (www.aaaai.org)
- ✓ **American College of Allergy, Asthma & Immunology** (www.acaai.org)
- ✓ **American Academy of Pediatrics** (www.aap.org)
- ✓ **American Board of Medical Specialties** (www.abms.org)

Other local medical societies may be able to provide additional recommendations.

Getting in to see your allergist

Rank the allergists on your list from first choice to last choice based on qualifications, reputation, and location, and then start calling around to make an appointment. Unfortunately, many allergists have a long waiting list, often several months. If you feel that you can't wait that long, you may need to go with your second or third choice.

Still having trouble getting in to see the allergist? Here are some tips and tricks from seasoned patients:

- ✔ **Set up appointments with two or more allergists.** When you finally get in to see one allergist, you can cancel the appointment(s) with the other(s). Don't cancel unless you're happy with the first allergist you see.

- ✔ **Ask your GP to call the allergist directly to see if she can fit you in sooner.** Your doctors may agree that waiting until the next available appointment could be dangerous.

- ✔ **Ask to be placed on the allergist's cancellation list.** If a patient with a scheduled appointment calls to cancel, the allergist can give the appointment to you. My co-author, Joe, who works at home (that lucky dog), has had great success using this strategy to get his kids in to see their specialists.

After you see your allergist for the first time and assuming you're happy with the allergist, don't leave the office without setting up at least one appointment in advance. This can trim your wait time in the future. If you don't need the appointment, cancel it a week or so in advance as a courtesy to other needy patients.

Teaming up with your allergist for optimum results

No matter what kind of healthcare issue you have, you get the best results when you team up with your doctor. To effectively team up with your allergist, here's what you do:

- ✔ **Be open and honest.** If you smoke or drink alcoholic beverages, for example, let your allergist know. If you have other health conditions, even if you think they're unrelated, inform your allergist. This is no time to be hiding important details.

- ✔ **Write down any medications you're currently taking.** Although medications don't typically trigger allergic reactions, they assist your allergist in painting a more accurate portrait of your condition, and your allergist needs to know of those medications in order to safely prescribe other medications.

- ✔ **Ask questions, even if they seem dumb to you, and express your concerns.** Keep those lines of communication open.

- ✔ **Listen carefully to what your allergist says and follow her advice.**

> ✔ **Keep in touch between appointments either over the phone or via e-mail, so your allergist is privy to any problems or questions that arise.**
>
> ✔ **Work with your allergist to develop an emergency back-up plan, in writing, in the event that you experience a severe reaction.** (Chapter 10 provides additional information on planning and equipping yourself for emergencies. Check out Chapter 7 for a form you can fill out to get your emergency action plan in writing.)

Getting the Skinny on Allergy Workups

Diagnosing a food allergy is about as challenging as finding an allergist who can see you the next day. Your allergist is likely to take a detailed history, perform a physical examination, and proceed with a battery of diagnostic tests to figure out what's going on and which foods are the prime suspects.

The diagnostic process is more complicated if your food allergy is not IgE-mediated, since the most common allergy tests — skin tests and RASTs — both rely on the presence of IgE antibodies. These tests are useless in diagnosing non-IgE mediated food allergies.

In the following sections, I lead you through the diagnostic process step-by-step, so you know what to expect along the way.

Making the most of your medical history

Your medical history is of tremendous value in diagnosing food allergy, so don't forget to bring the self-screening test you completed in the section "Self-Screening for Food Allergies," to your first appointment. In addition to what you've already recorded, your allergist is likely to ask you a series of probing questions to determine whether true food allergy is likely, and whether the allergy is likely to be IgE mediated.

Preparing to have your history taken

You can prepare for the doctor to review your medical history by jotting down your answers to the following questions:

> ✔ What foods do you suspect you are allergic to?
>
> ✔ At what age did the suspected food allergy begin?

✔ What were your specific symptoms?

✔ What was the timing of the suspected reaction(s)?

✔ Did your reaction occur soon after eating the suspect food?

✔ Does a reaction always occur when you eat that food?

✔ Had you previously tolerated that food? How often have you eaten it?

✔ How much did you eat before you had a reaction?

✔ Did anyone else who ate the same food get sick?

✔ How was the food prepared? How likely is it that the food had hidden ingredients?

✔ Were any medications used to treat the reaction? If medications were used, which meds were used and were they effective?

✔ What were you doing prior to or during the time you had the reaction? Just eating? Exercising? Taking a bath?

✔ Have similar reactions occurred on prior occasions?

Using your answers to these questions, your allergist formulates your medical history — one of the most important and useful diagnostic tools. Your allergist may also ask you to keep a food diary to find out even more about your diet and symptoms in an attempt to identify any consistent pattern to your reactions.

Investigating your history for clues

Although your history is the most important diagnostic tool, its usefulness varies depending on the results. Typically, the history leads to one of the following two common scenarios:

✔ **Bingo!** The history is precise and virtually diagnoses your specific food allergy all on its own. If you break out in hives the first time you eat an egg, for example, it's pretty obvious that you're allergic to eggs. In this case, further testing usually confirms the suspicion.

✔ **I dunno.** With more subtle symptoms, especially eczema and some of the non-IgE mediated gastrointestinal food allergies, reactions may be quite delayed. You may have had three or four meals and several snacks before you started feeling ill, making any clear link between cause and effect very difficult.

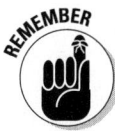

Several studies show that further testing confirms a history of suspected food allergy only about 30 to 40 percent of the time. Your allergist must interpret your history, including food diaries, with great caution.

Getting physical with a physical exam

You could place a pretty safe bet that by the time you get in to see the allergist, your symptoms will have magically disappeared. Your allergist asks to see the hives, and your skin is perfectly clear. Your tummy, which was as bloated as a beach ball two days ago, is as flat as an ironing board today. Even your sinuses are clear.

Even so, your allergist is going to perform a physical exam to look for signs of a possible food allergy, such as eczema and other rashes and symptoms of other allergic reactions, such as hay fever. What does hay fever have to do with food allergies? Well, food allergy is more likely to occur in those who have other types of allergy, and this can be an important clue.

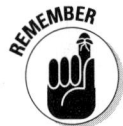

The physical exam, in and of itself, is not always conclusive. Your exam may reveal no abnormalities, even if you have severe reactions to multiple foods. After all, the only good thing about food allergy is that you usually look and feel fine as long as you're abstaining from the problem foods. One important bit of information a normal exam provides is that it reassures you and your allergist that you're probably okay with your current diet.

Poking around with skin tests

Once your allergist commences testing, you may begin to wonder if you mistakenly stepped into the acupuncturist's office. Allergists commonly perform skin-prick tests in which they poke or scratch the skin with an extract of the suspect food and observe any reactions on the surface of the skin. Your allergist may use any of the following three methods:

- ✔ The allergist places a tiny drop of food extract on the skin and pricks the skin through the drop with a small needle or plastic probe.
- ✔ Using a pricking device soaked in the food extract, the allergist pricks the skin.
- ✔ The allergist inserts a small amount of the food extract into the skin using a small needle. This method, called *intradermal* skin test, is rarely, if ever, indicated for food allergy diagnosis.

A positive skin test results in a mosquito bite-like reaction at the site of the test within minutes, indicating the presence of histamine, which causes the skin to swell. After 10–15 minutes, your allergist takes a reading and compares all tests to a control prick (to test your reaction to salt water, which shouldn't cause a reaction). A larger reaction — a larger bump on your skin — typically shows an increased likelihood that you're allergic to the tested food.

Guesstimating the number of pin pricks

How many times can you expect to get poked? If you're presenting symptoms of a nonfood allergy, such as hay fever or asthma, your allergist performs a fairly standard set of tests consisting of 20 to 40 skin pricks.

With food allergy the number of tests is typically based on patient history, so you can't expect a set number. An allergist usually performs skin prick tests for only suspect foods. If you've had only one reaction to milk, for example, your allergist is likely to test only for milk to confirm suspicions. If the history identifies no particular problem food — you have eczema, for instance, but no specific food reactions — then, your allergist is likely to test for only the five or six most common food allergens, including milk, egg, soy, wheat, and peanut.

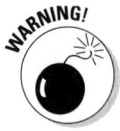

Be cautious of any allergist who recommends dozens of tests for food allergies. A few allergists out there routinely test every patient who walks into their office for 120 different foods, even if they have no reason to suspect a food allergy. Studies show that in children with eczema, if the skin prick tests or RASTs results are negative for the most common food allergens, the children are highly unlikely to be allergic to less common allergens.

Acknowledging the challenges of interpreting skin tests

Interpreting a skin test seems like a snap. Either it's positive or negative. What's so tricky about that? Actually, it's tougher than it sounds.

The easiest result to interpret is when the test is completely negative. When you test negative for a particular food, the likelihood that you have an IgE-mediated reaction to that food is next to nothing. The main exceptions occur in babies in the first six to nine months of life, during which time occasional false negatives occur.

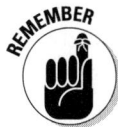

Skin tests are positive only if you have IgE antibodies to the food being tested. Skin tests do not detect non-IgE mediated allergies.

Interpreting positive food skin test results is more problematic. Positive tests indicate that IgE is present but do not, without confirmation from other sources, prove that a reaction will occur when you eat the food. In other words, the test can show a positive result or a *false positive* (a skin reaction even though you don't react to the food when you eat it). False positives occur in the following scenarios:

- ✔ You have a small amount of IgE antibody to a food but are not be truly allergic to that food. You can eat the food and experience absolutely no reaction to it.

- ✔ Some proteins in foods are cross-reactive with similar proteins in other foods or even environmental allergens like pollens. This *cross reactivity* can lead, for example, to a falsely positive skin test for soy in a person with peanut allergy, or a positive test to wheat in a person with grass pollen allergy. See the next section, "Accounting for cross reactivity," for details.

Take the results of skin tests with a dose of salt. Overall, up to 60 percent of all positive food skin tests turn out to be incorrect (falsely positive) upon further evaluation. Some studies show that the larger the skin test (the bigger the bump on your skin at the site of the test), the more likely a true allergy is at work, although this has not proven true in other studies. Skin test results are only one component of the diagnostic picture, allergists should evaluate them carefully and in the context of the big, clinical picture, as demonstrated in the following sidebar.

Accounting for cross reactivity

Cross-reactivity can occur when your immune system confuses one protein for another one. This typically happens with members of the same food family, but can occur between two allergens you may not imagine are related. A person who's allergic to tree pollen, for example, may not be able to eat apples or cherries. Someone who's allergic to ragweed may be sensitive to cantaloupe or banana.

Allergists remain vigilant of cross reactivity for two reasons:

- ✔ Cross-reactivity can often provide clues to other foods you may be allergic to or may become allergic to in the future.

- ✔ Cross-reactivity can thoroughly confuse test results.

When evaluating skin tests, your doctor needs to be aware of the possibility of cross reactivity, because the test may return a false positive result for a food you can safely eat.

Weighing the minor risks of skin tests

Allergy skin testing is generally a very safe procedure. However, because it exposes you to a food that you may be highly allergic to, caution is always in order. An occasional patient may in fact be considered too allergic for administering a safe skin test. Incidence of systemic (whole body) reactions, however, are very low — estimates run at about 30 reactions per 100,000 tests.

Confirming the results with other clues

Skin tests alone rarely prove much of anything. In a single week, I saw three patients, all of whom were diagnosed with egg allergy and came to me for a second opinion. Each had tested positively and had reactions of similar size to egg. Their cases illustrate the complexities of interpreting skin tests:

✔ **Patient 1:** The first patient had experienced two severe allergic reactions after eating scrambled eggs. In this case, the skin test confirmed the history and the diagnosis of egg allergy was virtually certain. This patient must avoid eating eggs.

✔ **Patient 2:** The second patient (a child) had severe eczema and was eating eggs regularly. He had never experienced an apparent reaction to egg and no evidence linked the eczema to a particular food in his diet. Since about 40 percent of children with severe eczema have underlying food allergy, and since egg allergy is the most common food allergy in children with eczema, this patient requires additional tests, as explained later in this chapter, to determine whether he is truly allergic to egg or not.

✔ **Patient 3:** The third patient was being evaluated for seasonal hay fever, and his allergist performed food tests for no particular reason. He eats eggs regularly and has never had any difficulty. Yet, his allergist told him to strictly avoid eggs, solely because he tested positive to egg. In this patient the history won. My colleagues and I felt safe assuming that the skin test produced a false positive result and that the patient could safely resume eating eggs.

Only allergists trained in the treatment of severe allergic reactions should perform skin tests, just in case you experience a severe reaction. Your allergist must have emergency equipment and drugs on hand for the treatment of anaphylaxis whenever performing a skin test. Chapter 2 provides more detailed information on anaphylaxis.

Hunting for IgE with RASTs

Another test that requires a needle is the RAST, a test that measures the amount of allergen-specific IgE in your blood. This test doesn't require an allergist; your GP can perform the test, but an allergist may be more qualified to interpret the results and is usually the doctor who performs the test. RAST consists of drawing a small amount of blood and then having the blood tested — by sending it out to a lab. Doctors can perform RASTs for almost any food or airborne allergen.

RAST terminology defined

RAST (short for *radioallergosorbent test*) is a term that actually refers to an older test method, one that allergists rarely use any more. The term stuck, however, and doctors still commonly the term to describe all the test methods that measure specific IgE antibodies in the blood. A more accurate term would be *immunoassay for specific IgE* but I use RAST throughout the book, because it's more common and a heck of a lot easier to type.

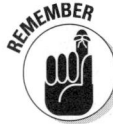

The most important point about RASTs is that they're not all the same. Some types of RASTs are more accurate than others, and the results of one type of RAST are not interchangeable with the results of another type. For diagnosing food allergies, the type of RAST that has the best track record is the Pharmacia CAP fluorescent enzyme immunoassay. Wrap your mouth around that one! To simplify the nomenclature, doctors refer to this type of RAST as CAP-FEIA or CAP-RAST.

As with skin testing, negative RAST results are quite accurate in ruling out an IgE-mediated food allergy, but positive RAST results do not necessarily mean you have a true food allergy. False positive results occur with RASTs for the very same reasons they occur with skin testing. However, because the RAST is more of a true measure of the amount of IgE in your system, differentiating a true positive test from a false positive test is generally easier than it is in the case of skin tests.

When your doctor gets the results, she looks at your *RAST score* and interprets the results based on the following criteria:

- ✔ The higher the RAST score, the more likely that the results represent a true food allergy.
- ✔ More importantly, for some of the most common food allergens, the doctor may compare your RAST levels to predetermined cut-offs, above which a true food allergy is almost certain. For example, using the CAP-RAST, which gives results on a scale from 0 (zero) to 100, an IgE level of more than 7 to egg, over 15 to milk, 14 to peanut, and 20 to codfish is highly predictive (greater than a 95 percent chance) that you're allergic to that food.

Your doctor can often use RAST results to track your levels of specific IgE antibodies over time. RAST levels that decrease over time are an excellent indication that you're outgrowing your allergy to a particular food. My colleagues and I typically decide when to try to re-introduce a food into a patient's diet based on the RAST result. (See Chapter 15 for details about outgrowing food allergies.)

Weighing the pros and cons of RASTs and skin tests

As you probably realized by now, neither skin tests nor RASTs are the perfect tests. Results can range from highly successful at best, to inconclusive, to misleading at worse. When discussing with your doctor which test would be most useful in your case, weigh the pros and cons of each.

Skin tests have a couple advantages over RASTs:

✔ A skin test is cheap.

✔ Skin test results are available almost immediately.

✔ Skin tests generally produce fewer false negatives. However, in food allergy testing, false negatives are uncommon with either test method, so this is not a huge issue.

RASTs have several advantages over skin testing:

✔ Certain medications, such as antihistamines, can interfere with skin testing, so you have to stop the medication beforehand. If you have trouble stopping your antihistamines, a RAST is an attractive alternative.

✔ Widespread skin conditions, especially hives or severe eczema, may preclude accurate skin testing.

✔ RASTs are less risky for patients who are susceptible to severe anaphylaxis.

✔ RASTs may be better at discerning a true positive from a false positive test.

✔ RASTs provide more information on the progress of an allergy over time.

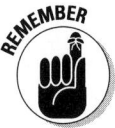

Neither skin-test nor RAST results are very good at predicting the type or severity of an allergic reaction. Although higher RAST levels generally indicate more severe reactions, numerous exceptions prevent RAST results from functioning as accurate predictors of a future reaction. This is due in part to the dose effect described in Chapter 3, but even with the same dose (amount of a problem food) three people with the same skin-test or RAST result may have hugely different reactions with exposure to the food. One person may eat peanuts regularly without symptoms, the second may experience minor hives, and the third may experience severe anaphylaxis.

Looking for Clues with Additional Diagnostic Tools

You've been interviewed, examined, and poked, and your allergist can provide you with no definitive diagnosis. It happens, especially when you're experiencing delayed reactions. Hope, however, remains. Your doctor has some additional tricks up his sleeve, including both eating the food (a *food challenge*) and not eating the food (an *elimination diet*). The following sections present additional diagnostic tools that can dig below the skin to unearth more mysterious causes.

Daring a food to make you react: Food challenges

When your allergies prove too elusive for skin tests and RASTs, your doctor may try to dare the allergies out of hiding by challenging them to react to suspect foods. This test, commonly called an *oral food challenge*, consists of feeding you increasing amounts of the suspect food under your doctor's supervision, while observing you for symptoms. Food challenges are considered the only foolproof test for most food allergies. In addition to identifying elusive allergies, food challenges serve three useful purposes:

- ✔ **Verify the accuracy of a positive skin test or RAST.**

- ✔ **Determine if a patient has outgrown an allergy.**

- ✔ **Diagnose cases of non-IgE-mediated reactions.** An oral challenge may be the only definitive way to diagnose a non-IgE mediated food allergy.

Don't try this at home. Food challenges carry a risk of serious reactions. Only trained personnel with emergency treatment immediately available should perform these tests.

Your doctor can choose to perform a food challenge using either of the following three methods:

- ✔ **Instruct you to eat the suspect food in increasing doses while observing you for signs of a reaction.** (With this method, unlike the following two methods, you know what you're eating.) This is the most common way to do a food challenge.

- ✔ **Have you to eat something that contains the suspect food without your knowing that you're eating the suspect food.** Your doctor mixes samples of the offending food with another food or adds it as an ingredient to another food, so you can't recognize it by sight, smell, or taste.

> ✔ **Have you swallow a capsule containing the allergen.** In some cases, the doctor uses placebo tablets, as well, to keep you in the dark about whether you're eating the suspect food or some inert substance.

The ideal way to perform a food challenge test is to do a "double-blind, placebo-controlled challenge." With this method, neither the allergist nor the patient is aware of which capsule or food contains the suspected allergen. In order for the test to be effective, you must also take capsules or eat food that does not contain the allergen (*placebos*). This ensures that any observed reaction is due to the allergen and not some other factor, such as stress or anxiety.

Discovering your allergens by avoiding them

When you eat something and it makes you sick, the logical thing to do is stop eating it. This is essentially what you do with an *elimination diet*. When you have a food allergy, your doctor often places you on an elimination diet permanently, or until you've outgrown the allergy (if you do outgrow the allergy), but doctors often use elimination diets on a temporary basis to diagnose allergies.

Challenging a food when the time is right

My colleagues and I often struggle to determine the right time to do a food challenge, especially to see if a patient has outgrown an allergy. If a patient has not experienced any recent reactions (recent reactions would guarantee that the patient is still allergic), we base most food challenge decisions on the CAP-RAST IgE level. If the CAP-RAST IgE level is low enough, we decide to move forward with a food challenge to verify that the patient has really outgrown the allergy.

A few years ago we published our experience with this method and were able to more clearly define the IgE levels at which a challenge may be reasonable. After all, we do not want to take the risk of a challenge if the odds of success are too small, but yet don't want to restrict the diet more than necessary. In our study, we reported on 604 food challenges in 391 children to the five most common food allergens. Our goal was to establish the IgE level at which we could expect a 50 percent pass rate, and we determined a cutoff level of 2 kUA/L (kili-units per liter) for milk, egg, and peanut. Data were less clear for wheat and soy where determining a definitive cut-off was more difficult. We concluded that IgE concentrations to milk, egg, and peanut and, to a lesser extent, wheat and soy, serve as useful predictors of challenge outcome and should be routinely used when advising patients about oral challenges to these foods. See Chapter 15 for additional details on working with your allergist to determine when conditions are relatively safe to proceed with a food challenge to determine if you have outgrown an allergy.

Cracking a tough case

Some patients have extremely challenging food allergies that defy the detection efforts of even the most determined and well-trained allergist. To demonstrate just how challenging the diagnostic process can be, I offer a case that typifies the usual patient that I see in my food allergy clinic on a daily basis:

Kyle is a two-and-a-half-year-old old boy who had severe eczema in the first weeks of life. His mother was breast-feeding him at that time, and he seemed to react to whatever his mother was eating. He underwent his first allergy testing at six months of age, and the results showed positive to milk, egg, and peanut. He was weaned to a soy formula, which he appeared to tolerate. By the time he saw me for the first time, he had been skin tested three more times, each test picking up more positive results. A detailed diet history revealed that his only obvious allergic reactions occurred with exposure to egg and milk. He had never ingested peanut or tree nuts and had seemed to tolerate wheat and soy.

Kyle's previous doctors told his parents that he was truly allergic to all the foods to which he tested positive. By the time I saw him, his diet was limited to seven foods — rice, apple, pear, chicken, squash, sweet potato, and carrots. Although his eczema was now well under control, he was losing weight and was miserable. The elimination diet had worked to improve his

eczema and had been helpful, diagnostically speaking, by showing that his eczema was due to food allergy, but it had truly put him at risk of malnutrition. Given the likelihood that many of his skin test results were falsely positive, I was hopeful that we could expand his diet.

I began by performing RASTs to a large panel of foods. With these results we could put the foods he was avoiding into three categories — almost definitely allergic, possibly allergic, and almost certainly not allergic. I felt that the foods in the last category — almost certainly not allergic — could be safely introduced at home. We were able to quickly expand his diet to include several major foods, including wheat, soy, and corn, as well as many new fruits and vegetables, with no worsening of his eczema. For the foods in the middle category — possibly allergic — I recommended that food challenges be done to further define his true allergies. This allowed us to introduce pork, oat, and potato into his diet. Food challenges to milk and beef were unsuccessful. For the foods in the first category — almost definitely allergic — including egg, peanut, tree nuts, sesame, peas, and fish, I recommended continued strict avoidance.

At this point, while his diet is still very restricted, his life and nutrition are both vastly improved. He will now be retested annually and his diet hopefully will expand further with time.

You may have already performed this test on your own by avoiding a particular food and then re-introducing it to your diet and finding that your symptoms returned. If you've already done this, your doctor should have included this piece of information in your history. If you haven't performed the test yet, your doctor may recommend it to confirm skin test or RAST results or simply as a logical next step — "we can't figure this out so let's avoid certain foods and see what happens."

An elimination diet typically spans the course of several weeks but consists of only two steps (plus a step that's sometimes recommended):

1. **Eliminate specific foods and ingredients from your diet, typically over a period of two to three weeks.** During this time, you carefully read food labels and find out about food preparation methods when you're dining out. See Chapter 6 for details about reading labels. Over the course of the elimination period, your doctor monitors symptoms, all of which should disappear in three weeks if you're following the right diet.

2. **With your doctor's okay, you begin to gradually reintroduce the foods that were eliminated, one at a time, while carefully recording any symptoms that arise when you partake of each food.** If your symptoms return, your doctor can usually confirm the diagnosis.

3. **In some cases, your doctor may direct you to once again eliminate the remaining suspect foods from your diet to reinforce the diagnosis.**

Maybe you're thinking that elimination diet is just a fancy term for food challenge, and it sort of is. You eliminate the food and then challenge it.

The elimination diet is not foolproof, and it can be risky. Psychological and physical factors can affect the diet's results. For example, if you think you're sensitive to a food, a response could occur that may not be a true allergic one. And if you've experienced severe reactions to certain foods, your doctor should consider reintroducing the food only in the controlled setting of a food challenge.

Pursuing the causes of non-IgE mediated allergies

As described in Chapter 1 and elsewhere, some types of allergy involve other parts of the immune system and are undetectable with the most common allergy tests — skin tests and RASTs. These are mostly gastrointestinal reactions, although occasionally eczema and other rashes may occur due to non-IgE mediated food allergies.

In such cases, allergists typically have to fall back on your history, which may range from tremendously helpful to completely misleading, especially if you experience delayed reactions or you and your doctor can't pin down a specific food. If the history reveals little useful information, your doctor may recommend one of the following next steps:

✔ The first next step is usually an elimination diet followed by either an oral food challenge or a gradual re-introduction of the food(s) at home.

✔ The second diagnostic approach is to perform a biopsy of the esophagus, stomach, or intestine (obtained through a scope by a gastroenterologist). To obtain the most definitive results, your allergist (with the assistance of your gastroenterologist) may repeat the scope and biopsies after an elimination diet or after you've re-introduced the food into your diet.

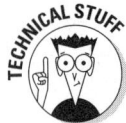

Another type of skin testing called *patch testing* has shown some promise in the diagnosis of non-IgE mediated food allergy. When used for food reactions, small amounts of a pure food are placed in tiny cups, which your doctor tapes to your back. The foods are chosen based on diet, knowledge of common allergens, and previous reactions. Your doctor removes the patches after 48 hours and reads them at 72 hours. During the writing of this book, no standardized reagents, application methods, or guidelines for interpretation are available, and patch testing is still finding its place in the diagnosis of food allergy.

Avoiding the untested and unproven

Admittedly, skin tests and RASTs, are less than perfect, but some allergy tests, often purported to be superior, are untested at best, proven to be worthless at their worst, and are usually pretty costly (and not covered by insurance). I commonly see patients who have spent thousands of dollars of these tests and who have been placed on broad avoidance diets based on totally inaccurate test results. Remember those quackologists I talked about earlier in this chapter. They're typically the misinformed, misguided souls who mislead their patients with these phony tests. Here's a list of the most common dubious tests to watch out for:

✔ IgG and IgG4 tests

✔ Sublingual or intradermal provocation tests

✔ Lymphocyte activation tests

✔ Kinesiology

✔ Cytotoxic tests

✔ Electrodermal testing

For details about unproven tests and treatments you need to watch out for, skip to Chapter 8.

Ruling out food intolerances

Certain foods can make you miserable even though you're not allergic to them. If your doctor examines your body, your history, and your test results and rules out food allergy, he may begin to suspect a *food intolerance* — an adverse food-induced reaction that does not involve the immune system.

Lactose intolerance is one example of a food intolerance. If you have a lactose intolerance, you lack an enzyme (*lactase*) that's essential for digesting milk sugar. In this case, the milk sugar is the culprit. In the case of a milk allergy, a milk protein is the perpetrator. When a person with lactose intolerance consumes milk products, symptoms such as gas, bloating, and abdominal pain may occur. Your doctor can perform a specific test for lactose intolerance called a *breath hydrogen test*, but for most other food intolerances no specific diagnostic test is available.

To diagnose an intolerance to other foods, such as wheat, your doctor is likely to re-examine the data he's already collected:

- **History:** A history that shows a predominance of gastrointestinal symptoms and a tolerance of small doses of the food commonly points to food intolerance. With food intolerance, symptoms typically occur when you eat larger quantities of the suspect food. While this can occur with food allergy, allergic reactions tend to occur at much smaller doses than food intolerances.

- **Test results:** If your skin tests and RASTs show no signs of food allergy, a food intolerance may be triggering your symptoms.

Treatment for a food intolerance is very similar to food allergy treatment. Your doctor is likely to instruct you to avoid the offending foods or at least limit your consumption. The same food substitutes can often help you vary your diet without missing the foods you love. In the case of lactose intolerance, your doctor may prescribe lactase supplements to help you digest the milk sugar.

Chapter 6

Concocting Your Own Avoidance Diet

*A*fter visiting your food allergist, you may feel as though you just stepped out of an old Henny Youngman joke: Patient tells his doctor, "It hurts when I do this . . . ." Doctor replies, "Stop doing that."

Much of the medical advice your allergist offers boils down to just that — avoid the foods that ail you. If you react to peanuts, stop eating them. If you break out in hives whenever you eat fish, order the roast beef, instead. If you get an itchy rash after gulping a glass of milk, stop drinking the stuff.

Ahhhh, if only it were that easy. Unfortunately, it's not, because people don't eat that way, chefs don't cook that way, and food manufacturers don't think that way. People mix and match foods and spices to create an infinite variety of flavorful foodstuffs. Almost every recipe for a tasty dish calls for several ingredients. Almost every processed food you find on the shelves contains a complex combination of constituents.

To further complicate matters, foods commonly go by several pseudonyms to cloak their true identities. Eggs hide behind labels like "albumin" and "simplesse." Milk sneaks around as "casein." Peanuts and soy slip past the guards under the alias of "hydrolyzed vegetable protein."

In this chapter, I take you beyond the recommendation to stop eating the stuff that ails you. I uncover the aliases of common allergens, show you how to decipher food labels, offer tips on meeting your nutritional needs while avoiding nutritional foods, show you how to design and manage your own avoidance diet, and reveal the pros and cons of rotation diets.

The Cheat Sheet that tears out in the front of this book gives you the Food Label Crib Sheet. Take it with you while grocery shopping. It helps you decipher those food labels so you can avoid the foods that ail you.

Setting Sensible Goals

You've just learned that you're allergic to one or more foods and that the foods can be hiding in the most unsuspected places. At this point, you probably feel a mix of shock, fear, anxiety, and depression. Your first impulse may be to resign yourself to a lifetime regimen of rice and water and whatever you can manage to grow in your vegetable garden.

I recommend a less radical approach, one that enables you to enjoy a bountiful buffet of foods safely. The first step is to set sensible goals:

- **Avoid the foods that ail you without avoiding anything you're not truly allergic to.** See "Drawing Up Your Avoidance Diet," below.

- **Read and understand food labels.** See "Decrypting Food Labels: Allergen-Savvy Grocery Shopping," later in this chapter.

- **Design a diet that contains a wide variety of foods you love, excludes your allergens, and enables you to maintain proper nutrition while retaining your sanity.** See "Feeding Your Nutritional Needs," later in this chapter.

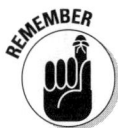

Don't overdo it. Anxiety may drive you to avoid more foods than necessary. An accurate diagnosis can tell you which foods you're allergic to, giving you a wider selection of foods you can safely enjoy.

Drawing Up Your Avoidance Diet

Describing an allergen-free diet as an "avoidance diet" sounds more gloomy than it really is. Sure, you want to avoid the foods that make you sick, but in the process, you often discover a cornucopia of cuisine that pleases your palate and more than satisfies your appetite. Consider creating an avoidance diet as a quest to discover more exotic foods, to become self-sufficient by cooking your own meals, and to wrest control from an illness that has, up to this point, burdened you with restrictions. Consider it liberating.

Maximizing your choices

At this point, you should have an accurate diagnosis in hand. If you haven't yet obtained a diagnosis, check out Chapter 5. The diagnosis is key, because it provides you with a list of foods you can't add to your grocery list. With your list of forbidden fruits (or nuts, milk, fish, or whatever you're allergic to) and the guidance and information provided later in this chapter (on how to read labels and address your nutritional needs), you're well equipped to set out on your quest.

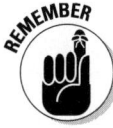

Your avoidance diet is unique to you and as varied as you choose to make it.

Your goal is to develop a diet with a variety of tasty foods, so that you don't miss the foods you love . . . at least not much. With that in mind, here are some important suggestions to keep you on track and maximize your food choices:

- ✔ **Design a diet that's right for you.** Create a list of everything you eat or would like to eat that contains the food you're allergic to, and then carefully seek substitutes based on age, nutritional needs, and tastes. If you love cheese, for example, but are allergic to milk, I'm not about to recommend soy cheese, because most soy cheese contains milk protein, and you may not even find it appetizing. Explore alternatives that you find appealing. Chapter 18 offers a list of tasty substitutes for some common allergenic foods.

- ✔ **Bolster your buffet.** When allergies are limiting your choices, fight back by trying different foods. Just make sure you read the labels carefully before testing the waters.

- ✔ **Be resourceful.** Your neighborhood grocery store may not be the best place to explore the multitude of available options. Visit health food stores, online specialty food stores, and stores like Whole Foods and Trader Joe's.

- ✔ **Hunt for bargains.** Healthy foods are typically more pricey than the highly processed foods that crowd the shelves of most grocery stores, so if you're on a tight budget, you may have to adjust your diet accordingly, clip coupons, and hunt for bargains.

- ✔ **Start cooking.** Learning to cook, if you're not an expert already, can increase your options tenfold while providing you with a new, rewarding hobby. By preparing your own meals from scratch, you can eliminate a host of processed foods from your diet.

Determining how strict you need to be

When I recommend an avoidance diet to my patients, one of the first questions they ask is "How strict do I need to be?" The short, safe answer is that you need to adhere to the strictest guidelines that you and your doctor establish. I recommend strict avoidance for two reasons:

- ✔ **Strict avoidance limits the risk of reactions.** Highly allergic people can experience allergic reactions, even severe and fatal reactions, when exposed to minute amounts of the offending allergen.

- ✔ **Strict avoidance, especially in young children, may improve your chances of outgrowing the allergy.** (See Chapter 15.)

I recommend strict avoidance of any foods that contain or are at a risk of containing a food that triggers an allergic reaction. However, I realize that all people are different. Work with your doctor to formulate a plan that ensures your desired quality of life while minimizing the risks.

Decrypting Food Labels: Allergen-Savvy Grocery Shopping

When you're allergic to a food, every trip to the grocery store is like a clandestine mission to identify and avoid the enemy. Before you step behind enemy lines and walk into your local grocery or convenience store, brief yourself on the following precautionary protocol:

- ✔ **Know all the ways that manufacturers can label the food you're avoiding,** as revealed in the following sections.

- ✔ **Read the ingredients on every package, the warnings, and the fine print.**

- ✔ **Re-read the label every time you buy the product.** Ingredients can change at any time, and the label does not have to announce "new and improved."

- ✔ **Master the oddities of food labeling.** For example, "dairy free" has nothing to do with being milk free. "Dairy free" refers to the presence of milk fat but not milk protein.

- ✔ **Avoid bulk foods, because they have a higher risk of contamination.**

- ✔ **Beware of the deli counter, especially if you have a milk allergy.** The worker at the meat counter may use the same slicer for meat and cheese.

Making sense of FALCPA

One of the great challenges in avoiding foods you are allergic to comes from the complexity of food labels. Unfortunately, foods may show up on a label under a variety of names. Fortunately, reading labels is becoming easier as a result of the Food Allergen Labeling and Consumer Protection Act (FALCPA), which went into effect on January 1, 2006.

FALCPA requires that manufacturers label the eight most common food allergens — milk, egg, peanut, tree nuts, soy, wheat, fish, and shellfish — in simple, unambiguous terms. Before the law, manufacturers could label milk as a "natural flavor" and label wheat as "starch." Now, manufacturers must call any form of milk "milk" and any form of wheat "wheat," usually in bold letters.

This new labeling law has been a major breakthrough, but reading labels is still a challenge, especially for the foods not in the top eight. "Starch," for example, may still mean "corn," and manufacturers can still call sesame a "natural flavor." To obtain reliable details about the more ambiguous terms, you still may need to call the manufacturer, or just avoid that product.

Going on an egg hunt

When you're allergic to eggs, a trip to the grocery store can be more challenging than your typical Easter egg hunt. Food labels hide eggs behind a host of names, and can show up as glaze on unlabeled bakery items, as clarifying agents in soups, or as a fat substitute.

What do you do when you have a recipe that calls for eggs? Provide a substitute. Chapter 18 suggests tasty substitutes for the ten most common foods that trigger allergic reactions.

Identifying the many faces of milk

Milk morphs into several food products that look nothing like milk, including cheese, butter, sour cream, yogurt, and pudding. It can also show up in a host of foods under an assortment of names.

A peanut by any other name . . .

In the world of food allergies, peanuts are in a class of their own. They're extremely allergenic and can cause severe reactions with minimal exposure, so if you're allergic to peanuts, you need to avoid foods that have even trace elements of the offending food.

Whipping the milk allergy

The parents of a two-year-old boy with a previously diagnosed milk allergy came to see me. They were frustrated beyond belief. When their son was first diagnosed, they were overwhelmed by the thought of removing milk form his diet. After all, he seemed to live on milk, cheese, and other dairy products. They ventured to the grocery store and were relieved to find a wide variety of milk substitutes. Within the first few minutes, they had filled their cart with lactose-free and dairy-free desserts and soy-based yogurt and cheese.

Over the following weeks, they became dismayed that their son continued to have frequent allergic reactions. They were convinced that he must be allergic to other foods, so they came to see me for further advice. After they described the milk-free products they had purchased, I immediately knew what was going on. All the milk substitutes they were feeding their son contained milk.

In reality, "lactose-free" indicates that only the milk sugar (lactose) has been removed; it doesn't refer to the milk protein that was triggering their son's reactions. Similarly, "dairy-free" refers to the source of fat in the product and has nothing to do with milk protein. To make matters worse, most soy cheeses contain casein, a very potent form of milk protein, and the soy yogurt had no milk ingredients but had a big "D" on the front of the package, indicated a likely milk contamination. Needless to say, the parents were a little shocked.

I provided the parents with the information they needed to accurately identify milk on food labels, which made their trips to the grocery store considerably more difficult. With a little practice, however, they became master label decoders and were overwhelmed with pride when they conquered the task and their son miraculously stopped having allergic reactions.

Spotting soy and soy products

Over the years, soybean products have become somewhat of a staple in our diets and the bane of anyone who has an allergy to it. It can hide in everything from the ubiquitous hydrolyzed vegetable protein to tofu and tamari.

Studies show that most individuals who have a soy allergy can safely eat soy lecithin and soy oil, but check with your doctor before you decide to indulge.

Shaking the tree nuts out of a label

Like peanuts, tree nuts can cause severe reactions with minimal exposure. If you have a tree nut allergy, you're likely to be allergic to several but not all tree nuts, but avoidance is most effective if you avoid all tree nuts.

Recognizing wheat's many aliases

For most people in the West, wheat is the bread of life. For those who have wheat allergies, however, wheat and the many food products that contain it are pesky troublemakers that are tough to spot

Smelling the fish on a label

When you've been diagnosed as having an allergy to fish, your first question is likely to be: "Which fish? Cod? Salmon? Sturgeon? Freshwater? Saltwater?" Although all fish are not created equal, most people who have a fish allergy are allergic to several types of fish, so I generally recommend that if you're allergic to one type, avoid them all — both freshwater and saltwater varieties, canned, fresh, sushi, you name it.

Allergic reactions to fish and shellfish can be severe and are often a cause of anaphylaxis, so if you're allergic to fish, be prepared to identify and avoid them.

Although canned fish tend to be less of a problem, avoid canned fish, as well, unless your doctor instructs you that a specific fish is okay for you to eat.

Cracking open mysterious shellfish labels

Shellfish are notorious for triggering severe allergic reactions and even anaphylaxis. If you're allergic to shellfish, you already know to avoid shellfish at home, but you should also remain aware of any risks from eating out and any hidden sources of shellfish.

Sifting out hidden sesame

Sesame is becoming increasingly popular in Western diet and increasingly a problem for those who are allergic to it. Sesame seeds contain extremely potent allergens and can cause severe allergic reactions and anaphylaxis. Although the sesame allergy gets less press than peanut and shellfish allergies, allergic reactions to sesame can be just as severe. Because sesame is such a versatile food, it can show up in a host of unsuspected places.

Sesame can show up in non-sesame products, especially bread, due to cross-contamination from other bakery items that use sesame.

Approaching Warning Labels with Caution

More and more food manufacturers are sticking precautionary labels on their packaging. You pick up a granola bar, and it says, "May contain peanuts." You'd think that the people making the granola bar would know if they put peanuts in it, but apparently they forgot. More of these precautions are showing up since FALCPA was passed, and I can speculate on only three reasons for this increase:

- ✔ Changes in manufacturing processes have introduced more opportunities for cross-contamination. (Machines used to produce a food that contains common allergens is used to produce food that doesn't.)

- ✔ Companies are becoming more allergy aware and conscientious in their labeling.

- ✔ Manufacturers are covering their posteriors to adhere to the new laws, even though FALCPA doesn't require it, contrary to popular belief.

The problem with these umbrella precautions is that they often and unnecessarily increase the anxiety of those who suffer from food allergies, and they slap additional restrictions on diets. They end up warning consumers of food items that are perfectly safe and add confusion and uncertainty to a labeling system that's sufficiently confusing.

In the following sections, I translate these precautions into plain English, identify the ones that suggest the greatest risk, and caution you to avoid the common mistake of assuming that just because you haven't reacted to a particular item in the past you won't react to it this time.

Deciphering the "This package may contain . . ." warning

Manufacturers often label products with cryptic precautions, such as "This product may contain . . ." or "Produced on shared equipment" or "Product may contain traces of . . . ." These phrases can signal anything from a nonexistent to a serious risk, so you have no choice but to take them seriously. Such precautions usually indicate that the manufacturer produces more than one product on a single machine, as described in the following scenarios:

✔ **Scenario 1:** A peanut product and a non-peanut product are produced on separate equipment, but the company says that if the peanut butter cookie line breaks down, they could start to make those cookies on the vanilla cream cookie equipment. This may never happen but the label appears anyway because of that theoretical possibility.

✔ **Scenario 2:** A peanut and a non-peanut product are produced on the same equipment but the equipment is thoroughly cleaned before switching from one product to the other. Some products may be more amenable to cleaning than others. A liquid food (ice cream is a great example) is quite easy to clean as long as sufficient care is taken. Dry products (cereals, crackers, cookies) may be harder to completely remove from machinery.

✔ **Scenario 3:** A peanut and a non-peanut candy are produced on shared equipment and no cleaning is done between runs. This could be deadly!

In the end, you can't truly know what these precautionary words mean, so you have to avoid any products that contain these vague warnings.

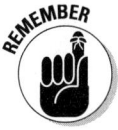

Virtually no ice cream is made on dedicated, peanut-free equipment, but most ice cream from large manufacturers is likely to be safe, whereas ice cream from small companies is commonly contaminated, often with no warning on the label.

Decoding the "Produced in a facility . . ." warning

Slightly less vague than "This package may contain . . ." is any precautionary label indicating that the product was made in a facility that produces another product that contains a common allergen. In some cases, the facility may manufacture the two products a quarter mile away from each other. The products may not even cross paths until they reach the distribution center, in packages, which is really no different from how they meet at the grocery store.

That doesn't mean you should ignore the precaution. It's not worth the risk, so the best recourse is to simply pass on such products and avoid them all. If you have a serious craving for the food and can't track down a safer alternative, then give the manufacturer a call and ask for details.

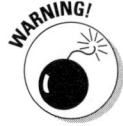

Always err on the safe side when it comes to precautionary labels. Risks of cross-contamination are certainly less with large companies than with smaller ones, but you should always check with the manufacturer to be sure.

Taking warning labels seriously

For lifelong label readers like me, the recent flood of precautionary labels has become an enormous source of frustration. Prior to the late 1990s these precautions were as rare as a bag of peanuts at a food allergy seminar. Now they're cropping up on the labels of the most innocuous foods. And the worst part of it is that they're starting to show up on lots of stuff I used to love to eat!

So, what's a food allergy sufferer to do? You have no choice — once the precaution appears, the product is off limits. As soon as the manufacturer splashes this warning on a product, the company is perfectly free to stop cleaning its equipment. A product that was previously safe may now pose a deadly risk.

Remaining cautious of foods you haven't reacted to . . . yet

Say you ate a couple candy bars before noticing the new precautionary warning, and they didn't make you sick. Can you safely assume that the warning is bogus and you're free to continue consuming the product without a care in the world?

Nope.

Even if you haven't reacted to the product, *yet*, continuing to consume it places you at risk. Why? Here are two good reasons:

- First, the company may have changed the way it cleans its equipment, especially now that it has a warning on the label that protects it.

- Second (and more importantly), the nature of contaminated food is entirely inconsistent. For example, if the plant produces a non-peanut candy after producing a peanut candy on the same equipment, the first 100 bags of non-peanut product may be loaded with peanut, while the next 100 have less, and the last 10,000 have none. Eating this candy is like playing Russian roulette — you may get away with it the first 49 times and then get burned by bag 50.

Feeding Your Nutritional Needs

Avoidance diets are like being caught between a rock and a hard place, especially with some of the major food allergens like milk, egg, and wheat, that comprise such a large part of our diets. You may not be able to eat one or more of these foods because they make you sick, but if you don't eat them you risk becoming malnourished.

To remain healthy, work with your doctor to devise a strategy that meets your nutritional needs while ensuring that you avoid the foods that trigger reactions. This is especially true for infants and young children and for certain specific nutritional requirements, including calcium. Improper nutrition, especially during the early years of development, can lead to serious health problems, including weight loss, poor growth, and weak bones. It may even affect brain development in young children.

The following sections reveal strategies for meeting nutritional needs while avoiding problem foods for specific stages of development. Because milk and milk-based formulas are the most serious concerns during the early stages of development, the examples we provide in the following sections focus primarily on nutritional issues that arise when infants and children must avoid milk.

Attending to your infant's needs

From birth up to approximately two years of age, infants require a diet rich in fat and protein, so a milk-free diet can be particularly risky for infants. Failing to meet the minimum requirements for fat, protein, calcium, vitamins, and other nutrients can have serious long-term consequences, even the loss of IQ points, so finding a suitable replacement is essential. The following list offers a few options along with important points to keep in mind when searching for a solution:

- ✔ Breast feeding is best, although in some instances the mother must avoid foods in her diet that the baby is allergic to.

- ✔ If breast feeding is not an option, use an infant formula that doesn't contain cow's milk. Alternatives to cow's milk formulas, including soy and extensively hydrolyzed formulas, may be appropriate alternatives to breast milk.

- ✔ Breast feeding or a suitable infant formula may be needed up to 18 to 24 months of age to ensure adequate intake of fat, protein, calcium, and vitamins.

- ✔ Soy is often a good substitute, but many infants who are allergic to milk are allergic to soy.

- ✔ Rice milk is not an adequate substitute.

If you have questions or concerns, consult a nutritionist, no matter what the age of the child.

Keeping your toddler on the right track

After age two or three, meeting a child's nutritional needs gets a little easier, at least theoretically. As a toddler, the child is more capable of ingesting and digesting a wider variety of foods. That's the easy part. The tough part is that toddlers are more capable of resisting your efforts to keep they away from the foods that make them sick, and they're generally pickier about the foods they choose to eat.

Toddlers still require lots of protein, but their fat needs become easier to meet. (Most pediatricians normally switch a child without food allergies from whole milk to a milk with a lower fat content at age two.) The approach for meeting the vitamin needs of a toddler with food allergies is much the same as meeting the needs of a toddler without food allergies — the child should eat a variety and a sufficient amount of fruits and vegetables.

For toddlers with milk allergy, getting enough calcium is especially challenging. Try the following options until you find something that your child likes or at least doesn't fuss about too much:

- ✔ Milk substitutes, such as soy milk or rice milk (rice milk is okay for older kids, because they can get their protein from other sources)
- ✔ Calcium-fortified juices, such as orange juice with calcium
- ✔ Calcium supplements

How much calcium does a toddler need? About 600 mg of calcium per day. Fortified juices typically have 200 to 300 mg per cup, but don't count on the label to tell you that. Labels typically express the amount of calcium in percentages, not milligrams, where 100 percent equals an outdated adult recommended daily dose of 1,000 mg (the current recommendation is 1300 mg for adults).

Some people think they can eat enough green vegetables to meet calcium needs but you would literally need to eat a head of broccoli daily to accomplish this.

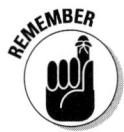

Getting a sufficient amount of calcium is critical for development and health, so keep trying different sources of calcium until you hit on something that your child can live with.

Maintaining a healthy diet with children and adolescents

Follow the average kid around for a day and watch what he eats, and you get a pretty clear idea of the challenges you can expect when trying to meet the nutritional needs of a child or adolescent, even one who doesn't have a food allergy.

At this stage, you either have an ally who's ready to take on more responsibility for taking care of herself and meeting her own nutritional needs or a child who prefers a more liberal lifestyle with lousy eating habits and a penchant for increased risk taking — cheating on the diet. Guess which one is more common. In Chapter 14, "Empowering Your Adolescent or Teenager," I discuss the challenges in greater detail and provide tips on how to effectively overcome them . . . with the assistance of your child, of course.

Focusing on calcium intake for adults

As an adult, you're capable of attending to your own nutritional needs, so I won't lecture you on the benefits of a varied diet, including plenty of fruits and vegetables that you're not allergic to. I will, however, stress the importance of getting your RDA of calcium.

By weight, calcium is one of the most plentiful minerals in the human body, accounting for 1.5 percent to 2 percent of body weight. And, as the milk commercials claim, it builds strong teeth and bones. The average adult requires about 1,300 milligrams of calcium, and people who don't have a milk allergy have little problem meeting this goal through a variety of milk products, including milk, cheese, yogurt, and ice cream. When you're on a milk-free diet, however, you need to explore other sources:

- ✔ Milk substitutes, such as soy milk or rice milk
- ✔ Calcium-fortified juices, such as orange juice with calcium
- ✔ Calcium supplements.
- ✔ Green leafy vegetables, including broccoli, collards, kale, mustard greens, turnip greens, and bok choy or Chinese cabbage
- ✔ Canned salmon or sardines, shellfish, almonds, Brazil nuts, and dried beans, assuming you're not allergic to those foods

Taking Turns with a Rotation Diet

Unlike an avoidance diet, which calls for the elimination of offending foods from your diet, a rotation diet allows you to eat some of the food some of the time. In other words, you limit the amount of the food that causes problems, but you don't completely eliminate it. For example, you may consume a tolerable amount of milk products, once or twice a week.

Sounds good, huh?

Well, it is good for some people — mostly for people with food intolerances rather than true food allergies. Food intolerances tend to be much more dose-related than food allergies, which can often be triggered by exposure to a very small amount of the problem food. Only by consulting with your doctor can you decide whether a rotation diet may be right for you.

Consult your doctor and get permission before attempting any sort of rotation diet, and check in regularly with your doctor. Your doctor may need to adjust your diet over time, as the food allergies may fluctuate in either direction.

Knowing when a rotation diet can benefit you

If you have a severe food allergy, I have one word of advice about trying a rotation diet: forget-about-it. Nobody with a serious food allergy or a risk of anaphylaxis should attempt it. It's just too risky. Consider it only if you meet all four of the following conditions:

- ✔ Your food allergy is mild.
- ✔ Your doctor tells you that you're at absolutely no risk of experiencing anaphylaxis.
- ✔ Your doctor gives you permission.
- ✔ Your doctor creates and monitors your diet, and you check in regularly for any necessary modifications.

Charting your game plan

An effective rotation diet is like a good golf swing. It requires a careful backswing, a smooth forward stroke, and an effective follow-through:

- ✔ **Backswing:** Plan in advance so you know exactly how much of each food you can eat on which days. Keep a calendar or food diary.
- ✔ **Forward stroke:** Follow your calendar, and don't try to fudge on the amounts of food you eat or the days on which you eat them.
- ✔ **Follow-through:** Log the foods you eat and note how you feel after eating them (on your calendar or food diary), and check with your doctor regularly to make necessary adjustments. In some cases, your doctor may need to do follow-up allergy tests to ensure that increased exposure to certain foods is not worsening your allergies.

Chapter 7

Making It Stop: Finding Symptomatic Relief

*A*t the core of every food allergy treatment plan are evasive maneuvers to steer you clear of the foods that commonly trigger reactions. In a world with so many foods and where certain ingredients pop up in the most unsuspecting places, avoidance can be nearly impossible 100 percent of the time. Even my most careful and vigilant patients occasionally experience reactions, sometimes severe.

For immediate relief and when avoidance is not 100 percent effective, the best available option is to treat the symptoms. In this Chapter, I cover the most common symptoms triggered by food allergies and help you stock your arsenal of medications to fight back when all attempts to avoid the foods that ail you aren't enough.

Pro-Acting and Reacting to Anaphylaxis

Anaphylaxis is a sudden, severe, and potentially life-threatening allergic reaction. You can minimize the severity of anaphylactic reactions by reacting to them in the following ways:

  ✔ Recognize the symptoms early.

  ✔ Self-treat immediately with the proper medications.

  ✔ Seek emergency medical care promptly.

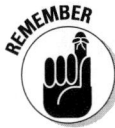

Effectively preventing future anaphylactic reactions hinges on avoiding the triggers. Whenever you experience a severe reaction, try to identify the specific trigger.

The following sections present preventive measures and emergency treatment instructions to avoid severe reactions and cut them short when preventive measures fail. See Chapter 2 for a more complete discussion of anaphylaxis — its symptoms and risk factors.

Defending yourself against anaphylactic episodes

Anaphylaxis is a frightening experience for the person who suffers the reaction, as well as for anyone in the near vicinity. Dreading future reactions is normal, but you can take a few simple measures to reduce the risk and calm your fears, as I explain in the following sections.

Obtaining an allergy workup

If you've experienced an anaphylactic reaction, visit an allergist for a workup. Your allergist can perform skin or blood tests to help identify your specific allergies, offer guidance on the treatment of future reactions, and provide you with a treatment plan in writing. (See Chapter 5 for details.)

Avoiding triggers

Avoidance is key to preventing future severe reactions. If you've experienced an anaphylactic reaction in the past, try to identify the food or foods that triggered the reaction, and strictly avoid those foods. See Chapter 6 for details about avoidance diets and for food allergy sheets that can assist you in identifying allergens in processed foods. The Chapters in Part III provide avoidance maneuvers that you can take at home and away from home.

Wearing an allergy alert bracelet or necklace

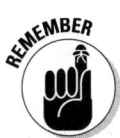

If you have a severe or even potentially severe food allergies or have experienced an anaphylactic reaction, wear an allergy alert bracelet, necklace, or similar alert tag at all times. If you experience another reaction and are too ill to explain your condition, your tag can help responders provide proper treatment as quickly as possible. This measure is especially important in children.

The alert tag should include a list of known allergies, as well as the name and phone number of an emergency contact. One device, Medic Alert, provides a toll-free number that emergency medical workers can call to obtain your medical history, list of medications, family emergency contact numbers, and healthcare provider names and numbers.

Drawing up an anaphylactic treatment plan well in advance

Once you've experienced an allergic reaction, particularly a severe reaction, the last thing you want to think about is a future reaction that may be even worse, but that's exactly what you need to do to save your life.

In the following sections, I cover the essential components of an effective emergency plan. Team up with your doctor to iron out the details and formulate your own plan using the form shown in Figure 7-1. This form can function as a great tool to include in your home emergency station, described in Chapter 10 and to keep on file with the school nurse.

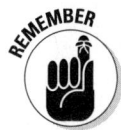

Because anaphylaxis can be life-threatening, you must treat it as you would treat any absolute medical emergency, including heart attack, stroke, or a severe diabetic reaction.

An effective plan can save your life, minimize the severity of an anaphylactic reaction, and get you feeling a whole lot better a whole lot sooner.

Stocking up on epinephrine . . . and knowing how to use it

Patients with a history of anaphylaxis or who are at risk of future anaphylactic reactions should always carry two *epinephrine autoinjectors* (EpiPen or Twinject). Epinephrine is the most effective drug. It treats all the symptoms of anaphylaxis, including the most threatening symptoms — low blood pressure, chest tightness or wheezing, and throat closure.

Your doctor can provide you with a prescription for epinephrine autoinjectors, but you also need to know some critical facts about autoinjectors to maximize their potential benefit:

❏ Fill your epinephrine autoinjector prescription immediately.

❏ Read the instructions provided with your autoinjector and review them with each refill just in case the instructions have changed.

❏ Make sure you're getting the right dose. Autoinjectors come in 2 doses — a *junior* for young children and a *regular strength* for everyone else. Officially, the full strength devices are approved for use for anyone over 66 pounds. The junior strength is a perfect dose for someone who weighs 33 pounds, but for every pound above that it underdoses more and more. For this reason most experts, including me, recommend switching from junior to regular strength somewhere between 45 and 55 pounds.

❏ Store epinephrine at normal room temperature away from cold and heat sources.

❑ Examine the epinephrine cartridge window periodically to ensure that the solution is colorless and contains no floating particles. Replace solutions that are discolored or contain particles.

❑ Check the expiration date on your autoinjectors regularly. (An expired autoinjector is better than no injector, so if all you can find during an emergency is an expired one, use it.)

❑ Keep at least two epinephrine autoinjectors with you at all times. Having an additional autoinjector at work, school, and home is a great idea.

❑ Store the home injector in a convenient location, and let family members and friends know where it is. Sticking it in the "junk drawer" or a cluttered medicine cabinet is a bad idea.

❑ Get up to speed on how to use your injector, as explained later in this chapter.

❑ Train family members, close friends, teachers, and co-workers on proper use in preparation for a possible emergency. In the midst of a reaction, you may panic and be unable to assist with your own injection.

❑ Act quickly when you first notice symptoms. A quick response is essential in preventing serious complications. Few, if any, known fatal reactions have been due to food-induced anaphylaxis when epinephrine was given promptly.

❑ A second dose may be needed if symptoms are worsening or not improving within 10–15 minutes or if symptoms return before emergency personnel and equipment are available.

Both the EpiPen and the Twinject offer trainer devices for practice and to demonstrate proper use to others. Anyone who may need to use it must practice with the trainer first. Most people end up with lots of expired injectors and I find it helpful to shoot an orange or grapefruit with one of these to see what a real one feels like. This is also a great practice tool for adolescents who are getting ready to take over responsibility for their medicines.

If you have a history of severe reactions, grab you autoinjector and give yourself a shot as soon as you notice the telltale signs of a reaction. As a general rule, administer epinephrine immediately if you:

✔ Have any two systems involved in a reaction, such as hives and stomach pains, or any other combination of two or more symptoms that affect different parts of your body

✔ Are having trouble breathing

✔ Feel tightness in your throat

✔ Feel faint . . . as though you may pass out

Food Allergy Emergency Action Plan

Patient's Name: _____

Allergic to: _____

Asthmatic: Yes* ☐   No ☐   *High risk for severe reaction

Accidental ingestion could lead to a severe allergic (anaphylactic) reaction. Signs of an allergic reaction include:

- **Mouth:** Itching or swelling of the lips, tongue, or mouth
- **Throat:** Itching or sense of tightness in the throat, hoarseness, or a hacking cough
- **Skin:** Hives, itching, or swelling of the face or extremities
- **Gut:** Nausea, abdominal cramps, vomiting, or diarrhea
- **Lungs:** Shortness of breath, repetitive coughing, or wheezing
- **Heart:** Lightheadedness, fainting
- **Anxiety:** Panic or sense of impending doom

Treatment Plan

- If an accidental ingestion is suspected or mild symptoms of a reaction begin, give diphenhydramine (Benadryl) _____ teaspoons (_____ mg) by mouth.
- If hoarseness, a sensation of tightness in the throat, difficulty breathing, or any symptoms from two or more of the above systems develop, give epinephrine (_____) and then call 911 to arrange transport to the nearest medical facility.
- If _____, provide the following treatment: _____.

Contact Information

Call for additional advice and instructions:

- Mother's phone: _____
- Father's phone: _____
- Other emergency contacts:

  Dr. _____ at _____

  Name: _____ at _____

  Name: _____ at _____

Note: Do not hesitate to administer medications or call 911 even if the parents or doctor cannot be reached. The severity of a reaction can change quickly and any of the above symptoms can potentially progress to a life-threatening situation.

Figure 7-1: Create your own custom food allergy emergency action plan.

Tragic delay

James, a 19-year-old patient of mine with peanut allergy and asthma, ate a chocolate chip cookie at his girlfriend's home that was supposed to be safe. He immediately felt itching in his mouth and throat and told his girlfriend that he must be having a reaction. He had never had a severe reaction before and was sure that a dose of antihistamine would work. They found some Benadryl in the medicine cabinet, and James took some, but a few minutes later he felt an asthma attack coming on, so he took several puffs of his inhaler. He looked scared, and his girlfriend knew something terribly bad was happening. She asked whether she should call 911 but James told her that they should wait a few minutes.

Where was his epinephrine? Unfortunately, since he had never had a severe reaction, James and his girlfriend had stopped filling the prescriptions I had been giving them each year. All my advice about this deadly combination of asthma and peanut allergy had gone unheard. Over the next 10 minutes, James began to swell, had increasing trouble breathing, turned blue, and passed out. By the time the paramedics arrived, his heart had stopped and no amount of epinephrine could save him at that point.

I met with his parents at the emergency room that evening and then again a few days later. They wanted to know whether this could have been prevented. Of course it could have been prevented if James had not trusted that the cookie was safe. That point is very important, but it's not the take home message. The real message here is that severe reactions can happen, even if you follow the strictest avoidance measures, so you must be prepared at all times. If James had had his epinephrine with him and had taken it promptly, he would still be with us and may well be married to the young woman who instead had to watch him die before her eyes.

Some people refuse to use epinephrine for fear of the needle. Others, including some doctors, won't prescribe it because they fear the side effects. Epinephrine is a very safe medicine. For a huge majority of allergy sufferers, the benefit far outweighs the risks. Discuss any concerns you have immediately with your doctor, and if your doctor is reluctant to prescribe epinephrine, you may need to do a little convincing or switch doctors.

Reviewing additional treatments for anaphylaxis

Although epinephrine is the first and best response to the onset of an anaphylactic reaction, other treatments are often used in addition to epinephrine to provide added relief:

- **Antihistamines:** Diphendydramine (Benadryl) and other antihistamines, given by mouth or by injection, can help symptoms subside during anaphylaxis.

- **H2 blockers:** Another class of antihistamines, called H2 blockers, may also be effective when added to the usual antihistamines — the H1 blockers. H2 blockers include medications like ranitidine (Zantac) and cimetidine (Tagamet), which are commonly used to treat ulcers and acid indigestion.

✔ **Inhalant medications:** Albuterol and other asthma medications can help if you have difficulty breathing, chest tightness, or coughing.

✔ **Corticosteroids:** Prednisone and other corticosteroids can help prevent a recurrence in the hours following an anaphylactic reaction and prevent late reactions, but they don't work rapidly enough for emergency treatment.

Other treatment in the emergency room should address any life-threatening respiratory and cardiovascular symptoms. ER personnel may need to give you additional doses of epinephrine and possibly oxygen or a breathing tube (to keep your airway open) for severe breathing problems. Treatment may also include medications to treat low blood pressure and cardiac arrhythmias (irregular heart beat). Even if symptoms are completely under control, your doctor should keep you under observation for a minimum of four hours due to the possibility of biphasic reactions.

Dealing with Itchy Stuff: Eczema

Eczema is a condition that may or may not involve food allergy. As I discuss in Chapter 2, food allergy is responsible for about 40 percent of the cases, and even when food allergy is the prime suspect, it is almost never the sole suspect. I always tell my patients that some part of eczema is literally the skin you were born to have. Even in the perfect environment and on the perfect diet, some people's skin is just too dry, too itchy, or too sensitive.

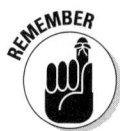

When food allergy is involved in eczema, the five most common food allergens are the most likely culprits: egg, milk, peanut, soy, and wheat. Other foods can certainly be involved but these top five are the most important to remember.

When food-allergy-induced eczema is itching to drive you crazy, avoiding the foods that trigger reactions is the first and most effective course of action, but symptoms can linger long after you stop consuming the food. If dryness and itchiness persist, treat the symptoms:

✔ **Moisturize, moisturize, moisturize.** Use a cream rather than a lotion, and apply it at least once a day, particularly immediately following a bath or shower. Most people with eczema discover that taking a long bath in warm or tepid water provides much needed relief, but if you don't follow up with moisturizer, that comforting bath can lead to drier and itchier skin later. If your eczema is severe, apply moisturizing cream multiple times per day.

✔ **Apply medicated creams.** Medicated creams or ointments — usually steroid preparations such as hydrocortisone — can control skin inflammation. While some steroid creams are very potent and may be unsafe to use on a regular basis, especially in children, low-potency creams are very safe and can be used on a regular basis, if needed. Two nonsteroidal anti-inflammatory creams/ointments for treating eczema are presently on the market. Their safety, however, has recently come under scrutiny, and the FDA requires a black box warning on these products until further research ensures their safety.

✔ **Soothe the itch with oral antihistamines.** Oral antihistamines can be valuable in relieving eczema's severe itching. The older style antihistamines, including Benadryl, are particularly beneficial at bedtime, since their sedative side effect can help you sleep through the itch. For daytime itching, opt for a non-sedating antihistamine, such as Zyrtec, Clarinex, or Allegra.

Identify and avoid anything that further irritates your skin, including any clothing, soap, detergents, or lotions that exacerbate your eczema.

Dealing with More Itchy Stuff: Hives

People who have hives know all too well what they are. If you itch inside and out, are covered with red splotches, and haven't been camping in a cloud of mosquitoes, you probably have hives. What caused them? I discuss that topic and describe the telltale signs of a hives outbreak in Chapter 2, but if you have hives you probably don't care where they came from. All you want to know is how to shake them.

The good thing about hives is that they typically go away much faster than a mosquito bite. They can be severe, but in most cases, a single dose of antihistamine leads to quick, long-lasting relief. If someone comes to me complaining of a week or two struggle with hives, I rarely suspect that food allergy is playing a major role.

To send your hives packing, I recommend the following medications, depending on the severity of the outbreak and the likelihood that the outbreak signals the beginning of a more severe reaction:

✔ Old-style, fast-acting antihistamines like diphendydramine (Benadryl) are a tried and true treatment for hives, although other antihistamines might be equally effective.

✔ Liquid forms of antihistamines are great for treating food reactions, because your body tends to absorb them more quickly, but chewable or fast-melt tablets may be equally effective.

✔ Epinephrine is the drug of choice if you believe that your hives are a sign of a potentially dangerous reaction. Consult your doctor.

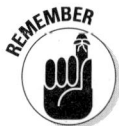

Other conditions, including anxiety, can cause hives, so if your hives appear to be unrelated to the foods you eat, consult your doctor about other possible causes and their treatment. Chapter 2 discusses the most common other causes.

Alleviating Gut-Retching Food Allergies

Your gastrointestinal (GI) tract is like a pipeline, starting at your mouth and ending at your... well... you know. Gastrointestinal food reactions can occur anywhere along this pipeline, and symptoms vary depending on where the reaction hits. As I explain in Chapter 2, reactions can be acute (occurring soon after exposure) or chronic, sometimes low-level reactions.

The GI tract is frequently involved in anaphylactic reactions. While a single episode of vomiting may not be cause for extreme concern, other GI symptoms, such as repeated vomiting or abdominal pain, are often a sign of a more severe reaction, so keep your epinephrine handy.

In the following sections, I introduce the most common GI tract conditions often attributed to food allergy, starting with the mouth and traveling down the pipeline.

Treating oral allergy syndrome

By definition, oral allergy syndrome is a reaction restricted to the lips and mouth and is characterized by itching (sometimes severe) and swelling (usually mild). Because the reaction is localized to the lips and mouth, it's not dangerous in and of itself, but sometimes, oral allergy syndrome can foretell the onset of a more severe reaction, in which the term "oral allergy syndrome" no longer applies.

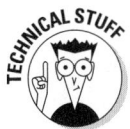

Another name for the oral allergy syndrome is the *pollen related allergy syndrome*. This name refers to the fact that the allergies that cause the syndrome — usually triggered by fresh fruits and vegetables — occur because of cross-reactivity with certain pollens. People with allergy to tree pollens, for example, may experience oral symptoms after eating apples, cherries, or peaches, while those with ragweed allergy may react to melons or carrots.

The allergies commonly associated with oral allergy syndrome are unique in the following ways:

- ✓ These allergies begin to show up in later childhood, only after the pollen allergies are strong enough to trigger cross-reactivity to the related foods.

- ✓ As opposed to most food allergens (peanut allergen becomes stronger with roasting), the allergens in these foods are largely destroyed by cooking. So someone with a reaction to fresh apples can usually eat apple pie or drink apple juice without experiencing a reaction. (Apple cider is another story.)

- ✓ Symptoms may vary with the season. Some people know that their apple allergy will become more intense in the spring (tree pollen season) and then begin to wane by the summer or fall.

- ✓ Allergy shots for the pollens associated with the allergenic food may make the related food allergy go away.

- ✓ The skin of some fruits contains more allergen than the meat of the fruit.

Preventions and treatments for oral allergy syndrome vary, depending on the approach you decide to take:

- ✓ **Do nothing.** Most people don't even tell their doctors about the allergy and decide to live with it. If you enjoy the fruit or vegetable more than you dread having an itchy mouth and lips, then you may decide to partake of it.

- ✓ **Avoidance.** If having an itchy mouth and lips isn't worth the enjoyment, then you may choose to forego the food.

- ✓ **Strict avoidance.** If eating these fruits or vegetables causes more severe reactions beyond those considered to be oral allergy syndrome, stricter avoidance is obviously needed.

- ✓ **Medicate.** Most reactions, however, resolve on their own within 20 or 30 minutes with no treatment.

Easing the effects of eosinophilic gastroenteritis

An eosinophil is a type of blood cell commonly found at the crime scene — the site of any allergic reaction. These cells are responsible for much of the inflammation that occurs in most chronic allergic conditions, including those that affect the skin (eczema), the nose (allergic rhinitis), the lungs (asthma), and the GI tract.

When eosinophils set course for your GI tract, they can cause a condition called *allergic eosinophilic gastroenteritis* — a chronic inflammation in the GI tract, sometimes localized and sometimes involving the entire GI tract. When the upper GI tract is involved, such as with *eosinophilic esophagitis* (swelling in the esophagus), symptoms include pain, reflux, poor appetite, and difficulty swallowing. Swelling of the lower GI often results in pain, diarrhea, or weight loss. Food allergy causes most cases of eosinophilic gastroenteritis.

In many cases, eosinophilic gastroenteritis is not an IgE-mediated allergy, meaning that the usual blood and skin tests may turn up negative for food allergy. Even so, your doctor may recommend a standard food allergy treatment:

- **Avoidance diet:** Many of those who suffer from eosinophilic gastroenteritis have multiple food allergies, so a complicated avoidance diet may be needed. See Chapter 6 for details on avoidance diets.

- **Change in formula (for infants):** In babies, sometimes a simple change of formulas may be sufficient for stemming future reactions.

When food avoidance is ineffective, steroids are the only medicines that clearly work. You may respond to a type of asthma medication called montelukast (Singulair) or other newer medications. Antihistamines are of little use. Other immunosuppressive agents may offer some relief, but they all carry risks and need to be monitored carefully, usually with the combined efforts of your allergist and gastroenterologist.

Muting the symptoms of eosinophilic esophagitis (EE)

Eosinophilic esophagitis (EE) is a form of eosinophilic gastroenteritis that's localized to the esophagus — your food chute. This condition is usually triggered by a food allergy, although environmental allergies can also contribute. In some cases, food allergy doesn't even play a role.

When food allergy is the cause, avoidance is the key to feeling better. When the cause is something more than food allergy, I've had excellent success using steroid-based asthma inhalers. Instead of having patients inhale the medicine, however, I instruct my patients to spray it in the mouth and swallow it.

Checking out remedies for allergic proctitis

Allergic proctitis (or allergic colitis) is a pain in the . . . well . . . end of the intestinal tract. The condition is especially common in young babies with symptoms of blood and mucous in the stools. Milk or soy allergy is typically the cause, although other foods may be involved in breast-fed babies.

Because allergic proctitis is not IgE mediated, it generally responds well to one of the following treatment trials:

- **Formula fed:** If the baby takes formula, then a milk-free or soy-free trial may clear up the condition.

- **Breast fed:** If the baby is breast feeding, the mother may need to avoid soy, milk, and possibly other suspect foods on a trial basis to identify the problem food.

Allergic proctitis is a rather benign condition in which the babies tend to feel and grow well. Half the babies who have it are fine by the time they reach their first year, and most others can eat all foods by the age of two or three.

Caring for enterocolitis syndrome

In young babies, a food allergy can cause a condition called *enterocolitis syndrome*, characterized by severe, repetitive vomiting that may lead to dehydration. Skin and blood tests are of no help in identifying food allergy, because the allergy is not IgE-mediated, but cause and effect usually provide a clear link to the food that's triggering the reaction.

Milk and soy allergies are most common but these reactions also occur with a large number of other foods. Food avoidance is the only treatment, and most children outgrow the allergy by two to three years of age. During these latter years, your doctor may recommend re-introducing the problem foods, but you should proceed with extreme caution, because reactions can be severe.

Alleviating the symptoms of celiac disease

Celiac disease, also known as *gluten sensitive enteropathy*, is a form of food sensitivity in which people can't tolerate any form of gluten — a protein found in wheat, rye, and barley. Symptoms typically include abdominal pain, vomiting, diarrhea, and weight loss (or poor growth in young children).

Symptoms can be quite severe and appear very early in life or remain low-grade, flying well below your doctor's radar until adulthood. Although celiac disease is not IgE-mediated, your doctor can perform other blood tests to make an accurate diagnosis. In all cases strict avoidance of all gluten is essential and typically requires you to abstain from these foods for the rest of your life.

For details on how to create and manage your own tasty and varied gluten-free diet, check out *Living Gluten Free For Dummies*, by Danna Korn.

Catching Your Breath . . . Asthma Symptoms and Treatments

Short of breath? Coughing? Wheezing? If you are, you may have asthma, a chronic condition, and underlying allergies may be triggering the symptoms, but a food allergy isn't the most likely cause. When you have an allergy-induced form of asthma, environmental allergens are the most likely suspects.

When you consult your family physician and describe your symptoms, she's likely to offer a diagnosis based solely on your reported symptoms, or she may subject you to a series of breathing tests, assuming you're at least five or six years old. Your allergist may perform a series of allergy tests, but these typically don't include tests for food allergy, unless you report additional symptoms typical of food allergy.

Although food allergy typically plays only a minor role, if any, in asthma, if you have asthma and a food allergy, you're at risk for experiencing more severe allergic reactions when you ingest a food that triggers a reaction, especially a reaction in which the throat and lungs are involved. Antihistamines have no effect on these reactions. In such cases, the reaction qualifies as an emergency. (See "Pro-Acting and Reacting to Anaphylaxis.")

For details on the diagnosis and treatment of asthma and tips for living well with asthma, check out *Asthma For Dummies*, by William E. MD, MBA Berger and Jackie Joyner-Kersee.

Treating a Chronic "Cold": Allergic Rhinitis

Most people attribute runny nose and sneezing to the common cold or hay fever. Something in your nose — a virus or irritant — must be causing the problem, right? Well, that's usually true, but food allergies can also trigger symptoms in your snout, including a runny nose, sneezing, congestion, and itchy, watery eyes.

If an allergen is the cause, your sniffles and sneezes are probably due to a condition called *allergic rhinitis*. Rhinitis means nose — think rhinoceros.

Whether your allergic rhinitis is triggered by environmental allergens or by a particular food, the symptom relievers are pretty much the same:

✔ Antihistamines, including loratadine (Claritin) and diphendydramine (Benadryl).

✔ Nasal sprays that often contain the same steroid medications used for asthma.

✔ Leukotriene blockers, such as Singulair, can also be helpful in controlling nasal allergies.

✔ A combination of nasal sprays and antihistamines (for the most stubborn cases).

Chapter 8

Debunking Alternative Tests and Therapies

In This Chapter

▶ Getting the straight dope on alternative allergy tests

▶ Steering clear of time- and money-wasting homeopathy

▶ Avoiding the overblown claims of vitamin and herb peddlers

▶ Poking holes in the leaky gut theory

▶ Dismissing meditation and massage as cure-alls

Spend about a half hour on the Internet, and you can find hundreds of Web sites where quackologists spew forth untested theories about allergies, alternative allergy testing, and cures. Many of the worst sites claim that just about every health condition imaginable from cancer to psychiatric and behavioral disorders can be traced back to something you're eating or not eating. These sites may even attempt to convince you that the medical community is somehow conspiring to keep you ill.

I would love to tell you and the thousands of allergy patients I see that a miracle cure for food allergy is available, and I wouldn't care who discovered it. If I could cure my own peanut allergy by popping a fistful of vitamins, sitting for an hour a day in the lotus position, or drinking some magic herbal potion, I'd do it myself. The facts, however, prove that such therapies offer very little promise and even less scientific evidence of success. Some may even be dangerous.

I can save you a lot of time, money, frustration, and unnecessary risk through a few simple words of advice: Get to a food allergist, get tested, and stick with the best care currently available — proven medical tests and treatments. Follow that advice, and you don't even have to read this chapter.

I write this chapter only because I know that you're likely to research food allergies on the Internet. Research is great, and I encourage you to investigate the latest medical breakthroughs, but I know that your research is going to lead you down some dark alleys. To keep you from getting swindled by the people and ideas lurking in those dark alleys, in this chapter, I separate medical fact from quack, so you can spend your time, energy, and money pursuing tests and treatments that actually work.

Exposing Meaningless Tests and Other Mumbo Jumbo

One of the biggest crocks of quackery is the claim that allergy tests are simply not thorough enough to accurately detect food allergies and sensitivities. Most of the practitioners who denounce standard allergy tests promote their own supposedly superior tests to uncover hidden allergies and sensitivities that can cause everything from acne and fatigue to obesity and even cancer.

These dubious tests are risky at best and dangerous at their worst for several reasons:

- These tests and treatments have not been validated by sound medical research data and are not supported by the medical community.
- They're often expensive, and your insurance won't cover them.
- They're unreliable.
- Test results typically call for convoluted and costly treatment regimens that don't work.
- Testing and treatments may discourage you from seeking effective medical treatment, leading to the potential danger of a severe reaction.

In the following sections, I expose the most common and questionable alternative tests for allergies.

Polling your cellular reactions: Cytotoxic testing

Back in the early 1980s, alternative practitioners, nutrition consultants, and chiropractors got all excited about *cytotoxic testing* — also called Bryan's test, the Metabolic Intolerance Test, or "sensitivity testing." "Cyto" means "cell" and you know what "toxic" means, so the idea behind this type of testing is to discover substances that poison your white blood cells — the blood cells that primarily fight infection.

To perform the tests and recommend treatment, the practitioner does the following:

1. **Draws a sample of your blood and then separates out the white blood cells.**

2. **Applies samples of the white blood cells to a large number of microscope slides, each of which is coated with a dried food extract, such as those used for skin testing.**

3. **Examines the slides under a microscope at various intervals to see whether the white blood cells changed shape or disintegrated — supposedly signs of allergy or sensitivity to the particular food.**

4. **Diagnoses your symptoms and recommends a personalized diet program that includes vitamins and minerals, most of which are conveniently for sale at the clinic.**

Cytotoxic hype

One of the most blatantly over-hyped promotions for cytotoxic testing was put forth by a laboratory in California that charged $350 to test for 186 common foods and additives. One of its ads, posted with the headline "DISASTER LINKED TO THE FOOD YOU EAT!," claimed that "if you currently suffer from any health difficulties, this test is worth taking."

A brochure from the company suggested that cytotoxic testing could help solve the problems of obesity, headaches, stomach and intestinal problems, depression, stress, confusion, sinus problems, asthma, arthritis, and hypoglycemia. They put on quite a road show to appeal to patients who were ready to listen to anyone who held out the promise of a cure for any and all their unexplained maladies.

After the company's glitzy slide show presentation, a young man who claimed that he had undergone two years of special nutrition training gave a lecture. Among other things, he advised the assembled group that inhalant sensitivities are not important, so people allergic to cats would no longer have cat allergy if they simply stopped eating the foods that made them allergic to cats.

A well know allergist and his wife happened to be in attendance. The doctor and his wife actually had no allergies, but her test report, which arrived three weeks later, said that she was allergic to 25 foods, including wheat, cane sugar, corn, potato, beef, and milk, and she should abstain from eating all of them.

Not only were the test results blatantly wrong, but the recommendation to avoid all these foods would have led to a significant reduction in quality of life and perhaps even to malnutrition.

Advocates of cytotoxic testing claim that food sensitivities can cause acne, anxiety, arthritis, asthma, back pain, baldness, bedwetting, conjunctivitis, constipation, depression, diarrhea, eczema, excessive sweating, fatigue, headaches, hearing loss, hoarseness, hypertension, hyperactivity, insomnia, learning disorders, nosebleeds, obesity, rashes, sinus trouble, stomach disorders, susceptibility to cancer, and just about any other physical ailment you (or they) can imagine.

The American Academy of Allergy, Asthma and Immunology (AAAAI), the nation's largest group of allergists, has concluded that cytotoxic testing is ineffective for diagnosing food or inhalant allergies. Its position paper noted the following:

- ✔ One study found that white blood cells from allergic patients reacted no differently when exposed to substances known to produce symptoms than when exposed to substances to which the patients were not sensitive.

- ✔ Another study found that cytotoxic test results did not correlate with allergic reactions or other negative reactions to foods and that the results were inconsistent when repeated in the same patient.

- ✔ In a double-blind controlled study, positive cytotoxic tests were frequently obtained to foods that produced no clinical symptoms, and foods that tested negative in cytotoxic tests did produce symptoms.

- ✔ Another double-blind study found the test results varied from day to day.

Looking at your lymphocytes with ELISA/ACT testing

The ELISA/ACT test is another medically unproven test that its advocates claim can uncover hidden allergies. According to a brochure promoting this test, scientific estimates show that hidden allergies are responsible for as much as 60 percent of all human illness. The brochure states that any of the following conditions may indicate the presence of hidden allergies: chronic headaches, migraines, difficulty sleeping, dizziness, runny or stuffy nose, postnasal drip, ringing in the ears, earaches, blurred vision, irregular or rapid heartbeat, asthma, nausea and vomiting, constipation, diarrhea, irritable bowel syndrome, hives, skin rashes (psoriasis, eczema), muscle aches, joint pain, arthritis, nervous tension, fatigue, depression, mental dullness, and difficulty in getting your work done.

To perform ELISA/ACT testing, a clinician draws your blood; cultures the white blood cells (lymphocytes); and observes how they react to up to 300 foods, minerals, preservatives, and environmental substances. Upon receiving the test results, the practitioner (typically a chiropractor) recommends dietary modification and supplements. Sound familiar?

Valid scientific studies have shown the ELISA/ACT test to have no value in the diagnosis of allergy. Moreover, many of the symptoms listed in SPL's brochure are unrelated to allergy and require proper medical care rather than supplements for effective treatment. (SPL is short for Serammune Physicians Lab, the people who developed ELISA/ACT.)

Unclogging your energy fields with NAET

Nambudripad's Allergy Elimination Technique (NAET) is one of the more interesting and useless tests and treatments for food allergies and sensitivities. The idea behind NAET testing is that some foods can block your energy fields, thus weakening your body — sort of like the effect that kryptonite has on Superman. NAET essentially combines kinesiology (described in the next section) with acupuncture (discussed later in this chapter in the section "Solving Allergies Through Acupuncture or Acupressure").

To test for food sensitivities, the practitioner instructs you to hold a food or other suspect substance in your hand or brings the food or substance in close proximity to your body — supposedly in the path of your energy flow. You hold your arms akimbo, and the examiner pulls down on your arms. If your arms show little resistance, then the tested food or substance is deemed to be a problem. (Some practitioners use other ways to test the effects of foods and other substances on muscle strength, but you get the idea.)

Positive test results reportedly diagnose weaknesses in your energy field that can then be remedied through acupuncture or acupressure. Unfortunately, as your arms get more and more tired during the procedure, the tests often return more and more positive results. A positive result may indicate only that you need to spend a little more time in the gym.

Because NAET is such a kooky idea, any scientist worth her science degree won't even test it, so little reliable data is available to support or refute NAET's claims.

You can read more about NAET at www.naet.com, but after you read the hype, I encourage you to visit www.chirobase.org/06DD/naet.html to learn some interesting facts about NAET and its developer, Devi S. Nambudripad.

Discrediting the claims of other dubious tests

Cytotoxic testing, ELISA/ACT, and NAET are a small sampling of the tests and procedures that are routinely marketed as food allergy tests and treatments. Although not all these treatment approaches have undergone rigorous study, none has been shown to be of any diagnostic value. Following are some of the more common and dubious tests and treatments:

- **Pulse testing** recommends that you take your pulse soon after eating to determine if you're sensitive to the food you just ate. If your pulse rate increases, then you supposedly are sensitive to a particular food. Although your pulse rate may increase after eating something, an increased pulse rate can be due to other causes and certainly does not provide a reliable indication of food allergy or intolerance.

- **ALCAT testing** is very similar to cytotoxic and ELISA/ACT testing. It tests the changes in white blood cell count and shape when the blood is exposed to certain known allergens and other problem substances.

- **NuTron testing** supposedly measures the reactivity of white blood cells to food and other substances. Practitioners use the results of the test to design a diet that eliminates foods that cause white cell *activation*, whatever that is. Proponents claim that the diet can help overweight people lose weight and cure many other conditions "caused by the release of inflammatory chemicals from the activated white cells."

- **The LEAP Program** uses the *Mediator Release Test* (MRT) to identify "delayed food allergies." Treatment involves dietary changes and sometimes the addition of supplements or herbs.

- **Provocative testing** consists of injecting increasing doses of a potential allergen under your skin until you report symptoms. These tests are no more accurate and could be more dangerous than standard skin tests, although, the small doses typically administered during the tests are usually not all that dangerous.

- **Sublingual testing** consists of placing suspected foods under your tongue to see what happens. Again, sublingual testing is no more accurate and is more dangerous than standard skin tests.

- **Neutralization** progressively administers smaller doses of substances until you no longer react. This is similar to desensitization protocols, which I discuss as potentially useful in Chapter 9. Neutralization, however, is typically performed with ultra-low doses (such as those given with homeopathic remedies, discussed in the following section), and the treatments are typically used to cure conditions such as ADHD or chronic headaches. Neutralization is not effective in preventing future food allergy reactions.

- **Immune-complex and IgG tests** assess immune reactions that are common but not necessarily related to allergy. These include food-specific IgG and IgG4 tests, which typically yield multiple positive results (many false positives) and may indicate a normal immune response to food. They do not predict true food sensitivity and can lead to recommendations that result in malnutrition.

- **Electrodermal skin testing** uses a computerized galvanometer to detect supposed energy imbalances when you come in contact with a food or substance. Think of it as a hi-tech variation on the theme of applied kinesiology, described next.

- **Applied kinesiology** (used in NAET testing as discussed in the section on NAET) tests your muscle strength after foods and other substances are placed in your mouth or hand or held in close proximity to your body.

- **Iridology** practitioners claim that they can spot the cause of a wide range of health conditions simply by peering into your eyes. Although medical doctors can diagnose several medical conditions, including Wilson's disease, by peeking in your peepers, your eyes hold no hidden clues that you have a particular food allergy.

- **Hair analysis** studies the mineral content in your hair to supposedly determine whether you have mineral deficiencies or heavy metal poisoning that's causing your food allergy. Studies prove that no reliable connection exists between the mineral content of hair or the existence of heavy metals in your system and the presence or absence of food allergy.

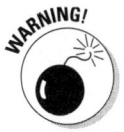

The list of bogus tests I provide here is certainly not all inclusive. New bogus tests and theories are always popping up, so remain vigilant and skeptical. When you see a new test or treatment that sounds promising, run it past your doctor before trusting your health and wallet to unproven theories, tests, and treatments.

Demystifying Homeopathy: A Little Hair of the Dog That Bit You

Homeopathy, founded by Hahnemann in the early 1800s, relies on the principle that the same substances that cause disease can cure it. Homeopathic remedies consist of ultra-diluted forms of the substance that's causing symptoms — so diluted in some cases, that the solution in which the substance is suspended contains only a "memory" of the substance.

Homeopathy is a holistic approach to medicine, with particular emphasis on the homeopath-patient relationship. The scientific interest in homeopathy for treating asthma, food allergies, and other chronic illness is considerable, as attested to by a large number of published studies, but clinical trials show no clear benefit of such treatments.

A recent review compared more than 100 clinical trials of homeopathy and conventional medicine in treatment of the same diseases and assessed the outcomes of the two types of treatment. After a detailed analysis, this review concluded that according to the results of the clinical trials, conventional treatments are much more effective than homeopathic remedies for the same diseases.

Deflating the Hype Surrounding Vitamins, Minerals, and Herbs

By eating a well balanced diet and perhaps supplementing it with a good multi-vitamin once a day, you provide for all your body's nutritional needs. Packing your body with mega-doses of vitamins and minerals doesn't make you any healthier, although it does help you lose weight as your wallet becomes lighter.

Flushing those allergies out of your system

Maybe you really don't have food allergy. Perhaps your digestive system is just so gummed up with toxic waste and parasites that it can't fully digest your food and effectively purge undigested foodstuffs, and that's what's causing your reactions.

That sounds plausible. Certain foods make you sick. Your gastrointestinal system is responsible for processing food. So maybe your digestive system just needs a thorough flushing to make it fully operational. That's the theory behind cleansing regimens that their advocates claim can cure a wide range of ailments, including "constipation, IBS, severe gas and bloating, weight gain, chronic fatigue, irritability, acid reflux, parasites, stomach pain, diverticulitis, skin and hair problems, and food allergies."

Proponents of the theory are convinced that you can flush these toxins right out of your system along with your food allergies and a host of other ailments. The following two body-cleansing treatments are the most popular:

- **Colon cleansing:** Practitioners often recommend a step-by-step cleansing regimen designed to flush your system with various herbal laxatives and other purgatives and then reestablish healthy functioning by replenishing your body's supply of friendly bacteria.

- **Chelation:** Chelation is a process of leaching the heavy metals — typically calcium, lead, and mercury — out of your body. A few practitioners claim that chelation can cure everything from arthritis to food allergies.

No clinical tests prove the effectiveness of these cleansing regimens in treating food allergy, and in some cases, they can deplete your system of essential vitamins, minerals, and nutrients.

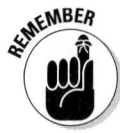

Herbal remedies may be effective in treating some diseases, even food allergies. In Chapter 9, I reveal a Chinese herbal formula that shows great promise.

The effectiveness of some medicinal herbs in treating some conditions is no surprise. Many common and effective drugs are derived from plants and herbs that often contain several active pharmacologic ingredients. Some medical systems (traditional Chinese medicine, Japanese, Kampo, and Ayurvedic) largely use herbs, often in fixed mixtures (for example, ma huang and saiboku-to) to treat diseases, including asthma and rhinitis.

The problems with herbal concoctions are that most of them are no more effective, no less prone to producing negative side effects, and often less safe than approved drugs that your doctor recommends:

- ✔ Contrary to what many people who choose herbal remedies over pharmaceuticals often think, herbal remedies can cause serious side effects and drug interactions. "All natural" does not mean "safe." Cyanide is a naturally occurring poison, and it's certainly not safe.

- ✔ Herbal remedies may not be as potent as manufactured medicines, so they're often not as effective.

- ✔ Herbal formulas don't have to meet the strict manufacturing standards of bona-fide medications, so they're more likely to be tainted by incorrect collection of plants, mistakes in preparation or manufacturing, variations in dosage, and contamination.

Addressing the Leaky-Gut Hypothesis

Another theory that attempts to focus food allergy on the digestive system rather than on the immune system is the hypothesis that people who have food or chemical sensitivities actually suffer from an over-permeable stomach lining that allows chemicals and allergens to pass through the stomach directly into the bloodstream and surrounding tissues. This condition, referred to as *leaky gut syndrome* has received a lot of press and generated far more attention on the Internet and in various articles and books than it deserves.

Some patients with eosinophilic gastrointestinal disease, which I discuss in Chapter 7, may truly get a leaky gut when their disease is out of control. This is pretty extreme though, and the notion that most of our maladies are due to leaky gut is primarily a fictitious diagnosis made on the Internet and in other publications by alternative practitioners. Don't fall for the hype that leaky gut syndrome is responsible for causing your food allergy or intolerance.

Healing Yourself through Mind, Body, and Soul Manipulations

Attending to your physical, emotional, intellectual, and spiritual needs is useful in preserving your overall health and improving your quality of life. Through proper nutrition and exercise, you preserve your physical well-being. Meditation and relaxation techniques can reduce stress — a common trigger for many maladies. Developing productive interpersonal relationships can further reduce stress and improve your emotional well being. And addressing your spiritual needs can provide you with a sense of interconnectedness and community interactions that can be very rewarding.

As a health professional, I encourage you to establish a healthy lifestyle and avoid unhealthy habits. Whatever improves your overall health can be a useful complementary therapy to proven medical treatments. As an allergist, however, I recommend that you avoid falling into the common trap of thinking that any combination of mind, body, and spiritual development can cure your food allergy. After reading the following facts, you should come to the same conclusion:

- ✔ **Chiropractic manipulation** of the spine may help you feel better overall, but any claims that chiropractic care can cure allergies is unproven. Done wrong, a spinal manipulation can even harm your body.

- ✔ **Breathing exercises,** including those practiced in Kundalini yoga can make you feel more relaxed and help with fatigue. Practitioners often recommend breathing exercises to help with asthma and food allergies, but no clinical test results prove that they're effective. At best, patients see some marginal improvement.

- ✔ **Yoga and other relaxation techniques** can have a positive effect on self-perceived well-being, providing an additional benefit, but they do not make food allergy go away.

- ✔ **Hypnosis and biofeedback techniques** have been tried to help asthma sufferers, but have not proven effective.

- ✔ **Reflexology and other massage techniques** attempt to physically manipulate your body in such a way to relax muscles, improve blood flow, restore the body's immune system to optimum functioning, and even rub out allergies. No clinical test results prove that any type of massage effectively reduces the incidence or severity of allergic reactions, including food reactions, but hey, if it feels good, don't let me get in the way.

> ✔ **Other treatments and procedures, including aromatherapy, chromo-therapy, Bach's flowers, anthroposophy, Hopi candles, hydro-colon, urine therapy, and clinical ecology** have no reliable data to support their effectiveness in treating allergy or asthma, although they may help you forget that you have it for awhile.

Solving Allergies through Acupuncture or Acupressure

Acupuncture is part of traditional Chinese medicine and is widely used for the treatment of chronic illnesses, including asthma. The theory behind the use of acupuncture is to restore the balance of "vital flows" by inserting needles at exact points of the body surface, where the "meridians" of these flows lie. If your acupuncturist is highly skilled, you don't even feel the needles going in . . . or so I'm told.

If you can't stomach the thought of being poked with needles, variations of acupuncture are available, including acupressure techniques, such as Shiatsu, and laser treatments.

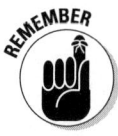

We can study acupuncture in a rigorous manner by using sham acupuncture as a control procedure. Several randomized controlled trials have assessed the efficacy of acupuncture in asthma, and no convincing evidence proves that acupuncture of any form is effective in treating asthma, rhinitis, or food allergy. Stick with proven diagnostic methods described in Chapter 5 and proven treatments presented in Chapters 6 and 7.

Chapter 9

Exploring Cures from Mice to Man: Current Research

After many years of research in mice and other animal models of food allergy, we (food allergy specialists including Bob) are now finally embarking on human studies investigating ways to truly treat food allergy and prevent its onset. This is very exciting since all we've had to offer until now is avoidance and symptom relief. I think I can safely say on behalf of food allergy sufferers the world over, "We want a cure . . . or at least some more effective treatments for preventing reactions."

Discovery of a treatment that can prevent food allergy or shut it down promises to be a long, slow process, but in the end, I am confident that eventually we will be able to treat food allergy such that the risk of anaphylactic reactions will be dramatically reduced or even eliminated.

In the long, long run — maybe 15 or 20 years down the road — I'm confident that we will be talking about *curing* food allergy, not just reducing reactions or their severity. Along with being the best doctor I can be to my patients, the quest for this cure will remain my focus until my eventual retirement.

In this chapter, I guide you on an exploration of medical treatment options and ongoing research that hold out some future promise for you or a loved one with food allergy.

Muting Allergen Sensitivities through Immunotherapy

When your immune system freaks out and starts attacking the food you eat, something is terribly wrong. Somehow, your immune system has been tricked into making some really bad decisions on what's good and what's bad for you. Your immune system is simply out of whack.

One approach to bringing the immune system back in balance is to retrain it, through immunotherapy, so it no longer identifies harmless foods as enemy invaders. In the following sections, I explain the concept of immunotherapy and describe several immunotherapies currently in development that show some promise.

Grasping the concept of immunotherapy

Immunotherapy attempts to correct your immune system's poor judgment (in some cases) and strengthen it to fight disease (in other cases). In other words, immunotherapy is any treatment that works to activate or deactivate the immune system:

- **Activate the immune system:** When the immune system lets down its guard, you become more susceptible to disease. Immunotherapy can kick your immune system in the pants, so it does a better job protecting you. For example, cancer treatments (sometimes referred to as *cancer vaccines*) are now available for stimulating the immune system to fight specific cancer cells.

- **Deactivate the immune system:** An over-reactive immune system can literally kill you when it's acting like some out-of-control overachiever. In allergy, immunotherapy has traditionally referred to treatments that involve intentionally exposing people to what they're allergic to — essentially desensitizing them to specific allergens over time. Medical professionals refer to this as "the development of immune tolerance" — making the immune system more tolerant of allergens.

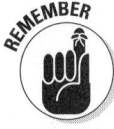

Taking a little hair of the dog that bit you may seem, at first, to be some quack homeopathic treatment for allergies, but medical doctors have successfully employed such treatments for almost a century.

Getting your allergy shots . . . but not necessarily for food allergies

Allergy tests reveal what you're allergic to: pollens, molds, or other allergens. Once your allergist identifies the allergens that ail you, she can prepare and administer allergy shots designed to make your immune system less sensitive to those allergens. Allergy shots have been available for years but are primarily used to treat environmental allergies, such as hay fever. Do they work on food allergies? I get to that question later in the section "Treating food allergies with allergy shots."

You or someone you know probably has had allergy shots to treat everything from hay fever to asthma. Following is a rundown of how a doctor typically determines which shots you need and administers the shots:

1. **Your doctor performs a series of allergy tests on you (see Chapter 5) to determine what you're allergic to.**

2. **Your doctor prepares the shots based on your allergy test results. In other words, not all allergy patients receive the same shots.**

3. **After a build-up period that normally takes 6 to 12 months, your doctor keeps you on a maintenance dose for the next 3 to 5 years.**

Overall more than 80 percent of people with environmental allergies experience improvement with allergy shots. Allergy shots also have proven very effective for people with allergies to bees and other stinging insects.

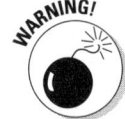

Allergy shots rarely work for eczema and often worsen the condition.

Recognizing the downside

The major downside of allergy shots is that they can cause allergic reactions, sometimes even dangerous anaphylaxis. This should not be surprising since you're actually being injected with the stuff you're allergic to. In addition to the risk of severe reactions, allergy shots often result in significant inconvenience:

- You have to get your shots at your doctor's office.

- You have to wait around for 20 to 30 minutes after each and every shot to make sure you have no reaction.

- The doctor's office must be equipped to deal with severe allergic reactions.

Food allergy immunotherapy's varied success

Doctors have used immunotherapy, in the form of allergy shots, to treat food allergy successfully on a few occasions, including one report published in 1930 of a child who was successfully desensitized to fish. In other studies, however, this form of treatment has proven too risky. In the best study conducted to date — about ten years ago at the National Jewish Hospital in Denver — researchers tested immunotherapy for the treatment of peanut allergy. The shots were successful in that patients in the treatment group were indeed able to tolerate increased amounts of peanut in food challenges after treatment. Unfortunately though, the patients also experienced a high rate of allergic reactions to the shots, and one patient who was supposed to be in the placebo group accidentally received a full dose of the peanut extract and died.

These results made it clear that standard allergy shots for food allergy would not be a practical option and that researchers needed to break new ground. Extensive research has now been conducted on the best ways to accomplish this, and we are now entering a new frontier, putting different methods that have thus far been tested only in animals to the test on people.

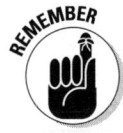

Some people cannot receive shots because their reactions are so severe, but most allergy patients tolerate the shots just fine.

Treating food allergies with allergy shots

When you see such the high success rate for allergy shots in treating environmental allergies (an 80 percent success rate), you may be tempted to jump to the conclusion that drug companies would be able to develop similar vaccines for food allergy.

Unfortunately, up to this point, the effectiveness of food allergy shots has proven less promising, (see the sidebar above, "Food allergy immunotherapy's varied success").

In the following sections, I describe the most promising new immunotherapy approaches, realizing that the medical community still has a lot to learn and that other methods may well be underway by the time you read these words. What's most promising is that food allergy research is accelerating at a very rapid pace.

Going under the tongue with sublingual treatments

The membranes in your mouth can sometimes absorb trace amounts of a substance without hitting you with a full dose. Researchers surmised that perhaps by placing a small amount of an allergen under the tongue, the patient could absorb just enough of it to help desensitize the immune system without a significant risk of serious reaction. In some cases, this ten-year-old-or-so theory has played out in practice through *sublingual treatments*.

Sublingual treatment consists of placing a tiny amount of allergen extract — in the form of allergen drops — under the tongue, where the patient typically holds it there for a minute or two and then either spits it out or swallows it.

Researchers have performed over 200 studies to explore the effectiveness of sublingual immunotherapy on environmental allergies, such as allergies to pollens and dust mites, with very encouraging results.

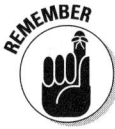

The great advantage of sublingual immunotherapy has been its safety record. Although an itchy mouth is common, *systemic reactions* (reactions that travel to other areas of the body) are so rare that patients can take these allergy drops safely at home. The allergy community has shown great interest in applying this form of immunotherapy to food allergy. The following sidebar describes one study performed on hazelnut allergy.

Finding hope in hazelnuts

A small but very important study published in 2005 focuses on the effectiveness of sublingual immunotherapy in patients with allergy to hazelnuts. Twenty-three patients enrolled in the study and were assigned to receive either hazelnut immunotherapy or placebo. Researchers assessed the effects of treatment by performing a controlled food challenge after 8–12 weeks of treatment.

Twenty-two patients reached the planned maximum dose at 4 days. Researchers observed systemic reactions in only 0.2 percent of the total doses administered. In challenge testing, the average amount of hazelnut it took to trigger a reaction in the group that received sublingual immunotherapy increased from 2.3 grams before treatment to 11.6 grams after treatment. Patients in the placebo group experienced no improvement, as you'd probably expect. Moreover, almost 50 percent of patients who underwent active treatment reached the highest dose — a whopping 20 grams of hazelnut — compared to only 9 percent in the placebo group.

This study, as well as several other small studies, have generated a great deal of excitement about this type of treatment. Many more studies are in the works in the U.S. and abroad, and we will be learning much more about this promising treatment in the next few years.

Chewing on oral immunotherapy

Oral immunotherapy is similar to the sublingual method — you take gradually increasing doses of an allergen to desensitize your immune system to it. Two key differences, however, set oral immunotherapy apart from the sublingual variety. With oral immunotherapy

- You actually eat the allergen rather than tucking it under your tongue.
- You eat the food (or at least some concentrated form of the food protein) rather than an extract of the food.

The basic procedure for administering oral and sublingual immunotherapy is basically the same, except that in the case of oral immunotherapy, you actually consume the allergenic substance. Here's how a typical oral immunotherapy treatment is done:

1. **Your doctor starts you on a miniscule amount of the food you're allergic to.**

2. **Over a period of weeks or months, your doctor gradually increases the dose.**

3. **Assuming you can tolerate the dose you consume at the clinic, you take that same dose daily at home for a period of days or weeks.**

4. **Assuming your symptoms don't recur at home over that time, you go back to the clinic for your next dose increase.**

5. **Once you've achieved the desired dose plateau, your doctor places you on a dose that you continue to consume daily at home for a period of months to years.** Hopefully, you eventually achieve complete and long-term tolerance.

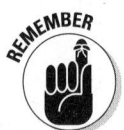

A few preliminary studies on oral immunotherapy have provided very encouraging results for milk, egg, and peanut allergy. We are currently conducting oral immunotherapy studies for both milk and egg allergy with high hopes that this method will prove to be both safe and effective.

So, where do you go for oral immunotherapy? Unfortunately, neither oral nor sublingual immunotherapy is likely to be approved for routine use in your allergist's office for at least five years, but I believe that someday one or both forms of treatment will be approved. We need at least 5 years though to work out the details, including how quickly to ramp up doses, how much of a food to recommend as a maintenance dose, how long to continue treatment before attempting a full-fledged food challenge, how to minimize the risks, and so on.

Battling back with modified protein vaccines

While allergy shots and sublingual and oral immunotherapy expose you to the complete proteins that cause your immune system to overreact, *modified protein vaccines* expose you only to pieces of the proteins to reduce the risks of severe reactions. A similar theory drives the development of other vaccines; for example, many anti-bacterial vaccines contain weakened or dead bacteria that can trigger your immune system to develop the required antibodies for fighting the disease without exposing you to the live, virulent bacteria.

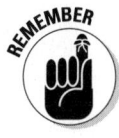

Allergens are proteins comprised of long chains of amino acids. What your immune system recognizes in a protein are small segments called *epitopes* rather than the entire protein. The epitopes, which bind to IgE (and therefore may be responsible for severe allergic reactions) are different from the epitopes that your T cells recognize. For a more technical discussion about the role that T cells play and how modified protein vaccines affect them, check out the following sidebar.

One food allergy treatment that uses a modified protein vaccine is called *peptide immunotherapy*, which uses small protein fragments (*peptides*) that bind to T cells. If appropriately designed, these peptide fragments would be unable to bind to the IgE (binding would cause allergic reactions), but the peptide fragments would still be able to stimulate suppressor T cells to render helper T cells unresponsive to subsequent allergen exposure.

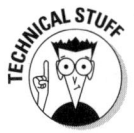

Researchers have studied peptide immunotherapy in people with cat allergy and discovered encouraging results. So far, however, researchers have tested peptide immunotherapy for food allergy only in animals. In one such study, two doses of a peanut peptide mixture were administered to peanut-sensitized mice prior to performing a peanut challenge, and the mixture effectively reduced the risk of anaphylactic reactions. More extensive desensitization protocols are being investigated in mice, and the first human trials will hopefully begin in the next few years.

Mutating proteins to use in immunotherapy

Molecular biology and chemical engineering have made great strides in the last few years. Humans can now modify genes, clone sheep, and engineer smart drugs. We can even modify proteins to create mutant food proteins unable to bind to IgE but quite capable of interacting with T cells.

Grasping the T-cell connection

T cells are white blood cells that fight infection. Think of them as the brains of the immune system. Anti-viral and antibiotic immunotherapy seek to stimulate the immune system's production of T cells to fight invading viruses and bacteria by improving your immune system's ability to recognize a specific bacteria or virus as an enemy invader. Allergy immunotherapy, on the other hand, seeks to make the immune system more tolerant of specific allergens in foods and discourage it from springing into attack mode.

When you develop an allergy, one group of T cells called *helper T-cells* instructs B cells to produce IgE. Another group of T cells called *suppressor T cells* turns off the immune response. The theory behind allergy immunotherapy, whether using complete allergenic proteins or modified proteins, works by stimulating the suppressor T cells to mute the immune system's response to specific food proteins.

Understandably, some people may be a little hesitant to be injected with a dose of mutant proteins, but the research shows some promise.

Here's how the genetic engineers managed to mutate peanut proteins to treat people with peanut allergy:

- The three major peanut allergens — Ara h1, Ara h2, and Ara h3 — were isolated and purified.

- IgE-binding and T-cell epitopes were mapped, and the DNA encoding these proteins was isolated, sequenced, and cloned.

- Engineered proteins were then created that differed by a single amino acid within each of IgE-binding epitopes. To IgE, this single amino acid tweak makes these engineered proteins like the surface of a non-stick pan, so very few of the proteins bind with the IgE antibody, but the proteins stick to T cells like Velcro, so they're still able to promote the immune system's suppressor T-cell responses, just like bona-fide peanut proteins.

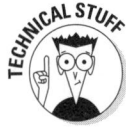

These engineered proteins have been tested on mice to determine their effectiveness in preventing peanut anaphylaxis. Researchers sensitize the mice to whole peanut and then desensitize them using the engineered proteins. Delivery by injection and both intranasal and rectal applications have now been studied with dramatic results, taking mice with severe peanut allergy and literally making the allergy go away. In fact, the rectal delivery appeared most effective in mice, and these proteins are now being produced in a suppository form to be tested in people, hopefully starting in 2007 or 2008.

Designing protein molecules that minimize IgE binding while preserving their ability to stimulate suppressor T-cells, should result in the availability of a well tolerated and effective food allergy treatment. While most of these pioneering studies focus on peanut allergy, we could apply the same techniques to other foods once the technology has been perfected. On the other hand, if treatments with intact proteins in sublingual or oral forms prove to be equally effective, then we may not need to invest the time, effort, and cost to create these bio-engineered proteins. Only time will tell.

Treating like with like: Homologous protein immunotherapy

Homologous is a fancy word for "similar." Researchers have known for a long time that peanuts and soybeans are similar — they share family ties, because they're both members of the legume family. This kinship is also reflected at the molecular level — their respective proteins share significant characteristics.

These molecular similarities led some clever researchers to wonder if they could create an immunotherapy treatment for peanut allergy out of soybean. After all, soybean proteins can be viewed as natural mutants of peanut allergens and therefore may function as effective desensitizing agents in allergen-specific immunotherapy.

To test this innovative theory, researches did what researches usually do: They rounded up some mice — in this case, mice that had peanut allergy. They then administered soybean immunotherapy to some of the mice, peanut immunotherapy to others, and a placebo to the third unfortunate group. What did they discover? Eureka!

✔ The placebo group still had the peanut allergy, which is no surprise.

✔ The mice that received peanut immunotherapy (using peanut rather than soy protein) experienced less severe reactions. Again, this is no surprise.

✔ The mice that received soybean immunotherapy were as equally well-protected as the mice that received peanut immunotherapy, and their clinical symptoms were significantly reduced compared with the placebo-treated mice.

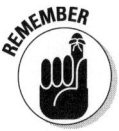

If soybean immunotherapy can be used in patients allergic to peanuts and is effective, the treatment would provide an immediate and better tolerated therapeutic option for patients with peanut hypersensitivity. In addition, the same strategy may be useful for treating other food allergies; for example, chicken proteins may be effective in treating someone with egg allergy.

Going sub-cellular with DNA vaccines

Another novel approach to the treatment of food allergy currently under investigation is called *DNA immunization*. DNA is the genetic material that makes everything in nature unique. DNA immunization triggers the body to produce the very proteins that it's allergic to, leaving most people sarcastically responding, "Yeah, that'll work."

The idea behind DNA immunization is that when the body produces the allergen from within, the immune system no longer views the allergen as a foreign invader, and hence has no reason to attack it.

Here's how it works:

1. Bio-engineers build DNA that codes for a specific allergenic protein, such as peanut.

2. This DNA is injected into the allergy sufferer — at this point a mouse, because we're not sure yet how risky it is for humans.

3. The immune system receives the DNA, and the body begins producing the allergenic protein.

This strategy has prevented the development of peanut allergy in mice, and some evidence suggests that it may be able to muffle existing peanut allergy in mice, as well. For food allergy, however, this therapy is far from ready for human experimentation, but similar strategies are being used to treat other diseases in people, including cystic fibrosis and sickle cell disease, so this may not be as far fetched as it sounds.

Treating Your Allergies to an Ancient Chinese Herbal Remedy

If you read through Chapter 8, you may think that I wouldn't even give the time of day to someone claiming that an ancient Chinese herbal remedy can cure food allergy. Actually, I'm pretty open minded until research fails to uphold the claims of snake-oil salesmen. In the case of a particular Chinese herbal remedy, research has upheld the claims of Chinese medical practitioners.

Herbal remedies have been used in Asia for centuries for the treatment of allergic diseases as well as for a huge number of other conditions. Several recent studies have tested whether these formulas — the most recent of which is called FAHF-2 (a combination of nine Chinese herbs) — are effective in treating peanut allergy in mice and to determine whether protection persists after therapy is discontinued. The following items summarize the results of various tests using FAHF-2:

- ✔ After challenges, all placebo-treated mice developed severe anaphylactic symptoms.

- ✔ In five separate experiments, no sign of any allergic reaction was observed in FAHF-2-treated mice.

- ✔ IgE levels were significantly reduced in FAHF-2-treated mice and remained significantly lower as long as five weeks after therapy.

How do FAHF-2 and other herbal remedies do their thing? At this point, we think that these herbal formulas contain some potent immunosuppressive properties. The actual mechanism of how they work is still being studied.

Herbal therapies are now close to human trials. Needless to say, both doctors and patients are showing a lot of interest in the results. Herbal preparations for allergies are now undergoing detailed analysis required by the FDA to ensure they do not contain any dangerous ingredients, but so far the safety profile looks reassuring. How well will this work in people? How much would an allergy sufferer need to take and for how long? These are all open questions at this point, but as we move closer to finding out the results of these studies, we have a lot of room for enthusiasm.

Fighting Back with Anti-IgE Antibody Therapy

The problem with most approaches to allergen immunotherapy is that they're allergen-specific — they treat only one allergen, making treatment complex and expensive for the many patients with multiple allergies.

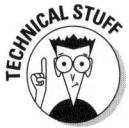

Wouldn't a single therapy, one that would be effective for multiple inhalant allergies as well as food allergies, be grand? Well, researchers are working on it. One such therapy, already in clinical trials, involves the use of *anti-IgE antibodies* — bio-engineered IgG antibodies that bind freely to IgE, rendering it powerless. Once the anti-IgE antibodies bind with IgE, IgE is unable to bind to mast cells and basophils, so the massive release of histamine never happens.

Several clinical trials involving patients with allergic rhinitis and allergic asthma have been completed and one form of this treatment (omalizumab, sold as Xolair) has now been approved since 2003 for treating allergic asthma in adolescents and adults.

The TNX-901 study

A study of 84 patients with peanut allergy treated with an anti-IgE product called TNX-901 was published in 2003. Patients received 150, 300, or 450 mg of anti-IgE or placebo by injection monthly for four months. All participants had a peanut challenge before and after treatment. In this study:

✔ Participants receiving the highest dose of anti-IgE experienced a significant decrease in their symptoms. Those receiving a baseline dose tolerated an average of about half a peanut, while those receiving the highest treatment dose were able to tolerate almost nine peanuts.

✔ About 25 percent of the participants, even in the high-dose group, had no change in peanut tolerance after treatment.

On the positive side, this study shows that anti-IgE would clearly provide protection to most patients with peanut allergy receiving the top dose. The other potential benefit of this medicine is that it is not specific for peanut allergy — it should work for other food allergies in the same manner and could also treat asthma and allergic rhinitis at the same time.

On the negative side, TNX-901 appears to be ineffective for about 25 percent of those with peanut allergy. Moreover, due to some complex legal issues, TNX-901 will never hit the market.

Results of studies on anti-IgE antibodies for food allergies show that the treatment is promising but not yet completely effective, as described in the following sidebar.

Would Xolair (the drug that's already available for asthma) work for food allergies? We don't quite know yet. Studies of Xolair for peanut allergy are in the works but will not be completed for several years, so no anti-IgE product will be approved for use for food allergy until these studies are completed.

Although theoretically Xolair and other anti-IgE therapies hold out some hope, they have a few things working against them:

✔ **Anti-IgE is not a vaccine or cure, merely a means of suppressing reactions.**

✔ **Anti-IgE needs to be given by injection at regular intervals — every two to four weeks — to be effective, and once it's stopped, the protection quickly disappears.**

✔ **Injections would be very expensive — about $1,000 dollars per dose with no guarantee insurance will cover them.**

✔ **If the total IgE level (all IgE to all allergens circulating in your blood-stream) is too high, anti-IgE therapy is ineffective.** For asthma, Xolair is not approved for use if the total IgE level is over 800. Unfortunately, many patients, including most patients with eczema and multiple food allergies, have levels far higher than that.

✔ **Possible side effects require further investigation.** Anti-IgE therapy has not been studied in young children or in those with more severe forms of peanut allergy.

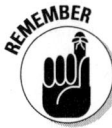

I feel strongly that anti-IgE therapy should be studied further and that it may be of great value to some patients. In the long run, however, one or more of the other forms of therapy described in this chapter are likely to have a greater ability to truly treat food allergy and do so without a lifetime of ongoing treatment.

Investigating Other Futuristic Treatments

Immunotherapy, especially the bio-engineered varieties, is hi-tech stuff, but other promising treatments are also being considered. In this section, I describe some of the hopeful treatments currently in research and development that you can expect to start hearing more about in the future.

Immunizing with immunostimulatory sequences

Another take on the DNA immunization technique under investigation is immunization with DNA that's *conjugated* (linked) to small strings of amino acids, forming what researchers fondly refer to as *immunostimulatory sequences (ISS)*. These ISS contain repeated sequences of two specific amino acids called *cytosine* and *guanine*. In animal models, ISS stimulate the immune system toward fighting infection while reducing its tendency to develop allergy. In addition, they clearly have the ability to turn down, and possibly even turn off, existing allergies.

No studies on the effectiveness of ISS therapy on food allergy in people have been done, but results from studies of ragweed allergy look very promising. Studies with ISS conjugation to peanut and other allergens are likely to begin in the next few years.

Going proactive with probiotics

Probiotics have proven more effective in preventing the onset of food allergy than in successfully treating existing food allergy. Two studies reveal their beneficial effects:

✔ In infants and young children with milk allergy, two-month treatment with probiotics, along with a milk elimination diet, decreased the severity of their eczema.

✔ In another study, expectant mothers were given either probiotics or placebo in pregnancy and during breastfeeding, as were

their infants for 6 months, starting on the first day of life. At 2 years of age, 23 percent of children were reported to have *atopic dermatitis* (dermatitis caused by food allergy) in the probiotic-treated group compared with 46 percent in the placebo group, indicating that the probiotic had some effect on the prevention of early atopic disease in infants at high risk.

Making the most of probiotics

Bacteria have a bad reputation. Commercials and news headlines constantly disparage them for the role that a few black sheep in the bacteria community play in causing infection. You rarely hear about the many good bacteria working to make the world a better place. But good bacteria do exist, and they offer some hope in preventing the onset of allergies.

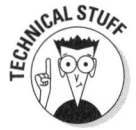

In scientific circles, these beneficial bacteria are often referred to as *probiotics* — live bacteria or their components that are reported to have beneficial effects on health by improving the balance of bacteria in the intestine. The major sources of probiotics are dairy products, including yogurt, that contain *Lactobacillus* and *Bifidobacterium* species.

Although the concept of probiotic foods was introduced more than a century ago, only recently have researchers evaluated probiotics in controlled clinical trials in the treatment of food allergy. The following sidebar presents the results of a couple of the more promising studies.

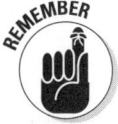

Most current interest in probiotics focuses on their potential to prevent food allergy rather than turning off existing food allergy. Even their effectiveness as a preventive is yet to be proven, but the theory makes sense and deserves further study. The likelihood that these products can actually turn off the immune system once the allergy has developed is small, especially compared to some of the truly exciting therapies discussed in this chapter.

Part III
Living Well with Your Food Allergies

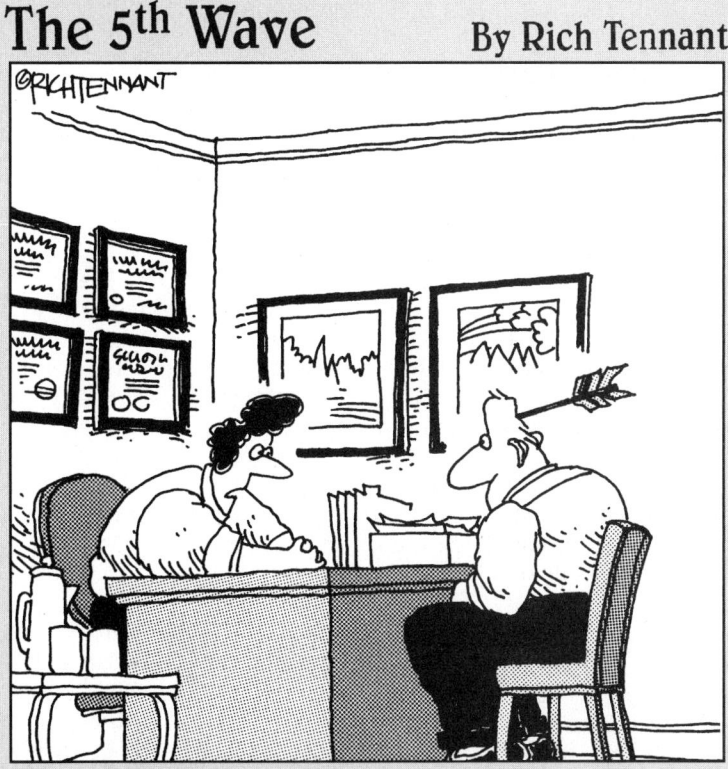

The 5th Wave   By Rich Tennant

@RICHTENNANT

"I don't mean to appear unenlightened, Mr. Grove, but I don't think this is the time to explore alternative forms of treatment."

In this part . . .

Your allergy tags along wherever you go — in your kitchen, your grocery store, at work, at school, on vacation . . . it even accompanies you on dinner dates and tells *you* what to order!

In this part, I show you how to apply the information you gathered at your doctor's office to your day-to-day living so you can more fully enjoy your life. The chapters in this part feature savvy strategies and tips from the trenches (supplied by yours truly, food allergy doctor and patient) on how to cope with your food allergies at home, on the road, in daycare, in preschool, and from kindergarten to your senior year in high school.

I also offer tips for parents of teens and tweens on how to encourage your children to take ownership of their food allergies and assume more responsibility for their own optimum health. Finally, I show you how to guesstimate the odds of outgrowing a food allergy and let you in on some tips that may improve your chances.

Chapter 10

Living at Home with Your Allergies

....

In This Chapter

▶ Ridding your house of allergenic foods

▶ Restocking the shelves with safer alternatives

▶ Brushing up on allergen-free cooking techniques

▶ Building your own information/emergency station

....

A good part of the time you spend at home, family members are munching on something. Whether they're grabbing a snack or sitting down for a seven course meal, family members must work together to prevent allergenic foods from finding their way into the family member who has the food allergy.

In this chapter, you discover ways to convert your home into a safe haven for you or your loved one who has a food allergy. Here I discuss the pros and cons of eliminating problem foods from your home. If you choose to keep the problem foods around, I suggest ways of shelving and labeling them to avoid accidental exposure and cross contamination. I show you how to stock up on non-allergenic foods and ingredients, equip your medicine cabinet with effective allergy treatments, and build an information/emergency station that has everything you need to prevent reactions and quickly respond in the event of any reaction.

Dumping the Bad Stuff . . . or Not

When a family member has a severe food allergy, the natural impulse may be to purge the household of all foods that can possibly trigger a reaction. While that is certainly an option, other options are available, and only you and your family can decide which option is best.

My personal preference

Most people develop beliefs based on their experience and how they were raised. The same is true for me. My views on how to manage a food allergy in the home are strongly influenced by the way my parents raised a child with a severe peanut allergy — me.

My peanut allergy was first diagnosed when I was still a baby. I grew up with seven brothers and sisters, most of whom ate peanut butter regularly. My father was, and still is, quite a fan of roasted peanuts. With all that peanut in the house, you may think I would be having reactions all the time.

Actually, despite the fact that peanut was a long-term resident in my house, I never had a single reaction at home. With eight children running around, my home was far from being a calm, organized environment, but a series of simple rules along with seven cooperative siblings kept me safe.

Some families choose to evict all problem foods from the premises. Others prefer eliminating only the riskiest foods. And some families opt for prevention and education rather than an outright ban. All these options are valid. As a family, you need to weigh the risks and benefits and decide for yourself, taking the following considerations into account:

- ✔ The severity of the allergy.
- ✔ The practical difficulty of eliminating one food versus another.
- ✔ The overall quality of life for all members of the family.
- ✔ The presence of other children in the home.
- ✔ The overall effects that a food ban may have on a child's ability to deal with food allergy in the real world.

In the following sections, I explore these deciding factors in greater depth.

Weighing the pros and cons of banning allergenic foods

When someone has a severe food allergy, and a miniscule amount of the allergen can trigger a dangerous reaction, you may decide to completely ban the food from your house. Most families with peanut allergy, for example, choose to remove all peanut from the premises, primarily for two reasons:

✔ Peanut allergy often engenders a greater level of fear, especially a fear that tiny exposures may lead to severe reactions.

✔ Most families find that they can give up peanut products without suffering any great hardship.

The situation for milk or eggs is often quite different. Although severe reactions certainly occur with these foods, they are somewhat less common than with peanut. More importantly, removing these foods from the home can cause significant hardship for nonallergic family members. Hence, few families living with milk or egg allergy choose to completely eliminate these foods from their homes.

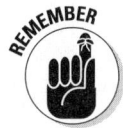

I never recommend that a family completely eliminate a food from the home. I understand why families choose to do this, but it is rarely, if ever, necessary. I believe that implementing reasonable precautions can create a safe environment even if the problem food remains in the home. I reveal the most effective precautions later in this chapter.

Reducing the fear factor

Keeping all problem foods in the home may even offer the additional benefit of alleviating irrational fears. When allergic children are accustomed to living around the foods that they're allergic to, they naturally develop a more rational respect for the possible danger. It's like having a gas stove or candles in your house. Children realize that the flame can harm them. They know not to touch the flame or play with fire, but when someone lights a match, they don't go running and screaming out of the house.

I see children every week who are completely paralyzed by the fear of an allergic reaction. They may panic when someone opens a candy bar across the room, truly fearing that this will cause a reaction or even kill them. If the same children had lived around the foods that they are allergic to, they almost certainly would not have this irrational fear.

Justified fear

In spite of my general advice to keep allergenic foods around the house, I understand why some families decide to eliminate a food from their home. Some families who've taken adequate precautions and still have witnessed severe reactions simply decide that the risk isn't worth it.

I recently saw a patient with severe milk allergy. The family had decided to keep milk in the home. The patient's brother, who is not allergic to milk, drank a glass of milk when he probably had some sort of stomach virus and proceeded to vomit all over the place, including all over his allergic brother. The milk-allergic brother turned into a massive hive.

No more milk in that home, and I really can't judge the parents for making that decision.

Other families have made the decision to ban certain foods because they always think the worst. They imagine that a babysitter will find the jar of peanut butter on the top shelf, where it is labeled with a skull and cross bones with Jimmy's picture on it, and decide to give it to Jimmy for a snack. As unlikely as this might be, I cannot promise them that such an event would never happen. This is exactly why the decision of whether to completely eliminate a problem food from the home is a choice that every family needs to make for itself.

Boosting the education factor

When families choose to keep a problem food in their home, they provide a valuable learning experience for the person with the food allergy and for other family members. The presence of the problem food creates a real-world environment in which family members must:

- ✔ Read and decipher food labels.
- ✔ Wash their hands before and after eating.
- ✔ Scrub down counters and tables.
- ✔ Practice proper food preparation.

In addition, the person with the food allergy is required to develop some level of self control to avoid problem foods that are readily available.

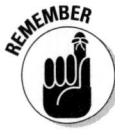

If you choose to eliminate problem foods from your home, and you have a young child with food allergy, provide other educational opportunities. Teach proper cooking techniques, practice reading food labels when you go grocery shopping, and stress the need for washing hands and scrubbing down counters and tables before and after eating.

Quarantining suspect substances

If you decide to let allergenic foods hang out at your house, you may decide to employ other strategies to protect the safety of the person who has the allergy. The following safe practices are not hard and fast rules, merely some ideas to consider implementing in your home:

- ✔ **Segregate safe and unsafe foods:** Designate a specific shelf in your cupboard or pantry for safe foods and be sure that everyone understands your system. You can similarly rearrange the items in your refrigerator.
- ✔ **Label the problem foods:** Special labels or stickers may provide an added measure of safety. You can purchase food allergy labels or use your computer or label maker to create custom labels that work best for you.

Labeling safe foods is often easier and more effective for a common food allergy, like milk. Labeling unsafe foods is often more efficient when unsafe foods are few as in the case of a peanut, tree nut, or sesame allergy.

- ✔ **Designate allergen-free zones:** Set rules that indicate where foods can and cannot be eaten. For example, if one child is allergic to milk, you may consider restricting the consumption of milk and other milk-containing foods to the dining room or kitchen table. Otherwise, family members are likely to spread milk all over the house.

- ✔ **Designate places at the table:** Consider establishing fixed seating arrangements at the table, especially if young children are involved. An allergy-free zone can reduce the chances that a child will share food or pick items off another family member's plate and lessens the chance of exposure to scattered crumbs, spills, and splatters.

- ✔ **Limit opportunities for cross-contamination:** If allergic foods are kept in the home, cross contamination is always a risk. All family members need to be especially careful with utensils. Grabbing the same spatula to serve a cookie that contains the allergen and using it to serve a cookie that's allergen free is a simple mistake that can lead to a severe reaction. Likewise, family members must learn to never dip the knife they used to spread their peanut butter into the jelly jar and to thoroughly clean the cutting board after preparing any allergenic food.

For additional tips and techniques to reduce the risks of cross contamination and other risks inherent in preparing and serving food, see "Cooking and Dining Safely in the Midst of Allergies," later in this chapter.

Stocking Up on the Essentials

Maintaining an allergen-free diet takes care, planning, and diligence. Not only do you need to make sure that your allergic family member has safe foods and beverages on hand, but you also must consider the nutritional value of the substitutes, especially for young children.

In Chapter 18, I suggest some nutritional substitutes for the most common allergenic foods, and in the Appendix at the back of this book, I include a selection of some of the most popular recipes from the Food Allergy and Anaphylaxis network. For guidance on basic nutrition, check out *Nutrition For Dummies* by Carol Ann Rinzler.

Running out to the corner store for a quart of milk when your child relies on soy, rice, or potato milk may not be an option. Stock up on any special substitutes for problem foods, especially when substitutes are available only in certain stores.

Once you get in the swing of things, living with food allergies does get easier. Ask and shop around for the stores that best serve you needs. A trip to a specialty store that has foods that you cannot find at your usual grocery store once or twice a month may be a great help in keeping your shelves stocked with nutritional goodies.

Before you head out to the grocery store, be sure to review Chapter 6, and consider copying and packing the field guide for each food that you or your family member is allergic to, so you are well-prepared to decipher the more cryptic food labels.

Cooking and Dining Safely in the Midst of Allergies

For families who rid their homes of allergenic foods, food storage, preparation, cooking, serving, and eating is of very little concern. The risk of accidental exposure is virtually eliminated along with the problem foods.

For those who choose to make the problem food part of their family, however, mealtime can be a real challenge. Not only do you have to sift through the grocery store shelves to find suitable substitutes and flip through food allergy cookbooks to discover recipes for palatable dishes, but you also have to master some techniques for preventing *cross-contamination* — an allergenic food tainting a nonallergenic food — and other opportunities for accidental exposure.

Preventive measures for cross contamination and accidental exposure apply to five areas (see the section, "Reducing the risks of cross-contamination" for more information on these preventatives):

- ✔ Storage
- ✔ Preparation
- ✔ Cooking
- ✔ Serving
- ✔ Eating

In the following sections, I briefly discuss the challenges of planning allergen-free meals and then reveal ways to lessen the risks of cross-contamination, airborne allergens, and other sources of accidental exposure.

Planning your meals

In some families, everyone's on a special diet. The doctor places dad on a low-cholesterol diet. Mom decides to try the Mediterranean diet to shed a few pounds. And teenage brother opts for the Atkins diet. The cupboards and fridge are packed with an assortment of special foods, and mealtimes take on the air of a food court, with everyone preparing their own special meal.

The same situation arises in many families living with food allergy. Many processed foods are eliminated from the diet, and certain ingredients that are staples for some family members become taboo for others.

Obviously, the most efficient solution is to round up the troops and convince the entire family to get on the same menu page. With all the available substitutes on the market and the allergen-free recipes provided at the back of this book and elsewhere, you may be surprised to find that the rest of the family actually prefers eating allergen-free. And, because allergen-free meals often rely less on processed foods, they're generally healthier than the meals you may be used to serving.

The process of planning and preparing allergen-free meals is especially bothersome for those who don't like to cook. For those who enjoy cooking, however, perfecting an allergen-free recipe can really be fun. Try to make meal preparation a family affair, getting everyone involved in picking recipes they'd like to try, and then team up to perfect the recipes.

Boning up on substitutions

One of the tricks to allergy free cooking is finding suitable substitutes for what you need to avoid. Over the past few years this market has grown tremendously, so that for the most common problem foods, you can usually find one or more excellent substitutes. Check out Chapter 18 for some of the more common food and ingredient substitutes.

Because food companies are constantly developing new substitutes, don't settle for only the substitutes listed in Chapter 18. Scour the grocery store and specialty store shelves for additional options. You may be pleasantly surprised at the wide selection.

Reducing the risks of cross-contamination

Families that eliminate allergenic foods have little concern over cross-contamination. Unless a neighbor, friend, or family member smuggles in a tainted dish, snack, or dessert, cross-contamination is a non-issue.

If your family has decided to establish a peaceful coexistence with the allergenic food, however, cross contamination becomes a significant concern. By setting a few rules and implementing proper preventive measures, however, you can establish a safe eating environment for your allergic family member.

One of the best ways to prevent cross-contamination is to focus on the areas where it's most likely to occur:

- ✔ **Storage:** Store all food in sealed containers. As long as the egg noodles and the egg-free noodles are in separate, sealed containers, they're highly unlikely to contaminate one another. Be careful of leaky packages or spills. A leaky milk jug stored on the top shelf can splash milk all over the place, especially if you have leftovers wrapped in cellophane or aluminum foil or stored in unsealed containers.

- ✔ **Preparation:** Food preparation is a common source of cross-contamination. Kitchen counters, cutting boards, knives, meat or cheese slicers, spoons, measuring cups, mixing bowls, spatulas, and a host of other food prep equipment can carry remnants of a problem food. To reduce the risk, thoroughly clean cutting boards between foods. Likewise, thoroughly clean all measuring spoons, mixing bowls, and other equipment and utensils between preparing the safe and unsafe foods.

A cutting board made of plastic or another hard surface may be easier to clean than a wooden cutting board. Some families use two cutting boards.

- ✔ **Cooking:** The biggest risk with cooking involves shared utensils, so clean utensils thoroughly between cooking safe and unsafe foods. As you're cooking, be particularly careful not to use the same spoon or spatula on a safe food that you used on an unsafe food. Contamination from spills or spatters is a lesser risk, as long as you keep the safe foods you're cooking a reasonable distance from the unsafe foods . . . and don't get too flip-happy with your spatula.

- ✔ **Serving:** With severe food allergies, even a trace of allergen on a spatula can trigger a reaction. Clean serving utensils thoroughly, and never use a utensil used to serve an unsafe food to serve a safe food. Remain extra vigilant when you serve safe and unsafe foods at the same dinner table to make sure the serving utensils remain with their respective serving dishes.

Grounding airborne allergens

When allergens take flight, they can cause inhalation reactions, as I explain in Chapter 3. Peanut dust, for example, can trigger even a severe allergic reaction particularly if a person is eating shelled peanuts in close proximity to someone with severe peanut allergy.

In the kitchen, airborne allergens pose a risk, because heat, spatters, splatters, and steam can launch allergens into the surrounding air. When cooking unsafe foods, the following conditions pose the greatest risk:

- **High heat on an open stove:** The greatest risk of a food allergen becoming airborne occurs when you cook the food at high heat on an open stove. The vapors and spatter that occurs can contain large amounts of food protein that can cause reactions if you are in close proximity to the cooking. Common examples of this would be frying an egg or hamburger or stir-frying fish or shellfish.

- **Steaming foods:** The process of steaming foods may also release large amounts of allergen. Steaming shrimp or crabs or boiling or roasting peanuts can pose a huge risk.

- **Prepping foods:** Some foods become airborne during the preparation process. Large amounts or wheat, for example, can cloud the air when you're baking a cake, kneading bread or pizza dough, or grinding up peanuts or tree nuts. Professional bakers sometimes fall victim to a condition called *baker's asthma*, triggered by a heavy exposure to wheat dust.

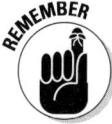

Airborne exposures are much less common when foods are baked or cooked at lower temperatures. So while reactions related to frying eggs are common, I have never heard of an airborne reaction from baking a cake.

To reduce the risks of airborne allergens, take the following precautions:

- **The person with allergies should keep a safe distance from the preparation or cooking area when unsafe foods are being handled.** Staying in the next room is almost always safe, and we rarely see reactions when the person with the food allergy is more than five or six feet away.

- **Install and use a well functioning exhaust fan on or above the stove.** This can make a huge difference.

- **Allow at least 30 minutes for the air to clear after a problem food has been prepared or cooked before the person with the food allergy re-enters the room.**

Cleaning the galley

Most household cleaners combined with a little elbow grease are sufficient for removing food allergens from countertops, tables, and chairs. Following are some tips for cleaning specific items, as well as a few potential problem areas:

✔ **Counters and table tops:** You can effectively clean these rigid surfaces with most household cleaners and elbow grease. Timing and diligence are most important — clean immediately after all food preparation and eating, and don't skimp on the elbow grease.

✔ **Sponges:** Patients often ask whether the kitchen needs to be equipped with two sponges, so an allergen-free sponge is always available. As a general rule, I do not feel that this is necessary. Using a sponge to wash dishes, even if the sponge is slightly contaminated does not pose a huge risk, as long as you thoroughly rinse the dishes after washing them. With counters and table tops, where rinsing is less of an option, thoroughly rinse the sponge after cleaning up potential allergens.

✔ **Dishes:** Thoroughly washing dishes either in the sink or dishwasher is usually sufficient for removing all allergens. When washing dishes by hand, diligence, elbow grease, and a thorough rinsing are the key ingredients to success. When using a dishwasher, carefully inspect all dishes as you empty the dishwasher to be safe — stubborn allergens clinging to dishes or a less powerful dishwasher can leave allergen residue on the dishes.

✔ **Cookware:** Practice the same techniques for cleaning pots, pans, and other cookware as you do for dishes. Some families choose to keep a separate set of allergen-free pots and pans, but this isn't really necessary. As for loading your cookware into the dishwasher, however, I'm less willing to trust the dishwasher unless you've done a pretty good job of pre-cleaning your cookware. Stoneware or other pieces that are more porous than the standard pot or pan may pose an additional risk, although this has never been proven.

✔ **Utensils:** In general, follow the same precautions as those for cleaning dishes and cookware, paying special attention to cooked-on foods and the nooks and crannies characteristic of most utensils. Be especially careful cleaning beaters and whisks, which are more likely to trap food remnants.

✔ **Dish rags, towels, and other fabrics:** Though easy to clean — one run through an average washing machine can loosen the grip of even the most clingy allergen — kitchen rags, towels, and other fabrics pose a significant potential risk. A dish towel used to dry a clean plate is certainly nothing to worry about, but if someone used the towel to wipe up a spill and then snuck it back on the hook, the towel could be very contaminated and transfer the allergen to that previously clean plate you're drying.

✔ **Tablecloths:** Vinyl or plastic tablecloths are best, because the surface doesn't absorb the gunk. If you use a cloth cover, it can pose a risk, especially in the case of liquid allergen spills, such as milk or egg. Again, the best way to clean a cloth tablecloth is to run it through the washing machine.

✔ **Grills:** For families who enjoy grilling out (or in), the grill is a potential hazard. Grilling a safe food along with an unsafe food — for example, a plain chicken breast alongside a breast marinated in soy sauce — could result in cross-contamination from spatter. As for any allergen residue remaining on the grill after cooking, I believe you can remove almost all food residue by heating the grill back up to burn off the remnants and then thoroughly scrubbing it with a wire brush.

Heating and wire-brushing the grill, however, is not 100 percent safe. I've seen a fair number of reactions traced back to a contaminated grill. Following are some safer alternatives:

- **Safe:** Place a double-thick layer of aluminum foil over the area on the grill where the allergic person's food is being cooked.

- **Safer:** For the more compulsive chef, a second, allergen-free grill grate offers added protection.

- **Safest:** For the ultimate in compulsive grilling, a two-grill system is the safest option. For all you grill cooks out there who want a new grill, tell your significant other that the doctor said you really need a separate grill for optimum safety.

Organizing an Information Station

Every family living with food allergy should have a minimum of one food allergy emergency kit, complete with instructions, stored in a convenient central location that everyone knows about. In addition, you may want to create an allergy information center where you store additional information, recipes, your doctor's phone number, insurance information, and this book for quick reference.

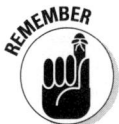

In a family in which the parents are often not present, educating family members and sitters and even perhaps neighbors is essential. Whoever's in charge needs to know the rules, emergency procedures, and where the medications are stored.

In the following sections, I lead you through the process of gathering the essential resources and medications, and making sure everyone knows where to find them.

Assembling an emergency kit

Once you and your doctor have decided which medicines you should have on hand in the event of a reaction, assemble an emergency kit with the following items:

✔ Medications, including an antihistamine and epinephrine autoinjectors if your doctor prescribed them.

✔ Your Food Allergy Emergency Action Plan from Chapter 7, providing clear, detailed instructions of what to do in the event of an allergic reaction. (Review the plan regularly to make sure all information is current, especially contact names and phone numbers.)

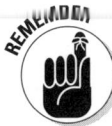

Store the emergency kit in a safe, convenient place, and make sure everyone in the house knows where it is.

Most families decide to keep two emergency kits — one that sits at home and one that travels with them. The travel kit may need to be a bit more compact but should still contain all medications and instructions. A similar kit may also make sense if your child spends lots of time elsewhere, such as at the grandparents' house.

Bringing your sitter up to speed

Leaving your child with a baby sitter is always a bit nerve wracking but this is multiplied by a thousand when your child has severe food allergies. Here are some guidelines for making parents' night out as safe and stress-free as possible for all involved:

✔ **Find a babysitter who may be more mature than the usual fare.** Sitting for a child with a severe food allergy is not an ideal entry-level position for a 13-year-old. If you're really lucky, you can find a college student or other young adult. If you're lottery-lucky, you may find someone who has a food allergy, a sibling with a food allergy, or best yet, a nursing degree.

✔ **Tell the sitter exactly what your child is allowed to eat.** Take-out orders, special snacks, and treats are strictly off limits. Set the acceptable food out as clearly as possible.

✔ **Describe the foods that your child is allergic to, and make sure the sitter understands the house rules on what she can and cannot eat around your child.** If you have two or more children, explain what they're to eat and not eat, point out the designated eating areas, and review clean-up policies.

✔ **Train the sitter on the treatment plan for a reaction.** Show her where the emergency kit is stored, and review the plan in detail, including how to spot symptoms. Show her the epinephrine injector and demonstrate its use with a trainer. Then ask her to repeat it all back to you and demonstrate the injector, until you're sure she "gets it."

✓ **Provide explicit details on how and when to contact you, as well as phone numbers for other people who may be able to help in the event of a reaction.** This often includes a trusted friend or neighbor as well as your doctor.

✓ **Stress the importance of calling 911 in the event of an emergency.** If your child has a severe food allergy, make sure the sitter knows to call 911. If the epinephrine autoinjector is used, a call to 911 is mandatory.

Put everything in writing, just in case your sitter needs a brief refresher course on what to do and what not to do. If your child is older, he or she can provide guidance. For younger children, consider using the form supplied in Chapter 12 as is or slightly modifying it for the sitter.

When you first hire a sitter, consider having the sitter come over to spend some time with your family and get a feel for the routine and the do's and don'ts. You may ask them to spend an afternoon as a "mother's helper" so they don't feel like they're being watched or interviewed the whole time. This gives the sitter a real feel for your kids and hands-on experience with safety routines. The visit is likely to make your kids feel more comfortable being left with the sitter, as well. Many parents find this useful, and it may even be more useful for parents with children who have food allergies. It can certainly put you more at ease.

Chapter 11

Eating Out and Traveling with Food Allergies

*H*ome may be your safe haven when it comes to food allergies, but life outside the confines of your abode is just too tempting to pass up. You gotta get out and enjoy yourself, let your hair down, relax. When you have food allergies, however, wandering far from the safety of home may bring more anxiety than relaxation, and that's perfectly understandable.

In this chapter, I try to relieve some of your anxiety by assisting you in preparing and packing for your excursion — whether you're walking down to the local diner to grab a bite to eat or flying across an ocean for business or pleasure. Here I show you how to pack your medications, find out about medical facilities available at your destination, become more aware of the challenges you'll face on the road, and read a menu and talk with the server before placing your order at a restaurant.

Preparing for Your Outing

A safe, anxiety-free outing requires some advanced preparation, especially if you're venturing out to an area where you're not so sure the natives have an abundant supply of foods and beverages you can safely consume.

In the following sections, I show you how to prepare for your excursion across town, country, or seas. I remind you to pack your emergency kit, advise you to stock up on staples (both food and beverages), and show you how to properly identify yourself as someone who has a food allergy (just in case you experience a severe reaction).

Toting your allergy emergency kit along with you

When you properly equip your home and educate family members about food allergies, as explained in Chapter 10, your food allergy becomes a less intrusive part of your life at home. You know that everyone knows the drill and that your emergency kit is readily available at a moment's notice.

Although you may not be able to establish the same comfort level for times when you leave the house, you can establish a good level of safety by planning and packing for emergencies. Make it a habit:

- **Pack a travel bag with your emergency medications.** See Chapter 10 for a list of items to pack.
- **Before you leave the house, grab your bag just as habitually as you put on your shoes.**

You can toss your emergency medical kit in your car, but make sure you don't expose the medicines to extreme heat or cold, which could make them less effective. Also make sure that if you park your car and then wander some distance from it, that you take the medical kit with you.

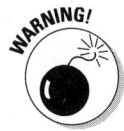

Any time you leave the house, even if you're not planning to eat out, *always* bring your emergency medicines with you. In the old days, people ate three meals a day, generally at scheduled times. Nowadays, food is readily available at any time of day or night . . . even in the wee hours of the morning. Eating — and a possible reaction — can happen *anytime*. Of course, you don't even have to be eating for a reaction to occur — airborne or contact exposure can trigger a reaction, so always be prepared. Travel and eating out, however, clearly add risk to the equation so it is even more important that you prepare for the worst in these situations. Many of the reported food-induced anaphylactic events and even fatalities have occurred in individuals with food allergy who did not have their emergency medications with them at the time of the allergic reaction or the medication treatment plan was not followed appropriately.

Packing a safe food stash

When wandering off to uncharted territory, you never know what the natives of that region eat . . . or which fast food restaurants are readily available, so pack some safe provisions just in case.

Safe foods to pack depend primarily on the food allergies you have and where you're going. If you have multiple food allergies, especially to common foods such as milk or egg, eating out can be a huge challenge and you may need to pack lots of food. For more isolated food allergies — even severe allergies like peanut or tree nuts — you can usually find plenty of safe foods no matter where you go, so you can pack light.

Wearing a medical ID bracelet or necklace

Venturing out on your own always increases the risk that you won't receive proper emergency treatment if needed. When traveling with others, always let your travel companions know about your food allergies and what to do in the event of a reaction. When traveling solo, wear a medical ID bracelet or necklace. If you have a severe reaction and can't tell others what's happening, they can quickly tell from the bracelet or necklace what's happening. The best feature of the bracelet is that it contains a toll-free (800) number that's accessible from just about anywhere.

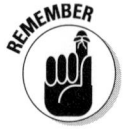

I recommend that you wear your medical ID bracelet or necklace at all times, so you don't forget to put it on before stepping out. If you prefer to wear it only in situations in which you may be taking on some added risk, eating out and traveling are at the top of the list. You can order food allergy ID bracelets on FAAN's Web site at www.foodallergy.org. ID bracelets and necklaces are available in a variety of styles and designs to satisfy the requirements of the most style-conscious patients. If you just can't bear the thought of wearing an ID bracelet or necklace, carry an emergency ID card in your purse or wallet.

Taking Your Allergies Out to Dinner

Eating out is a little risky whether or not you have a food allergy. In most restaurants, all the food preparation occurs in the back room. You never really know what the cooks and other staff are doing back there. You don't know where the food came from, how it was stored, or how it was handled.

All you know is that when the server sets the plate in front of you or hands you your to-go bag, the food looks and smells yummy.

When you have a food allergy, you place even more trust in the restaurant. Cooks and other kitchen staff must be particularly careful to avoid any ingredients that contain the allergenic food and to prevent cross-contamination via unclean cooking surfaces or utensils. Even a splatter or airborne particles of an allergenic food can land in your dinner dish if the cooks and servers aren't careful.

In the following sections, I guide you through the process of weighing the pros and cons of eating out and provide some guidelines to ensure a safer experience when you do decide to eat out.

To eat out or not to eat out . . . that is the question

The risks of eating out vary with your food allergy. If you have a severe milk allergy, even the most allergy-friendly restaurant may not be safe enough — it's just too easy during the hustle and bustle of a lunch or dinner rush for someone back in the kitchen to slip up. If, however, you can find a restaurant where the personnel take special care — down to using separate pans and utensils — you may be relatively safe.

I know of a few restaurants that have mastered allergy-free cooking, so I know that running such an establishment is possible. It just takes more time and work than most restaurants are willing to commit.

Even when you're eating out at a restaurant where you are completely confident that the chef is following all necessary precautions, keep your emergency medications close at hand.

If you own or work in a restaurant or the owner of your favorite eatery wants to learn more about allergy-free cooking, the Food Allergy and Anaphylaxis Network, the Food Allergy Initiative, and the National Restaurant Association have worked together to develop an excellent education program called *Food Allergy Training Guide for Restaurants and Food Services*. You can order it online at www.foodallergy.org or call the Food Allergy and Anaphylaxis Network at 800-929-4040. I believe that the rising prevalence of food allergies along with programs such as these and the growing willingness of restaurants to cooperate will lead to restaurants with increased allergy awareness where those with food allergies can dine more safely.

Locating allergy-friendly restaurants

Locating an allergy-friendly restaurant is often mainly a process of elimination. Allergic to fish or shellfish? Cross seafood restaurants off your list. Even if you're ordering off the Turf side of the menu, the chances of cross-contamination from the Surf foods is just too great. Allergic to peanuts or tree nuts? Avoid Asian restaurants. Nuts are all too common in Asian dishes. Don't let temptation overrule your natural avoidance instincts.

Because peanut allergies tend to cause more severe reactions, I provide a special restaurant guide for peanut avoidance in Chapter 4 along with other tips and tricks to avoid accidental exposure.

Taking the restaurant's attitude pulse

When it comes to food allergies, restaurant personnel have attitudes, either good or bad. Ideally, when you inquire about allergen-free foods, the server, cook, and manager are receptive, knowledgeable, caring, and sensitive. Many of the restaurants that fit this description are run by managers who have food allergies or have a close family member with food allergies.

Unfortunately, you may not be so lucky to find such a restaurant. Many restaurants would prefer that you never showed up. The servers and cooks may even act ignorant, rude, and otherwise uncooperative. When you find yourself in such a situation, the best response is usually to go elsewhere. You may be able to whip the restaurant into shape but, in the meantime, you may be taking unnecessary risks.

Avoiding the riskier eateries

Some restaurants and other eateries are simply not conducive to allergen-free dining. Following are several types of establishments that may pose a higher risk:

- **Buffets:** Observe a buffet for about two minutes, and you immediately know why buffets are high-risk areas for patrons with food allergies. The foods in the buffet line rub elbows. People can't find the spoon for the potatoes, so they serve up their spuds with a spoon that was sitting in the egg noodles. Messy patrons fling the food around as though they were having a food fight.

- **Bakeries:** In addition to the risk of airborne allergens, particularly for people with wheat allergy, bakeries are notorious for cross-contamination. Baked goods often sit next to or on top of each other in large display cases. Tongs and other serving utensils are often shared and reused. In such an enclosed environment, allergens easily spread from one food to another.

✔ **Restaurants that serve pre-made foods:** Restaurants that cook meals from scratch are best. You tell the chef which ingredients to use and which ingredients not to use, and that's what you get. Some restaurants get pre-made entrees that they slap together to create your meal. Call ahead and ask if the chef cooks the meals from scratch or uses pre-packaged meals.

Giving fast-food restaurants a thumbs up

Fast-food and franchise restaurants have gotten somewhat of a bad reputation lately, but they offer some advantages for those with food allergies:

✔ **Standardized food preparation and cooking procedures ensure that meals are likely to be the same at all locations.**

✔ **Most larger restaurants have Web sites where you can study the ingredients in detail before you go.**

✔ **Larger restaurants often share less equipment.** While most restaurants use the same deep fryer for multiple foods, many fast food joints use dedicated oils, at least for their French fries. So while another restaurant might be frying shrimp or mozzarella sticks in the same oil as the fries, at a fast-food or chain restaurant, your fries are more likely to be fried in fries-only oil, but ask to make sure.

Avoiding the risks of airborne exposures

With all the activity and the variety of foods at most restaurants, airborne allergens also pose a possible risk, particularly if you're sensitive to airborne allergens. To limit the risk, take the following precautions:

✔ **Be on the lookout as soon as you walk through the door.** The waiting area may have allergy-unfriendly snacks, such as peanuts in their shells.

✔ **Ask to be seated at a table far from the kitchen, especially if the kitchen is open to the dining room.** Sitting close to the kitchen exposes you to a higher concentration of airborne allergens, including milk, egg, peanut, wheat flour, fish, shellfish, and meats. Cooking launches most airborne allergens, but food preparation accounts for its fair share — chopping nuts, beating flour in a mixing bowl, kneading bread, or rolling pie crusts.

✔ **For those with milk allergies, steer clear of the cappuccino maker.** Patients can have airborne reactions in areas where milk is being frothed.

Chatting it up with the staff

Allergen-free dinners start out not with the food but with the restaurant's staff. When you book a table at a restaurant, tell the person who's reserving the table about your food allergy. Ask the person to ask the chef whether she can provide you with a meal that doesn't contain the food you're allergic to. If the person is not sure, consider eating at a more accommodating restaurant.

When you arrive at a restaurant, make sure the waiter or waitress knows about your allergy and how serious it is. If you are not confident that they understand how important it is for you to avoid a particular food, then look for another restaurant.

Despite careful planning, not all the pertinent information you provide may be accurately relayed to the chef. One way to ensure that the chef is made aware of your food allergy is to prepare a chef card. A chef card is a personalized card on which you list the foods you're allergic to and related ingredients, as well as ways to avoid cross-contamination from utensils, surfaces, and other dishes in the kitchen.

Use the sample chef card shown in Figure 11-1 as your guide. Make copies and keep the chef cards in your wallet or purse. You can personalize your chef cards by using bright colored paper, designing your own cards, or laminating the chef cards. When you go to a restaurant, give a chef card to your server and ask him or her to share it with the chef.

Table Number

I, Lillian Gray, am severely allergic to egg.

To avoid a life-threatening reaction, my meal cannot include any of the following ingredients.

Egg in any form	Globulin	Meringue	Ovovitellin	Lecithin
Egg substitutes	Livetin	Ovalbumin	Simplesse	Marzipan
Eggnog	Lysozyme	Ovomucin	Natural flavoring	Marshmallow
Albumin	Mayonnaise	Ovomucoid	Artificial flavoring	Nougat
Pasta				

Even a tiny amount of these foods can cause a reaction. Please clean any utensils, pans, counters, cooking surfaces, and other equipment thoroughly before preparing my meal, and do not prepare my food near any of these foods items.

Thank you for helping to keep me alive.

Figure 11-1:
Create a custom chef card to present at restaurants.

In the event of a reaction, take the following actions:

I carry an EpiPen. Grab tube in your fist with the gray activation cap near thumb. Remove gray activation cap. Jab tip firmly into my outer thigh (through my pants), hold there for several seconds, and then gently massage shot area. Call 911.

Ask before you eat

"Ask Before You Eat" is the advice that New Jersey's Department of Health and Senior Services (NJDHSS) and researchers at Rutgers University's Food Policy Institute and Department of Nutritional Sciences offer to people with food allergies.

That simple bit of advice is your best protection against accidental exposures and cross-contamination. Unless the restaurant staff is fully aware of your food allergies and is well informed on how to properly prepare food to prevent cross contamination, you can't really expect them to serve you a safe meal.

For more about the Ask Before You Eat program, check out www.foodallergy.rutgers.edu.

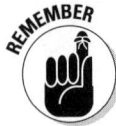

Your chef card doesn't take the place of asking questions or careful planning when you're ordering at a restaurant. Chef cards can't guarantee an allergen-free dining experience, but they can help make your meal safer.

A few Web sites have chef cards already made up. The Food Allergy Initiative offers several food allergy cards in several languages for eating out at more exotic restaurants. Most of these pre-fab cards are useful, but they often contain a list of the top allergenic foods — you place a check mark next to the foods you're allergic to. With so many foods listed on the card, this can be a little confusing. I prefer creating a custom card that shows only the foods you're allergic to. However, if you'd like to check out these other cards, visit the following sites:

✔ www.foodallergy.org/downloads/chefcardtemplate.pdf

✔ www.supermarketguru.com

✔ www.foodallergyinitiative.org (click the Downloads link)

✔ www.achooallergy.com/foodallergycards.asp

Studying the menu for safe dishes

A menu is not a cookbook. A menu usually tells you the name of the dish, a brief list of the main ingredients, and the price. Rarely can you tell from the brief menu description what the chef's secret ingredients really are. To safely order, be as selective when choosing an entrée as you are when choosing a restaurant, ask plenty of questions, and watch out for hidden ingredients:

✔ **Read the menu carefully.** If the food you're allergic to appears in the name of the dish, cross it off your list. Remember that the food might not be mentioned in the dish's name or description, so always check with the waiter or waitress.

✔ **Ask what's in it.** Tell your server what you're allergic to and then ask which items on the menu do not contain the problem food. Ask about the specific ingredients used to prepare a particular dish. If your server doesn't sound sure, ask to speak to a manager or chef. Ideally, let the restaurant know about your food allergy before you arrive.

✔ **Ask how the food is prepared.** The way the food is prepared often influences how safe it is to eat. Make sure the server and the chef know not to share cooking equipment, including deep fryers, or utensils between your food and other foods being prepared or cooked. Let them know the dangers of cross-contamination from spills or splatters.

✔ **Keep it simple.** Ordering pure, basic foods is best. A flame-broiled steak without sauce and some plain green beans are unlikely to cause a reaction. A casserole or anything else that contains a mix of ingredients is more likely to contain something you don't want.

✔ **Pass on the sauce . . . or get it on the side.** Sauces are great hiding places for allergens. A sauce is likely to contain peanuts, fish, milk, wheat, or any number of hidden ingredients. Order your sauce on the side. Better yet, forego the sauce altogether.

✔ **Ask about the dressing.** Most dressings contain oils, and many salads contain nuts or seeds, even if you can't see them. Ask which oils have been used in the dressings. If you have milk or egg allergy, ask if the dressings contain mayonnaise. Ask if the salad contains nuts or seeds. Even if you're ordering the fruit salad or chicken salad, you still need to ask these questions.

Be particularly careful around anything that contains a mix of ingredients, including sauces, crackers, and breads. These foods often contain hidden ingredients, such as:

✔ **Almonds** (in your marzipan; a sweet paste often used as cake filling or topping)

✔ **Fish sauce** (in Thai dishes)

✔ **Milk** (in some crisps)

✔ **Oyster sauce** (in Chinese food)

✔ **Peanuts** (in Satay sauce; an Indonesian sauce in which you typically dip your meat)

✓ **Sesame seeds** (in hummus)

✓ **Tree nuts or peanuts** (often used in sauces and in dessert toppings or fillings)

✓ **Wheat flour** (in soups or sauces)

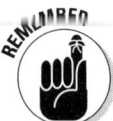

Explain to the server the seriousness of your food allergy. The server may not completely understand the potential danger until you stress it. Also, let the server know that allergens often exist in foods as hidden ingredients. Continue to talk with the server until you're confident that the person understands and is qualified to serve you safe food. If your server doesn't seem to "get it," and you're not confident that you're getting through to him, speak with the manager or chef to assure that the meal you are ordering will be safe to eat.

Stepping gingerly across the dessert menu

You made it through dinner without the slightest hint of a reaction. Now, you can kick back, relax, and reward your successful vigilance with a sinful dessert. Whoa! Not so fast. That dessert menu may tempt you with some of the riskiest foods in the building, whether you are allergic to milk, egg, wheat, peanut, tree nuts, or even seeds. They are risky for three big reasons:

✓ **Desserts frequently contain one or more key allergens, often as a hidden ingredient.** Very common examples would include finely ground peanuts or tree nuts in a pie crust, a cake that contains a nut extract, or a pastry that has been "washed" with egg whites. These could all produce deadly exposures.

✓ **Desserts are at high risk for cross-contamination, all the way from the mixing bowl to your plate.** Pastry chefs, particularly in small bakeries or restaurants, commonly bake like most people do at home — they use the same mixing bowl, cookie sheet, spatula, and serving utensils for all their desserts, without washing them thoroughly in between. Even if the dessert comes from a larger manufacturer, we see lots of reactions related to the serving utensil or ice cream scoop used at the restaurant.

✓ **Many restaurants do not actually make their own desserts and therefore often have no knowledge as to what they are really serving.** Restaurants often buy their desserts from pastry shops and others who specialize in desserts.

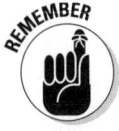

I always save dessert for home, where we can make something that we know will be safe. To some, this may seem unnecessarily cautious, but as a group, desserts count for far more reactions than foods from any other menu category. Why risk ruining a lovely, safe dinner by topping it off with a risky dessert?

Traveling with Your Allergies

Travel poses a challenge for everyone. You have to plan ahead, reserve accommodations at your destination, pack all the stuff you need, and, if you're flying, make sure you get to the airport in plenty of time to check in and weave your way through security.

For those with food allergy, travel is far more challenging, and the more severe and complicated the allergy, the more challenging it becomes. In the following sections, I act as your food allergy travel guide, to assist you in planning a safe and enjoyable journey.

Whenever you travel, consider carrying a signed medical release giving people permission to administer emergency medications, including epinephrine. Some people are so afraid of being sued if something goes wrong, that they refuse to intervene, even when someone is at risk of dying. You can pick up a sample release at www.foodallergyinitiative.org (the Food Allergy Initiative provides medical releases in several languages).

Plotting your course and itinerary

Your food allergy doesn't monopolize your travel plans, but it may influence them. In the following sections, I provide some general guidance on traveling that covers both domestic and foreign travel. Later in this chapter, I offer some tips on traveling with your food allergies to foreign lands.

Picking your mode of travel — by air or by land?

When you're traveling on a tight schedule to a distant destination, flying may be the only mode of travel that makes sense. When driving is an option, consider the benefits — you can pack more of your own food, choose your restaurants more carefully, and you don't have to risk sitting elbow-to-elbow with someone who decides to snack on a food that you're sensitive to in the middle of the trip.

Getting on the plane with your meds

If you decide to fly, be prepared for airline regulations that govern medications and foods you need to carry with you. Prior to your flight, ask your doctor to write a letter explaining why you need the items you've packed. Some baggage inspectors are sticklers, and they may require an official letter.

With my own epinephrine, in all the flights I've taken (and I'm a frequent flyer), I've only been questioned five or six times. Only once would I have been unable to carry the medicine on board without a letter. Still, you should always carry a letter to the airport, just in case. I've had to fax or email letters to patients all around the world to get them past security.

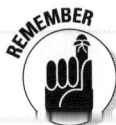

Make sure your medications are in their original packaging. Be particularly careful that prescription medications are in their prescription bottles.

Staying with family or at a hotel?

When you're traveling to see relatives, family accommodations are usually best . . . assuming, of course, that the family you're visiting understands food allergies and is supportive. With family, you have kitchen privileges for preparing your own meals and plenty of storage space for special foods.

On the other hand, some families just don't get it when it comes to food allergy. If you're family just doesn't get it, when every trip to their home is like navigating a mine field, you may be better off staying elsewhere (while you, of course, try to gently instruct them about food allergy).

Following the crowds or roughing it in remote destinations?

When you're going on vacation, you may have several destinations from which to choose. Some people enjoy the hustle and bustle of big cities, major attractions, and locations that attract tourists — places where emergency medical treatment is readily available. Others prefer the solitude of remote areas — some so remote that you'd need to aerial-drop emergency medications to the site.

Which do I recommend? It's pretty much a toss-up. You may think that populous areas are safer because of their better access to emergency medical care, but remote locations offer some benefits. Every year, I have a number of teenagers in my practice who want to go on camping or canoeing or outward bound trips. While this often causes outright panic for their parents, I remind them that if all their teenagers can eat is what their parents put in their backpack, they are much less likely to have a reaction than eating out at local restaurants.

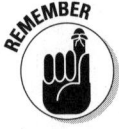

You may be dealing with other allergic conditions along with food allergy, such as asthma or eczema. If you have found that one climate or environment is particularly good or bad for your health, be mindful of this as you draw up your plans. I have several patients who travel to the same, family-favorite vacation spot year after year and call me every year to report a severe asthma attack. I wonder how this destination manages to remain a family favorite when they visit the local emergency room almost as often as they see me.

Planning your meals

When you're on vacation, one of your primary goals is to leave drab daily routines behind. With food allergies, however, your daily routines are often your best protection.

Although I don't want to ruin your trip by suggesting that you click back into your daily eating routine, some careful planning can enable you to vary your diet while remaining reaction free. Staying safe requires a combination of packing safe foods, reading labels when you go shopping, and carefully reviewing and choosing restaurants.

Scoping out allergy friendly grocery stores

When traveling to an unknown place that isn't exactly a thriving metropolis, you may have trouble finding a grocery store that carries the allergen-free foods to which you've become accustomed.

Consider scoping out such areas prior to departure. If you have a computer with Internet access, search Google for "grocery store" followed by the destination city and state or zip code to view a list of grocery stores in the area. You can also search online phone books, such as YellowPages.com at www. yellowpages.com.

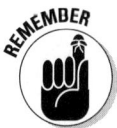

If you're traveling to a remote destination that has limited access to grocery stores, you may have to stock up on your own food supplies before departing. See "Packing a safe food stash" earlier in this chapter.

Lining up a motel with a kitchenette

Most families with food allergy, especially if milk, egg, wheat, or soy are involved, prefer to prepare most, if not all, of their own meals. If you cannot stay with friends or family, this is going to be much easier to accomplish if you can stay in a hotel or motel with a kitchenette. Thankfully, these have become more and more common in recent years and generally a whole lot nicer.

When you arrive, take a close look at the facilities and inspect for cleanliness. Food residue may be present on pots and pans, dishes, cutting boards, and so on. If the kitchen or the cooking equipment appears suspect, ask the hotel or motel personnel to clean it up prior to the time you plan on cooking your first meal.

Checking out the local restaurants

Researching a few safer local restaurants before departing on your journey is a good idea. Using a combination of guide books and the Internet, you can draw up a list of restaurants that sound good to you and then start calling the restaurants to get a feel for which ones would be most accommodating.

Follow the same guidelines for choosing restaurants at your destination that I provide earlier for selecting local eateries (see "Taking Your Allergies Out to Dinner"). When you arrive, take the usual steps described previously. By preparing in advance, you're much more likely to start your trip right, rather than having a total meltdown before you've even had your first meal.

Scoping out available healthcare providers

I have one family that travels everywhere they go with a map noting every emergency room on the route they are taking. While this is a bit extreme, and more than is necessary, having some knowledge of available healthcare facilities is not a bad idea.

Thankfully, in the United States, most hospitals are very capable of dealing with an allergic reaction. The biggest issue is having some idea of how far away from help you are so that you and your doctor can plan accordingly. For example, if you're far from medical attention, you may need to have additional doses of medicine available so that you can deal with a reaction as you wait for help to arrive.

Flying to foreign lands: international travel

When traveling in your own country, you're well-schooled in what you have to deal with and how to deal with it. Food labels, although they may be a little cryptic, are fairly standard. You're familiar with the protocol of communicating your needs to restaurant servers and chefs. You know who to call and how to call in the event of an emergency.

When you travel to a foreign land, however, you're journeying to unfamiliar territory. You're unfamiliar with the way they do things, and they're unfamiliar with you. Even more challenging is the fact that the food they eat may be entirely different from what you're accustomed to.

Confronting problems in foreign lands

The following items can make you more aware of the issues you face when traveling to foreign lands and bring you up to speed on some possible solutions:

- **The problem food is in everything!** In Asian countries, you're going to be dealing with a lot of peanut. In Israel, sesame permeates the menu. In Japan, fish is the staple. You may not need to cross a destination off the list, but you may need to pack a lot of your own food. Just make sure you can get through the customs check with the food you bring.

✔ **You don't speak the language.** Eating out safely requires an ability to communicate your allergy and your needs to the server and chef. If you don't speak their language, you may not be safe eating out at the local establishments. Sometimes, a chef's card in the local language can help — check out the cards at `www.foodallergyinitiative.org`. To further complicate matters, the locals may speak different languages or dialects.

✔ **You don't read the language.** Ever try grocery shopping in China, Japan, Germany, France, Russia? Those people have the gall to label their foods in something other than English! Well, that's obviously a problem, but even English-speaking countries can pose a problem with their food labeling. Food labeling in Canada, Western Europe, Australia, and New Zealand is typically excellent and in some instances better than in the U.S. Elsewhere, labeling may be limited at best. Stick with basic fresh foods.

✔ **Emergency medical care may not be very accessible.** Before you depart, meet with your doctor, tell her where you're going, and discuss your concerns. Stock up on special medications, if needed, and obtain a letter from your doctor stating that you need to carry these specific medications. Makes sure all medications are labeled appropriately.

Tweaking your emergency action plan

Chapter 7 provides an emergency action plan. That plan is designed for home, work, school, and local travel. If you're traveling outside the country or to a remote location in your country of residence, adjust your plan to treat reactions more aggressively:

✔ **Pack lots of epinephrine.** You should have at least three doses and maybe more depending on the length of your stay and your ability to obtain more. Prior to leaving on your trip, ask your doctor under what conditions you should administer a second or third dose.

✔ **Pack lots of antihistamines.** Benadryl is usually the antihistamine of choice, as discussed in Chapter 7.

✔ **Pack a steroid, such as prednisone.** In most cases, you don't get the steroid until you're in the emergency room. When traveling to a place where the emergency room is inaccessible, you should have your own supply ready to go. Consult your doctor about the use of the steroid — when to take it and how much to take.

✔ **Respond immediately to reactions.** Don't even think of taking the wait-and-see approach. Administer epinephrine immediately.

Surviving the long flight

A two- or three-hour flight can be a little uncomfortable, but when you're airborne in close quarters for 12 hours a more, the discomfort seems to rise exponentially. When you have a food allergy, the risk of reaction also tends to increase. When you're going to be on a long flight, take a few extra precautions:

- ✔ **Pack food.** I'm not about to bash airline food, but when you have food allergies, you can't trust it, particularly on international flights.

- ✔ **Carry on your medications.** Don't check the bags that contain your medications. Carry them on with you, so you have them on the flight, and, if your bags are lost in transit, you have the medications when you reach your destination.

- ✔ **Inform the flight crew.** The flight attendants should know that you have a food allergy, and they should be aware of what to do if you experience a reaction in flight. Often, the flight crew will ask if a doctor or other type of medical professional is on board the flight who would be willing to respond to your needs. This is another situation in which you should be prepared with extra doses of medicine and an appropriate action plan.

Flying with peanuts: avoiding peanuts on your next flight

Peanuts used to be as common on airplanes as they are at baseball games, making flying especially nerve wracking for people with peanut allergy. When passengers are packed tighter than sardines on a flight for several hours, and the attendant starts handing out bags of peanuts, you may start eying that emergency door and hoping you had a parachute handy.

In most cases, peanut on flights does not pose a significant risk. I fly often, frequently on international flights, and I've never had an in-flight reaction. Others have, however. Most of these reactions are caused by eating something that contains peanut on the flight. Far fewer reactions are caused by contact, and inhalation reactions are rare. Check out Chapter 4, where I discuss the risk of peanut dust in greater detail.

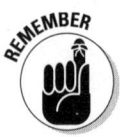

I've personally flown hundreds of times without any difficulty, and I have a very severe peanut allergy. To remain safe, however, always have emergency medication available. Although policies are forever changing, most airlines are willing to make some accommodations for those with peanut allergy, either by offering peanut-free flights or peanut-free buffer zones. Visit the FAAN Web site (www.foodallergy.org) for up-to-date information on specific airline policies. Even though I personally do not take these precautions, I think that peanut-free accommodations are a reasonable request for most families. If, however, you cannot find such a flight, or you find out at the last minute that the promised flight is unavailable, the reality is that airborne reactions on airlines are very rare in the spectrum of things and do not expose a major risk to most patients.

Cruising for a reaction

The cruise is becoming a more and more popular vacation choice, but if you've ever been on a cruise, you realize that the middle of the ocean is not the best place to experience a severe food reaction. Like most vacation options, however, cruises have their pros and cons:

- ✔ **Cons:** Most cruises have a doctor on board but the quality of the doctor, and the depth of the doctor's experience in treating food allergies, cannot be guaranteed. Have a detailed emergency action plan in place, as discussed in Chapter 7, and share it with the doctor and other personnel on board. Make sure they know where your emergency medications are stored and that they can get to them in a hurry. You should also tweak your emergency plan, (see "Tweaking your emergency action plan," earlier in this chapter), to treat reactions more aggressively. Also, make sure that you can contact your doctors, no matter where in the middle of the ocean you are. Fortunately, the development of satellite phones has made this much easier.

- ✔ **Pros:** Some cruises have a well-trained staff that's very willing and able to prepare special food just for you and is quite capable of responding effectively in the event of an emergency. Eating on a cruise ship with experienced chefs may certainly be much safer than dealing with a dozen new restaurants in a less controlled environment.

I have a large number of patients who have had great luck with cruises. It makes me a bit nervous, but if you do your homework and can identify a safe cruise line, your trip may be as safe as it is enjoyable. Plan ahead and talk with the right people. Ask other people you know with food allergy if they've taken a cruise, and see what they recommend.

Witnessing the miracle of Disney: A case study

Many restaurants and vacation spots have taken on food allergy as a serious issue and have proven that they can make it work. I do not want to lead anyone to believe that the Disney resorts are the only place that have made this work, but they do set the gold standard of how to do food allergies right.

Of all my patients and their families who've stayed at a Disney Resort, I have never heard a bad report, and most families are brought to tears by the thought that their child can go out to eat safely. The chefs go the extra mile and offer tours of the kitchen and anything else you need to make you comfortable, even if you prefer to read every label on every box yourself.

Chapter 12

Conquering the Challenges of Daycare and Preschool

*Y*ou can establish a virtual blockade around your home to prevent unfriendly foods from being smuggled across the border, but when you ship your toddlers off to daycare or your little tikes off to preschool, they enter a world where allergenic foods are often readily available, temptations are strong, and ignorance is rampant.

To safeguard your children when they leave your protective fortress, you often need to re-create the safe environment of your home wherever you choose to send your child — daycare, preschool, summer camp, or even at the home of a relative or one of your child's friends.

In this chapter, I provide the information and insight you need to make a well-informed decision whether to send your preschool children outside the safe haven of your home. I then provide guidance on how to work with your daycare provider, preschool personnel, and other caregivers to create a safer environment where your child can mingle with other children with less risk of exposure to potentially dangerous food allergens.

Making the Big Decision: To Send or Not to Send

Parents always face a few difficult decisions in which they seek to do what's best for their family and healthiest for their children. The decision of whether to send a child to daycare or preschool, especially a child who requires special care, can be even more taxing.

Some families have limited options. In single-parent homes or in homes where both parents must work to make ends meet, the option of one parent staying home is immediately off the table. Parents may consider asking a family member to provide child care, but if family members don't live nearby or don't exactly qualify for the job or want it, this option is off the table, as well. With no suitable choices, the decision to send junior to daycare or preschool has already been made.

In families that have multiple workable solutions, the decision-making process may be a bit more thorny, especially if your child is severely allergic to multiple foods. As with most decisions regarding food allergy, the bottom line is whether the potential benefits justify the risk.

Weighing the risks of daycare and preschool

You can significantly minimize the risks by following all the precautions I recommend in this chapter, but you can never completely eliminate the risk of accidental exposure, even in your own home. To accurately weigh the risks of sending your child to daycare or preschool, consider the following factors:

- **Age:** As children pass through their preschool years, they become more and more capable of assisting with their own care and managing their food allergy. Two-year-olds have virtually no self control or awareness of their allergy or their surroundings and require much more vigilance from the childcare providers. Three-year-olds typically have some understanding of their food allergy and may even have enough self-control to resist the offer of some tempting food. By the age of four or five, children with food allergy who are properly educated about avoidance at home have considerable understanding of their food allergy and can truly play some role in protecting themselves.

- **Place and providers:** If you've been fortunate enough to locate a daycare provider or preschool that seems to be very knowledgeable about food allergy, this may make your decision easier. On the other hand, if you're not really comfortable with any of the preschools available, then foregoing preschool or at least waiting another year may make more sense. See "Finding the Right Daycare Center or Preschool," later in this chapter, for guidance on selecting a suitable childcare facility.

✓ **Allergy types and severities:** Finding a safe environment may be easier if your child has a single peanut allergy than if your child has multiple, severe food allergies. Although peanut allergy can certainly be deadly, preschools are often much more aware of peanut allergy, and you may even be able to find a peanut-free preschool. If your child is severely allergic to milk, egg, or wheat, accidental exposures certainly pose a greater risk, and you have almost no chance of finding a preschool that completely eliminates these common foods.

Considering the benefits of daycare or preschool

Daycare and preschool offer some valuable benefits in terms of social skills, but very little academic benefit. Personally, I think the academic benefits are minimal and blown way out of proportion. Daycare and preschool can, however, accelerate a child's development of social skills and, in some cases, lighten the load on the parents and enable them to pursue their own personal and professional goals. This, in turn, may improve the overall emotional well being of some families.

Only you can decide what's best for your family, but don't think you have to send your children off to preschool out of fear that they'll fall behind in school if you don't. Preschool offers little to nothing in the way of academic development that your child can't get at home.

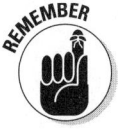

Social skills are important, however, so if you decide to keep your child home during the preschool years, seek out other opportunities for your child to interact with other children.

Finding the Right Daycare Center or Preschool

Generally speaking, the younger the child, the more care the child requires. By the time your child heads off to kindergarten, she can pretty much take care of the basics on her own. At this stage, most schools are pretty well equipped to deal with food allergies, especially now that food allergies are so prevalent.

Unfortunately, at the age when an allergic child requires the most care and vigilance — during the daycare and preschool years — providers are often ill-equipped to deal effectively with food allergies. Most daycare providers and preschools don't even have a food allergy policy or procedures in place to guide them.

During these early years, toddlers and preschool age children are at particularly high risk when it comes to food allergy because:

- They move fast.
- They put almost anything in their mouths and share food without concern.
- They're often messy eaters.
- Many can't keep their hands to themselves.
- Children under the age of three have little understanding of their food allergy and may even be more tempted to share food because they've been deprived of certain items at home.

Three- and four-year-olds usually start to gain an understanding of their food allergy and begin to protect themselves to some degree, but they still need lots of supervision. These factors make it especially important that you choose a daycare or preschool carefully and then work with the facility to establish all necessary policies and procedures to keep your child safe. In the following sections, I highlight the most important food allergy factors to consider when selecting a preschool or daycare center for your child.

Shopping for allergen-free schools . . . or not

When shopping for a daycare center or preschool, should you insist on an allergen-free environment? For children over the age of six, I'm generally not a big proponent of prohibiting peanuts or other common allergenic foods. When you're in the market for a daycare center or preschool, however, particularly if your child has a peanut or tree nut allergy, an environment void of all problem foods is, of course, ideal.

The question is, how accessible are allergen-free facilities? The answer depends on which foods your child is allergic to. In the past, allergen-free preschools and daycare centers were unheard of, but now I would estimate that about half of all preschools are peanut-free zones. As for other allergenic foods, including milk, egg, and wheat, you're unlikely to find any school that bans these foods or is even open to considering implementing restrictions.

Are allergen-free facilities really best?

One of the major arguments against allergen-free schools is that they may foster a false sense of security. Teachers, parents, and children sometimes get lulled into thinking that that jotting down a few rules and regulations prohibiting certain foods is 100 percent effective in keeping them off the premises. In practice, avoidance is rarely 100 percent effective, even for those who are very careful.

The ideal environment for preschool age children is one in which the most common and dangerous allergenic foods are banned from the premises, but teachers and caregivers remain vigilant, carefully read food labels, monitor the foods that children bring for lunch and snacks, and carefully supervise all eating activities to ensure a safe environment for everyone.

When choosing a daycare center or preschool, all other factors being equal, a school that restricts or prohibits the food that your child is allergic to is a better choice than one that allows it. However, finding such a facility can present a huge challenge, particularly if your child is allergic to something other than peanut.

Never get lulled into a false sense of security that allergen-free really means allergen-free. Peanut-free, for example, merely means other children are *less likely* to pack peanut butter sandwiches for lunch or snack on peanut butter crackers. It means your child has *much less* of a chance of being accidentally exposed to peanut, because a lot less of it will be spread around the classroom and cafeteria. Peanut-free, however, does not mean that all the other parents read every label as carefully as you do and that everything other kids bring in is completely peanut-free.

Assessing a facility's knowledge and experience with food allergies

As you go about investigating daycare centers and preschools, you may be shocked at the differences you find from one place to another. The knowledge and experience at childcare facilities generally falls into one of the following three categories:

- ✓ **Uninformed and inexperienced:** The facility has had few or no children with severe food allergy and has very little knowledge of food avoidance and emergency treatment. An uninformed, inexperienced staff is not reason alone to scratch the facility off your list. A facility that's excellent in other areas of childcare and willing to learn and implement effective food allergy policies and procedures may still be an excellent choice.

✔ **Misinformed:** The center has been thoroughly misinformed about food allergy and has a policy in place that's not even close to meeting your child's needs. A common example would be a policy and procedures inspired by a family who says, "my child only has a mild peanut allergy, so you don't need to worry too much. It's fine for him to eat cookies and candies as long as peanut is not a main ingredient. And since he has only broken out in hives before, my doctor says he does not need an epinephrine prescription." This school may approach your child with the same bias, which could create a very dangerous situation.

✔ **Well-informed and sufficiently experienced:** You luck out and find a center that has been whipped into shape by other families who've approached food allergy with the same vigor and vigilance as you.

Inexperience with food allergy is much less common today than it was just ten years ago. With the rising prevalence of food allergy, most centers that care for young children have had to deal with food allergy and develop at least a few standard procedures for dealing with it.

Even if the childcare facility you choose is well-informed and has had experience dealing with food allergies in the past, don't assume that the staff knows how to properly treat your child. In "Teaming Up with Your Child's Daycare Center or Preschool," later in this chapter, I guide you through the process of bringing the school up to speed on *your* child's food allergy.

Avoiding uncooperative facilities

If you have no option of whether to send your child to daycare or preschool or you decide that the social benefits outweigh any drawbacks, be sure to choose a cooperative facility. The problem with daycare centers and preschools is that no laws govern how they treat children with food allergies. When your child is older, if you choose to send him to public school, federal laws mandate that the school provides a safe environment for your child and address any special dietary needs.

Most daycare centers and preschools are not bound by these regulations and have the ability to say "No" if they don't agree with your requests or recommendations. The exceptions to this are centers that receive federal funding,

such as Head Start programs, where they are bound by laws similar to those in the public school system.

You may think that logic and compassion would rule the day and that you can persuade the facility's administration to enact effective food allergy policies and procedures, but some facilities are simply unwilling to cooperate.

Don't choose a facility that strikes you as uncooperative. You may end up fighting a battle for "the principle of the thing," in which your child is almost certainly destined to become the loser. Trust your instincts. Don't even consider leaving your child at a facility that seems unwilling to provide a safe environment.

Gauging the size factor

The size of a childcare facility is less important than the ratio of children to caregivers. For example, a preschool with a child-to-teacher ratio of 6-to-1 is typically safer than a preschool with a ratio of 12-to-1, even if the preschool with the 6-to-1 ratio is much larger overall.

During mealtimes, snack times, parties, and other activities when eating is involved, an adequate number of caregivers is particularly important to supervise the children and ensure that all food remnants have been cleaned from the tables and from the children immediately before and after eating.

 A cafeteria or other designated area for eating can help reduce exposure and food contamination by keeping food out of the classrooms where children spend the bulk of their time. Larger preschools and daycare centers are more likely to have designated eating facilities.

Consulting the school nurse (or whoever's in charge)

If you're lucky, you may stumble upon a daycare center or preschool that has its own nurse. This is only likely to happen in a larger facility, so if you opt for something smaller, a nurse may not come with the package. The following sections help you evaluate whether a nurse is a must-have at your facility as well as how to best evaluate the nurse or person in charge at your facility.

Knowing whether you need a nurse

Is the absence of a nurse sufficient grounds for crossing a facility off your list? Not really, as long as the facility has the following in place:

- A cooperative staff committed to maintaining a safe environment for all children.

- Information and training required to limit your child's exposure to allergenic foods. (You may need to become the trainer and resource person.)

- Instructions, training, and medicines to respond to allergic reactions quickly and effectively. (Again, you may be the main source for instructions and training.)

- A competent surrogate for the nurse — typically the school administrator — responsible for implementing and maintaining all the policies and procedures needed to keep your child safe.

Evaluating the nurse or whoever's in charge

When researching the best options for your child, speak to the nurse or who-ever's in charge of attending to health-related issues. This conversation can give you a much better idea as to whether this facility is the right place for your child. Engage the nurse or surrogate nurse in a discussion about your child's food allergy and try to get a sense of the following:

✔ Does this person really get it?

✔ Does this person understand food allergy and how dangerous it can be?

✔ How much experience does this person have caring for children with severe food allergy?

✔ Does the person fully grasp that even tiny food exposures can be deadly and that they need to be prepared to treat allergic reactions immediately?

Once you've selected a daycare or preschool, engage in a more detailed discussion with the nurse or administrator. The section, "Teaming Up with Your Child's Daycare Center or Preschool," guides you through the essential meetings and training sessions and provides additional tips on how to team up with your child's daycare center or preschool for optimum safety.

Teaming Up with Your Child's Daycare Center or Preschool

After you select a daycare center or preschool for your child, your real work as child advocate begins. Now, you must make sure that your child's care-givers are knowledgeable and skilled in caring for your child and that they understand specifically which foods your child needs to avoid and what sort of care to provide in the event of a reaction.

In the following sections, I provide guidance on how to educate your child's caregivers; select, train, and equip staff members to provide quick, effective emergency care; assist the facility in developing clear, comprehensive procedures for preventing accidental exposure to problem foods; and work with the facility and other parents to establish it as a peanut-free zone.

Food allergy organizations have developed a variety of educational materials specifically for schools and preschools. These can be very helpful, especially if you're dealing with a facility that has limited experience caring for allergic children. The Food Allergy and Anaphylaxis network has an excellent training program complete with a video and written materials. Visit www.foodallergy.org for details.

Educating your child's caregivers

Anyone you place in charge of caring for your child — daycare providers, teachers, school nurses, camp counselors, even grandma and grandpa — must be fully informed of your child's food allergy.

When sending your child off to preschool or daycare, provide a fact/instruction sheet with the following information, and make sure that everyone in the setting who will have contact with and responsibility for your child reads and understands the information:

 ✔ **Your child's name and photo:** Caregivers must know your child's name and face.

 ✔ **Type of food allergy:** Everyone should know that your child has a food allergy and be able to identify the foods and ingredients that your child must avoid. The food allergy sheets in Chapter 6 can assist you in providing detailed information.

 ✔ **The need for your seal of approval on any food items:** Specify that only the foods you approve are to be given to your child. In addition, encourage the school's staff to carefully read food labels prior to giving your child a particular food. They should know that manufacturers sometimes change the ingredients they use, so they must read the label every time.

 ✔ **The dangers of cross-contamination:** Cafeteria workers need to be aware of the potential dangers of cross-contamination, so they follow proper food preparation techniques. All cooking utensils and surfaces must be cleaned thoroughly before preparing and serving your child's food. Chapters 10 and 11 can help you lay out food preparation guidelines.

 ✔ **The necessity for cleanliness:** Cafeteria workers, dining room supervisors, your child's caregiver, and others must be aware that your child needs to eat off of a clean table with clean utensils. In addition, students should wash their hands with soap and water after eating. Refer to the following section, "Establishing some basic lunchroom policies," for details on lunchroom policies.

 Set up a face-to-face meeting with your school's nurse, administrator, and all other parties involved in your child's care, distribute your fact/information sheet at the meeting, and encourage staff members to ask questions. Follow up with regular reminders over the course of the school year and any updates from your child's doctor.

Figure 12-1 provides a form you can fill out and distribute to your child's caregivers. This form can assist caregivers in preventing your child from accidental exposure, but the form is no substitute for a treatment plan. See "Planning for possible emergencies," later in this chapter for details on preparing and training for possible reactions. Chapter 7 includes a form you can fill out to create a custom emergency treatment plan.

| Your child's photo | My name is: _____ |

I cannot eat or be exposed to the following foods and ingredients:

_____   _____   _____

_____   _____   _____

_____   _____   _____

_____   _____   _____

To avoid accidental exposure to these foods, please help me follow these rules:

- Don't provide food or snacks that my parents have not approved.
- Don't let me share food with other children.
- Scrub my table with a household cleaner before I eat.
- Sit me at a table with other children who are not eating the foods that give me problems, or make sure I have a seat between me and other children.
- Make sure all students thoroughly wash their hands before, and especially after eating.
- Even a tiny amount of a problem food left on a spatula used to serve my food can make me severely ill, so please prepare and serve my food on freshly cleaned surfaces with clean utensils, pots, pans, or bowls.

If I am exposed to the foods or ingredients that make me sick, I may develop the following symptoms:

- Hives, swelling, or itchy rash.
- Itching or swelling of lips, tongue, or mouth.
- Tightening, hoarseness, coughing.
- Abdominal cramps, vomiting, diarrhea, or nausea.
- Fainting or passing out, paleness, blueness, irregular heartbeat.
- Coughing, wheezing, difficulty breathing.
- Fear of impending doom, panic, chills, sudden weakness.

Figure 12-1:
Use this form to quickly bring childcare givers up to speed on your child's food allergy.

If I show any signs of a reaction, do not hesitate to get me help, because I may not be able to ask for help. Immediately contact one of the following staff members who are well-trained in providing my emergency treatment:

Staff member name: _____

Staff member name: _____

Staff member name: _____

Establishing some basic lunchroom policies

The lunchroom, whether it's a separate cafeteria, a designated eating area outside the classroom, or the same room in which your child spends most of his day, is the main battle ground for fighting accidental exposure to food allergens.

Fortunately, a good dose of vigilance, proper cleaning procedures, some common household cleaning agents, hand soap, and a little elbow grease can help your child's daycare center or preschool win the battle and provide your child with a safer place to eat. The following sections describe three simple policies and procedures for creating an allergy-friendly eating area.

Whenever requesting special arrangements for your child, attend to both physical and emotional needs. Even very young children are sensitive to being singled out, particularly if it isolates them from their classmates and makes them a target for teasing. When asking for special treatment for your child, make it clear that the accommodations are to be accommodating, creating a situation as close to "normal" as possible.

Scrubbing down the tables

After every meal or snack, a kitchen worker or staff member should thoroughly clean the tables, especially if children are eating in the room in which they spend most of their day. Following are some guidelines on proper cleaning:

- ✔ **Use common household cleaning agents.** As I explain in Chapter 3, these cleaning agents have been proven effective in removing even the most stubborn remnants of peanut butter and other allergens.

- ✔ **Clean carefully and thoroughly.** Rub hard, don't simply swipe a rag over the tables and chairs. Scrub any globs of food off the surface.

- ✔ **In a cafeteria, before eating, wipe down the table where the child with food allergies will sit.** This is especially important if the child is eating during a second or third lunch shift.

Washing hands . . . it's not an option

I recommend that all children wash their hands before and after eating. The pre-wash is primarily for sanitary purposes and to prevent your child from ingesting any food allergens she may have picked up from toys or other objects. The post-wash is more important for preventing allergic reactions — to reduce the likelihood that another child who ate a food that would make your child sick will spread it around the classroom or inadvertently rub it on your child. Remember, kids at this age can't keep their hands to themselves.

Caregivers must supervise the hand-washing ritual and make sure that the children wash their hands properly. Keep these tips in mind:

- **A thorough scrubbing with a moistened wipe does the trick.** A superficial swipe with a wipe is inadequate.
- **A good, thorough hand washing with soap and water followed by a thorough drying of hands with paper towel also works.**
- **Antibacterial gels are not effective in removing food allergens.**

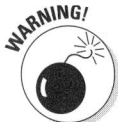

If the childcare facility has one of those cloth towel rollers for drying hands, it could pose a risk of accidental exposure. If your child dries her hands on the same portion of a towel that another child wiped her hands on, any allergens on that towel could wipe off onto your child's hands. Paper towels or a hot-air hand dryers are best.

Arranging for safer lunchroom seating

Distancing your child from other children who are eating the foods that can trigger reactions is an important measure for preventing accidental exposure, especially in daycare and preschool. The trick is to provide safe seating without unnecessarily isolating your child. Here are three effective options:

- **Designate a peanut-free table, as explained in Chapter 13.** If your child is allergic to peanut, chances are she won't have to eat alone. In some cases, the peanut-free table may be used for children with other food allergies, as well, because these tables are typically cleaned more thoroughly and supervised more closely.
- **Draw up a seating arrangement so children with the same food allergies are less likely to be accidentally exposed to the problem foods.**
- **Arrange the seating to provide a little buffer around your child.** Your child may need to be seated next to children who are not eating a problem food or be seated between two empty places to create a buffer zone.

Caregivers should also enforce a no-food-sharing policy during all eating activities. Preschool kids love to swap foods and try the exotic foods that they've never seen in their own homes, particular when they're young, but food sharing is a big no-no, and anyone supervising eating activities must strictly enforce the no-sharing policy.

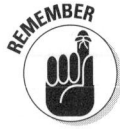

Kids move fast and can shoot across a table or across a room faster than a paper wad. The lunchroom may also have a fair share of sloppy eaters and kids who talk with their mouths full. Close adult supervision is key to preventing accidental exposure.

Making your childcare facility peanut-free

Because peanut is notorious for triggering potentially severe reactions, many daycare centers and preschools have formal peanut restrictions in place. If your child is allergic to peanut, and the facility does not ban or restrict peanuts, you can advocate for various restrictions:

- ✔ Formal peanut-free facility, in which the administration officially prohibits children from bringing in anything with peanut as an ingredient.

- ✔ Voluntary peanut-free facility in which parents are encouraged to pack peanut-free lunches and snacks for their children.

- ✔ Peanut-free tables, where your child can eat lunch and snacks. For more about peanut-free tables, skip to Chapter 13.

A peanut-free school can be achieved several different ways. If the administration agrees that peanut prohibition should be a universal policy, then they mandate this policy and communicate it to all the parents. In some instances, the school may be reluctant to enact a formal policy but will let it happen on a more voluntary basis. The administration may be willing to provide you a list of names and addresses of the other parents, so you can communicate with them directly.

Figure 12-2 shows a sample letter that I offer to parents who want to ask other parents for their cooperation in keeping a facility peanut free. You may need to modify the letter to better suit your needs, but the general tone of the letter has proven very successful in persuading parents to cooperate in creating a safer environment.

Planning for possible emergencies

One of the rules I stress throughout this book is that reactions happen, no matter how many theoretically-effective avoidance maneuvers you have in place. So even after taking all the steps to prevent reactions, you must provide the childcare facility with the training and medications it needs to treat your child effectively in the event of a reaction.

Storing medicines in a safe, convenient location

Every daycare center and preschool has some sort of policy or procedures in place for storing and administering medications. Find out where the medications are stored and who's in charge of administering the medications to your child.

Dear Fellow Parents:

As you may have heard, our child, Jane, has a severe allergy to peanuts. If she eats or even touches peanuts, peanut butter, or any food which may have been in contact with peanuts, she could develop a life threatening anaphylactic reaction. Because of this risk, we would be most grateful if you would refrain from sending peanut or nut snacks, or even any foods which are labeled as containing or possibly containing peanuts or other nuts, to school. In addition, please avoid sending in any home baked goods which may have come in contact with peanuts. Finally, if your child has eaten peanut products in the morning, please wash their hands and face so that they will be less likely to pass on traces of peanut when they come to school. Even a trace of peanut butter left on a toy might trigger an anaphylactic reaction.

We understand that these measures are burdensome and may be a tremendous imposition, particularly when so many children enjoy peanut butter. Unfortunately peanut allergies are becoming increasingly common these days, and although Jane is aware of her allergy, she is till too young to understand the consequences of eating peanuts and doesn't have the maturity to resist temptation. I think you would all agree that we must do whatever is necessary to keep our children safe, and by cooperating with these few requests, you will be contributing greatly to the welfare of our daughter. We thank you for your understanding and wish you and your children all the best during the school year.

I have also attached a list of safe snacks that may make your shopping a bit easier. If you have any questions, please feel free to call or email us at any time.

Sincerely,

Jane and John Doe
j&jdoe@genericaddress.com
(555) 555-5555

Figure 12-2:
Writing a letter to the parents often results in a safer environment for your child.

Because allergic reactions can become very serious very quickly, medications must be readily accessible at all times. In some cases, childcare facilities store all medications in a central area, such as the nurse's station or the administrator's office. In other cases, your child's teacher or primary caregiver is entrusted with the medications. Which option is best? That depends on several factors:

- ✔ How far away from the central location is your child during most of the day, and especially during and after lunch, snack time, and parties? If your child's primary caregiver has to run through long halls or to another building to get to the medicines, she may need her own supply.

- ✔ Is the central location accessible at all times? If the central location is off limits or locked at certain times, then the facility may need to store a set of spare medications in another room.

- ✔ Who's responsible for giving the medication? If responsibility belongs to both the nurse and the teacher or other caregiver, then the teacher or other caregiver should have ready access to their own set of medicines. If, on the other hand, the teacher does not even know how to administer the medications, having access to them makes little sense.

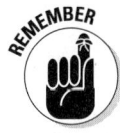

Clearly label and organize all medications and store your child's emergency action plan, as discussed in Chapter 7, with the medications to avoid any confusion in the event of an emergency. I prefer that medications not be under lock and key, simply because locks throw another obstacle in the way of a speedy, effective response. If medications must be under lock and key, make sure two or three people have a key immediately available at all times.

Appointing and training emergency responders

Almost every daycare center and preschool places someone in charge of storing and dispensing medications — typically the school nurse or the facility's administrator. To ensure that a competent individual is always on-call, establish a failsafe system with fully-trained staff members in place:

- ✔ **Appoint a minimum of two (preferably three) staff members to act as emergency responders in the event of a reaction.** Having only one fully trained individual on call is an accident waiting to happen. A single sick day or other staff member emergency would put your child at risk.

- ✔ **Provide each designated emergency responder with a copy of your child's Food Allergy Emergency Action Plan, as discussed in Chapter 7, and review the plan with your emergency responders in person.**

- ✔ **Train each emergency responder to administer medications.** They need to know how to spot signs of a reaction, how to assess the severity of a reaction, when to administer each medication, how much medicine to give, and how to give it. If you're sending in epinephrine autoinjectors, all emergency responders should be trained on how to administer the shots. Use a trainer device to demonstrate autoinjector use, and then have the people in charge of giving the shots demonstrate its use back to you to make sure they follow the proper technique.

- ✔ **Let all your child's caregivers know who the emergency responders are and how to contact them.** They should also need to know how to spot the early warning signs of a reaction and be aware of the importance of quick, decisive action.

- ✔ **Identify the nearest emergency medical facility, make sure their EMT's (Emergency Medical Technicians) carry epinephrine, and supply a phone number to call immediately in the event of a severe reaction.** Onsite emergency treatment coupled with immediate professional medical care is required for severe reactions. Sometimes one or two shots of epinephrine are not enough.

- ✔ **Meet with the emergency responders before the school year and intermittently during the school year.** Provide detailed information and instructions during the initial meeting. Subsequent meetings can be informal and brief but are still important.

And the medications are where?

A mother recently called me for a new prescription for her child's epinephrine. According to our records, she had already filled the prescriptions we provided for the epinephrine autoinjectors, so unless she already used those, she should have had a sufficient number of autoinjectors for both school and home.

The trouble was the school couldn't find the two autoinjectors she had brought in. When she visited the school at the end of the semester to pick up her child's medication, the staff members in charge of storing and administering the medications were unable to find the autoinjectors. Needless to say, the mother was shocked

and dismayed to find out that her child had been at risk in the preschool that she had come to trust.

The moral of this story is that follow-up meetings with the people in charge of storing and dispensing medications is essential. This unfortunate situation could almost certainly have been avoided with an occasional refresher course and perhaps a mini-drill to make sure all the pieces were in place for an effective emergency response.

Consider staging a drill in which your child's caregivers respond to a mock emergency situation, so they know just what to do, whom to contact, where the medications are stored, and how to administer them.

Chewing on Some Snack-Time Issues

For better or worse, snack time is often the highlight of the day in preschool. It boggles my mind why some people think that a child needs to eat every two or three hours, but apparently the majority of parents and preschools think that children will somehow pass out from hunger if they don't have something to eat every couple hours. Perhaps how snack time is handled should be one of the main considerations in your daycare or preschool selection.

In any event, the following list describes the most common snack-time scenarios:

- **No snack time:** Children simply don't bring snacks, which cuts down on opportunities for accidental exposure.

- **Fruits or vegetables:** Some "progressive" schools allow children to bring only fruits or vegetables, or the school serves fruits or vegetables for snacks.

✔ **Parent-approved snacks:** The school provides all snacks, but consults parents for input. If you can get on the snack selection committee, work with the school to choose snacks that are safe for your child. This could even work if your child is allergic to something other than peanut, such as milk, egg, or wheat.

✔ **Parent-provided snacks:** Parents send in the snacks with or without parental guidance. This isn't always the best-case scenario for a child with food allergies. Even if other parents know about the allergy, they may not be as careful as you are about making sure the snacks they buy or prepare are truly allergen-free. In this case, you may volunteer to be the go-to parent for snacks or to work with a team of other parents in the class to provide safe snacks.

✔ **Counterproductive snack suggestions:** Some facilities may actually recommend that parents send in snacks that contain the very allergenic food your child is allergic to. The facility may, for example, insist that peanut butter be a regular snack item. Here's where you need to step in and make your voice heard.

The key to safe snack- and meal time for your child lies in your ability to provide all your child's food or at least guarantee that the food being provided by the school and other parents is safe.

Keeping Parties Fun while Making Them Safe

Traditionally, parties provide an opportunity to let down your hair, break rules and routines, indulge your desires, and throw caution to the wind. Unfortunately, just about everything that many parents think makes a party fun increases the risks for people who have a food allergy:

✔ **Any activity that breaks the routine, including parties and field trips, increases the likelihood of accidental food exposure.**

✔ **Party foods — cookies, candy, cake, and other finger foods — are often too tempting for a child to resist.**

✔ **Well-meaning parents often send in risky foods that they fully believe are safe.** They often don't realize that the innocent sugar cookies they bought were contaminated by peanut at the bakery or that a benign looking candy, such as jellybeans or candy corn, might actually contain peanut or egg.

> ✓ **Lots of party foods contain peanuts or tree nuts.** This is especially true around the holidays. We always see clusters of reactions around the major holidays, especially Halloween and Christmas.

So how can you keep parties safe? Follow three rules:

> ✓ **No foods without the prior approval of the allergic child's parents.** This is the granddaddy of all party rules.
>
> ✓ **No exceptions to the first rule.** No matter how safe or innocent the food may appear, never break, bend, or otherwise misinterpret the meaning or importance of rule number one.
>
> ✓ **Send in a safe party food.** To make sure that your child is not pooped out of the party, caregivers must inform parents in advance of an upcoming party, so you can send in a safe party food — an allergen-free cookie, cupcake, or other suitable alternative.

If the school is planning a field trip or other outing off school grounds, work with your child's caregiver to ensure a safe trip and make sure the emergency medications travel with your child. For additional tips on ensuring a safe field trip, check out Chapter 13.

For the unplanned parties and activities, go with plan B. Ask the caregiver to keep an approved party food on hand in the event of an unplanned party or if you forget to send something in. This could be a cupcake stored in the freezer or box of favorite cookies with your child's name on it stored in the cupboard.

Chapter 13

Sending Food Allergies Off to School: K-12

. . . .

In This Chapter

▶ Considering the home-schooling option

▶ Teaming up with school administrators, teachers, and nurses

▶ Sitting down to a safe lunch and other eating activities

▶ Navigating field trips, bus rides, and parties safely

▶ Qualifying for special modifications under Section 504

. . . .

*A*lmost all parents experience a little fear and trepidation, in addition to some relief, when they send their children off to school. Your child may become the victim of cruel bullies, be exposed to infectious diseases, get in with the wrong crowd, or get hurt on the playground.

Parents of children who have severe food allergies have one more thing to worry about — their allergic children experiencing a severe allergic reaction.

As I explain in this chapter, one option is to home school your allergic child, but for many parents, home schooling is out of the question. For other parents, home schooling just doesn't fit into their plans for Junior; they want their child to attend the local school system, so he can be "like other kids."

What's the alternative? To find a good school where the administrators, teachers, and other staff are fully aware of the dangers surrounding food allergies and then work with the school to make it even safer for your child.

In this chapter, I provide you with all the advice, tools, and tips you need to create a safer educational environment for your child, from the time she steps on the bus in the morning until the time she bursts through the back door in the afternoon.

Selecting an Allergy-Safe Educational Environment

Parents want the best education for their children. What's best, however, varies greatly from one parent to another. Some parents simply don't trust the educational system to properly educate their children and keep them safe, so they choose to home school. Some parents believe that private schools offer superior educational opportunities. Others find that the combined value of academics and social-skills learning provided by their local public school systems are the perfect solution.

I can't tell you what's best for your children, whether or not they have food allergies, but in the following sections, I lay out your options and provide some guidelines, so you can make a well-educated decision in respect to your allergic child's safety.

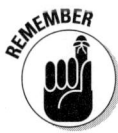 Public schools are required by law to make accommodations, even for the most allergic child. If you have trouble convincing your school to cooperate, which is hopefully not the case, refer to "Going Behind the Scenes with 504 Plans," later in this chapter, to find out more about your rights.

Calming your fears with the age factor

In Chapter 12, I discuss the pros and cons of sending younger children to preschool, and I point out that age plays a big factor in allergy safety. Younger children are much more prone to accidental exposure to food allergens. As your child moves on from one grade to the next, however, accidental exposure becomes less and less of a risk for the following reasons.

✔ Many children outgrow their food allergies when they reach school age, or at least the allergies may be less severe.

✔ School age children have a greater awareness of their food allergy and their

surroundings, enabling them to play a more proactive role in their own safety.

✔ Classmates are more mature — better able to keep their hands to themselves and follow proper etiquette in the lunchroom.

In addition, once your child is school-aged, if you send your child to a public school, the law is more clearly on your side — public schools are required by law to provide a safe environment for your child.

Home schooling: The ultimate in allergy safety?

For parents who are already considering home schooling their children, having a child with a severe food allergy may tip the scales in favor of home schooling. The decision is perfectly understandable. The parents, leaning toward home schooling their child anyway, factor in food allergy and choose home schooling as the best option.

Few parents who have children with food allergy, however, decide to home school based solely on the fact that the child has a food allergy, no matter how severe it happens to be. Even in cases when the parents do base their decision to home school solely on the food allergy, they often could have made arrangements with the school to provide an acceptable level of safety.

Assessing public versus private schools

If you're thinking about sending your child to a private school, you probably already have a lot on your mind, including the big question — "Can we afford it?" You're probably weighing the costs and benefits right now and considering various factors, including academics, athletics, religious beliefs, family tradition, and social benefits. When deciding whether to send a child with a severe food allergy to a private or public school, other considerations may influence your choice:

- **Legally protected rights:** Although most private schools are just as concerned about the safety of their students as public schools, laws and other regulations that govern medical conditions and disabilities, including food allergy, do not apply to most private schools. Establishing the right accommodations in a private school is a more voluntary process.

- **Cooperation:** Some private schools are unbelievably accommodating when it comes to food allergy, while others are abysmal. By speaking to other families and to school administrators, you can usually gauge the school's willingness to cooperate. Private schools typically fall into one of the following three categories:

  - **Experienced and proven:** The school has had many students with food allergies and has established an excellent track record in keeping them safe.

  - **Unproven but willing:** The school has little experience dealing with food allergy but is very willing to work with you to make their school the best possible place for your child.

- **Inexperienced and unwilling:** The school has little or no experience in dealing with food allergy and is unmotivated to change course. Administrators may see it as too bothersome or too much of a legal risk.

✔ **Size:** School size matters, but not in the way that many parents may think. Some parents think that smaller is better, especially if the school has a higher student-to-teacher ratio, because the school provides more supervision. A smaller school, however, is less likely to have a cafeteria, meaning that students probably eat in the classrooms. While the cafeteria may sound like a nightmarish place for someone with food allergy, it can actually be made quite safe, and I almost always prefer to get the food out of the classrooms as much as possible.

✔ **Nurse availability:** Having a nurse on staff is a big plus, but it shouldn't make or break your decision. Again, larger schools are more likely to have a full-time nurse, but some small schools have a nurse, and some large schools don't. I'm used to working with schools without nurses, and most schools can establish a safe environment even without a nurse.

✔ **Location:** Occasionally, the location of the school, especially the proximity to your home, is an important factor. Being closer to home can mean shorter bus rides, or no bus ride at all, and a shorter distance for you to travel in the event of a reaction.

In the final analysis, food allergy is not likely to be the deciding factor between public and private schools but these are all important issues to consider.

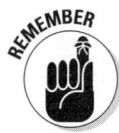

Although public schools are required by law to accommodate special needs, not all public schools are equally eager to conform to the legal requirements. In other words, certain public schools can be as uncooperative as a private school. With public schools, however, you have more legal leverage to force them into providing the necessary accommodations.

Making a Safe School Safer for Your Child

Even if you pick the safest school in your neighborhood, accidental exposure to a food allergen is always a possibility. To limit the risk of accidental exposure, you can work with your school to implement some proactive preventive measures.

In the following sections, I show you how to review and assist in modifying your school's food allergy policy, coordinate safety and emergency efforts with the school's nurse and other staff, and make school buses and lunchrooms safer.

Reviewing food allergy policies

No matter which school you choose, the school should have some sort of food allergy policy in place. As I discuss in Chapter 12, many schools have existing food allergy policies influenced or even established by parents of allergic children who've attended the school. These policies often range from dangerously deficient to very thorough and useful, so carefully review the school's existing food allergy policy in the light of the guidelines I lay out in the following sections.

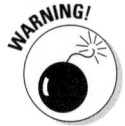

A school's food allergy policy merely sets out procedural guidelines. A policy is no replacement for specific information you provide to the school about your child's food allergy and detailed instructions on what to do in the event of a reaction. Refer to Chapter 7 to create a food allergy emergency action plan for your child, and keep it on file at the school. Chapter 12 includes a useful form you can fill out to provide basic information about your child's food allergy to teachers, coaches, and other school staff who have regular contact with your child.

General procedures

A school's food allergy policy must include general procedures to ensure medication is stored in a safe, convenient location and that staff members are properly informed. Review your school's food allergy policy to make sure it answers to the following questions:

- **Where are medications stored?** The school should store the medications in a convenient location accessible to all staff members at a moment's notice, and all staff members should be aware of the location.

- **Where is each student's emergency health care form filed?** In the event of an emergency, staff members should be able to pull up the form for immediate reference. Consider storing the form with the school nurse or administrator and having a copy available for your child's teachers. Storing a copy of the emergency form along with the medications is also a good practice.

- **Who should know about the food allergy and how will they be trained?** All teachers, coaches, cafeteria workers, office personnel, playground supervisors, bus drivers, and other staff members who have regular contact with your child should be informed of what your child is allergic to, how to prevent accidental exposure to a food allergen, and what to do in the event of an emergency. If your doctor prescribed epinephrine autoinjectors, two or more staff members should be properly trained on administering shots.

✔ **Who will train substitute teachers (if applicable)?** The food allergy policy should specify how substitute teachers are to be trained when your child's teacher misses a day of school.

Food handling and eating

During the day, most students have some sort of break for lunch and perhaps even a snack time. Every school's food allergy policy must answer the following questions:

✔ **Where do students eat their lunch and snacks?** A policy that keeps food out of the classrooms is best, but if your school does not have a central eating facility, this may not be an option.

✔ **Who provides the snacks?** School-only provided snacks are best. All snacks must have clear, understandable labeling of all ingredients. If the school has a policy in which students can bring their own snacks, then you may need to deal with this issue with your child's teacher. See "Protecting Yourself without Becoming a Party Pooper," later in this chapter.

✔ **Can the classroom be allergen free (for example, peanut free)?** Although your school's food allergy policy may not ban a particular food, it should include a statement that a particular classroom can be made allergen free at the parent's request.

✔ **What are the specific cafeteria procedures?**

• Peanut free tables and other seating arrangements should be spelled out. See "Designating peanut-free tables and other seating arrangements," later in this chapter for details.

• If the school prepares and serves its own food, preparation and serving procedures should be in place to clearly identify foods that may contain ingredients that your child is allergic to and to prevent cross-contamination. Chapter 10 details proper food preparation techniques.

• The policy should describe who's in charge of cleaning the tables, when tables need to be cleaned (before the first lunch room shift and after each shift), how tables are to be cleaned (scrubbed thoroughly), and what cleaning solution to use.

✔ **How and when are students to wash their hands?** The school should require that all students wash their hands before and after eating.

Food allergy reaction emergency procedures

Prevention is not always 100 percent effective, so your school's food allergy policy must have a plan B in place that details the following:

- **Where should the student go for help?** If your child begins to experience a reaction, she needs to know ahead of time where to go for help — the teacher, the main office, nurse's office, or somewhere else.

- **Who should accompany the child?** When experiencing a reaction, even if it appears mild at first, your child should never be left alone. A teacher or fellow student who knows what to do if the reaction intensifies should accompany the child to seek help.

- **Who is to stay with the other students?** Most schools do not allow students to remain unsupervised, so a plan should be in place for another teacher or staff member to remain with the other students should the teacher need to leave the room immediately.

- **What should be done if the student is in the lunch room, classroom, or gym?** The food allergy policy must specify a separate plan for any scenario in which your child may find himself in at school, including the gym or lunch room. Who's the go-to person in each scenario?

- **Who's responsible for calling the nurse?** If your school has a nurse, who's in charge of contacting her — the teacher, administrator, or someone else? What does this person need to do to contact the nurse in an emergency?

- **If the nurse is not present, who's next in line for action?** A backup emergency person should always be in place in case the nurse is out for the day or cannot be contacted.

- **When should the person in charge call 911?** Instructions should spell out the conditions under which the person handling the situation should call 911. Whenever epinephrine is administered, a call to 911 is mandatory.

 Schools have drills for fires, tornadoes, and even, unfortunately, school ground intruders. Very few schools have drills for treating medical emergencies. Consider staging a drill for a severe allergic reaction. A brief rehearsal or two can ensure that everyone knows the role they play, that the medications are accessible, and that the people administering the medications are able to do it properly.

Field trips

A field trip transports your child out of the relative safety of the school grounds and places him in a challenging, less-controlled environment. Your school's food allergy policy should address this challenge:

✔ **Who's responsible for carrying and administering the medications?** When your child is away from school, her regular emergency treatment person may not be readily available. In such a case, who's going to play that role on the field trip? The teacher or the parent in charge of chaperoning your child's group may need additional training.

✔ **Are you able to attend?** If you're able to go on the field trip with your child, this may be the best option. You can ensure proper prevention, carry the medications yourself, and you know what to do in the event of a reaction.

✔ **What steps can be taken to minimize risks?** As with other activities, the key issues revolve around eating. Make sure you know what snacks or meals may be needed and what food exposures may inadvertently occur during a specific trip. Packing your child a lunch for the field trip may reduce much of the risk.

For additional details on handling field trips, see "Taking Your Allergies on a Field Trip," later in this chapter.

After-school activities

After school, your child may be involved with extra-curricular activities, such as the school newspaper, yearbook, sports, or student government. Another teacher or a parent may be supervising this activity. Your school's food allergy policy should address how food allergies are handled during after-school activities:

✔ **Who's in charge if a reaction occurs after school?** The most important step in ensuring safety after school is to inform the person in charge of the after-school activity about your child's food allergy and what to do in case your child experiences a reaction. The food allergy policy should specify that the coach or other activity supervisor is to be properly trained. In addition, whoever may substitute for the coach or activity supervisor also requires proper training.

✔ **Where are medications stored?** If medications are normally stored in the nurse's office, which may be locked after school, the policy must specify a convenient, readily accessible location for the medications after school, or the activities supervisor should be required to carry a separate, fully stocked emergency kit.

✔ **Who should the activity supervisor report a reaction to?** When other emergency personnel leave the school at the end of the day, who should the activity supervisor contact in the event of a reaction?

✔ **What steps should be taken during a reaction?** The policy should lay out the specific steps the activity supervisor needs to take if your child experiences a reaction. Use the emergency action form in Chapter 7 as your guide.

Pow-wowing with the nurse, administrators, and other staff

The best food allergy policy, if not properly implemented, is useless. As a parent of a child with food allergy, your role is to ensure that everyone in the loop remains well-informed. In the following sections, I show you how to meet with key school personnel and pass along the necessary information to them.

Preparing for your food allergy meeting

Before the school year is scheduled to kick off or preferably near the end of the previous school year, prepare for a meeting with teachers, administrators, and other school personnel. In preparation, gather the following materials:

- **Food allergy policy:** Make a copy of the school's food allergy policy for each person who's planning to be at the meeting. Staff members may not even be aware that the school has a food allergy policy. On your copy, highlight and annotate the areas you want to focus on.

- **School-required forms:** Most schools have their own forms you must complete and keep on file with the school. Obtain these forms early, so if they require your doctor's signature, you can have the forms completed before your meeting.

- **Your child's food allergy sheet:** Every staff member at the meeting should know your child's face, what she's allergic to, and the basic rules to follow to prevent exposure to the problem foods. See Chapter 12 for a sample food allergy sheet. Complete it and make a copy for each person planning to attend the meeting.

- **Food allergy emergency action plan:** Whoever's in charge of administering medications and treatment should have a food allergy emergency action plan customized for your child. Chapter 7 provides the form you need, unless your school requires that you file a different form.

- **Medications:** Have all the medications you plan on storing at the school with you at the time of the meeting, especially if your doctor prescribed epinephrine autoinjectors. Bring a copy of the instructions for the autoinjector and one or two trainers to demonstrate their use.

- **Food preparation and serving instructions:** Cafeteria workers must get up to speed on proper food preparation and serving procedures to prevent accidental cross-contamination. See Chapter 10 for tips.

For additional materials that can help a great deal with educating school staff members, visit the Food Allergy & Anaphylaxis Network Web site at www. foodallergy.org.

Scheduling your food allergy meeting

In the spring near the end of the school year is typically the best time to meet with school administrators and staff. Gathering all required personnel during the summer is nearly impossible. If you miss the spring and summer vacation, try to set up something just prior to your school's opening day. Meet with the principal or other school administrator and request a meeting with all staff responsible for keeping your child safe:

- The school administer responsible for developing and implementing the school's food allergy policy.
- The school nurse or nurse's aide and anyone else responsible for dispensing medications and providing emergency treatment.
- Your child's teacher(s).
- Food service personnel if the school prepares its own lunches. (If your child is going to brown bag it, include food service personnel in the meeting to discuss the need to thoroughly clean the table your child will be sitting at. See "Packing for Lunchtime: Cafeteria or Brown Bag?" later in this chapter for details.)

Delivering your food allergy presentation

With food allergy information and medications in hand, you're well prepared for your food allergy presentation. You can handle the meeting however you think is best, but many parents have found the following agenda useful:

- Discuss food allergies in general.
- Discuss your child's particular food allergy, highlighting preventive measures and what staff members can do to help ensure your child's safety.
- Review your child's food allergy emergency action plan, emphasizing the role that each person plays in providing immediate, effective treatment.
- Review the school's food allergy policy, highlighting meal times, allergen-free tables, hand washing, and how you expect snacks to be handled.
- Open the floor to questions and keep notes in case staff members request additional information or instructions that you don't have with you.

Feel free to make special requests of administrators or staff members for any additional safety measures not already in place. In most cases, you can simply negotiate a solution that works for everyone. In other cases, you may need to supply a letter from your doctor or resort to more formal, legal action, if the school is unwilling to cooperate, which is rare.

Don't make your food allergy meeting a one-time event. Do an encore performance at least once a year, even if all the personnel are the same as last year and everything worked to perfection. Review policies and procedures; provide updated forms, if needed; and check on the medications. When problems arise, a follow-up meeting is a must, but even when everything is running smoothly, schedule a meeting to provide reassurance, say thanks, answer any questions, and, perhaps, even treat the staff to a batch of cookies — allergen-free, of course — for a job well done.

Not all staff members may be willing or able to attend your presentation, so be prepared to contact staff members individually to set up meetings. With unwilling staff members, a non-confrontation approach is best. By explaining the seriousness of your child's food allergy and mentioning that the staff member may need the information to keep your child safe and alive, you can usually gain the person's full cooperation. People are usually uncooperative simply because they don't fully understand how important this is. If the staff member is still unwilling to cooperate, contact the principal — one of the principal's main jobs is to attend to parent concerns, and they're usually well aware of their legal obligations to do so.

Dealing with medications on school grounds

Every school stores and dispenses medications for students who require them during the day. In most cases, the school requires that you send medications in their original package, clearly labeled, and often with your doctor's instructions or a permission slip signed by the doctor.

With most medications, a missed dose doesn't pose any risk to the student's life. In the case of food allergies, however, if sufficient quantities of the medication are not readily accessible, and the staff member in charge of administering the medication is unavailable, the situation can pose a significant risk to your child.

In the following sections, I recommend procedures to minimize the risks.

Ensuring the medications are accessible

Prior to the beginning of the school year and a couple times during the year, check to make sure that your child's medication supplies are fresh and fully stocked. If the school keeps medications under lock and key, which I recommend against doing, find out who has the key, and make sure your child's teacher knows who's holding the key.

Don't just call into the school. Ask to see where the medications are stored. By asking to see the medications yourself, you can get a pretty good idea of how accessible they are. If the office has to hunt around for the key to the medicine cabinet for ten minutes, you've just observed a problem that the school needs to address. In addition, you may discover that the school has misplaced your child's medications. Inspect in person with your own two eyes.

Naming the keepers of the medications

Storing your child's medications in an easily accessible, central location may be adequate, but if your child is stuck out in a satellite classroom at some point during the day, then you may need to supply a second or even a third set of medications to provide easy access at any point during the day.

In some cases, having your child carry his own medicines may be best, but it's not always the optimum solution. See "Working toward independence: Carrying your medications," later in this chapter for details.

Establishing a strategy for dispensing medications

Work with your doctor to fine-tune the Food Allergy Emergency Plan provided in Chapter 7 or to complete whatever emergency treatment form your child's school requires. Some forms are better than others, and some doctors take more care than others to complete these forms.

If the school's generic forms are inadequate or your doctor provides only sketchy instructions, don't be shy to ask for something more detailed.

Working toward independence: Carrying your medications

Some schools allow older students to carry their own medications, as long as the school has this in writing signed by your doctor. In fact, many states have laws that give students the right to carry their own medications, assuming the situation requires it.

Carrying medicines obviously has the advantage of guaranteeing that the medicines are immediately available. This approach, however, is not ideal in all situations. Consider the following:

- ✔ **Can you trust your child?** Some kids lose everything and others can't resist the temptation to show other kids what they have in their bag. I've seen several inadvertent injections of epinephrine with this sort of show and tell.

- ✔ **Can your child administer her own medications?** Pre-teens may not be able to give themselves their own medication, particularly an epinephrine autoinjection. In such cases, the medicine does no good unless a responsible adult is immediately available.

- ✔ **Is your child willing to carry the extra baggage?** Toting around fanny pack or some other bag with medications may cramp your child's style. As long as the medicine is readily available in a matter of minutes, which usually is the case at most schools, then burdening your child with this responsibility may not make sense.

Riding the school bus with food allergies

The school bus has become an icon of Americana — a relatively safe mode of transportation that carts the kiddies off to school every morning and drops them back at home in the early evening. For students with food allergies, however, even a relatively safe bus ride can be a source of anxiety.

If your child is a responsible teenager and the school allows its students to carry medications, your child can carry his own medications and take most of the worry off your plate. If not, then you may face a tricky predicament due to the following complications:

- Few school systems require their bus drivers to carry or be responsible for administering medications.

- If the bus driver agrees to take care of the medications, you still have the hassle of handing the driver the medications in the morning and having the driver pass the medications to the school, pick them up after school, and return them to you.

- Storing epinephrine on the bus is not a good idea, because it would be exposed to hot or cold weather.

- A substitute bus driver may show up who's heard nothing about the food allergy or the medicine.

That being said, here are your options:

- Drive your child to school yourself to avoid the whole situation.

- Pick up and move to one of those rare school systems that have trained all their bus drivers to treat an allergic reaction.

- Lobby your school system to train their bus drivers and organize a system to store and transfer medicines.

- Make the bus safer by putting the following precautions in place:

    - Be certain your child knows about her allergy and can be trusted to never, ever share food with other children.

    - Inform the bus driver of your child's allergies.

    - Have your child routinely sit in the front seat where the bus driver can keep a better eye on her.

    - Make sure the bus driver has cell phone access at all times to call for help if needed.

Even if you have no other option than to send your child on a bus without medications and without a bus driver who's fully equipped to deal with a severe reaction, I believe it is an acceptable risk, especially if the bus ride is relatively short. Over time this situation will hopefully improve in more and more school systems.

Designating peanut-free tables and other seating arrangements

Peanut-free tables are now an option at many schools, and most schools are willing to provide one if requested. Should your child's school have designated peanut-free tables or special allergen-free seating arrangements? This is for you, your child, and the school to decide, based on the following considerations:

- ✔ **Do peanut-free tables help?** Yes, especially for children younger than nine years old. By the time a child is nine or ten years old, I believe that these allergen-free tables no longer provide much benefit.

- ✔ **What does your child want?** Peanut-free tables and other seating arrangements may add to the stigma of having a food allergy. Ten years ago, I wrote letters requesting that schools provide peanut-free tables. Now I write a lot more letters to liberate kids from their peanut-free isolation wards.

- ✔ **Does the school mandate peanut-free tables for students with food allergies?** To protect the school from lawsuits and ensure safety, some schools require students with food allergies to sit at peanut-free tables. In other schools, the choice is up to the student and parents.

The specific arrangements for peanut-free tables vary widely from school to school. The more isolating the arrangement, the more distasteful it is for the child. In fact, this is the main reason that families ask to remove their child from peanut-free purgatory. Following are a couple examples of allergen-free table arrangements that schools have implemented:

- ✔ Students are allowed to invite one or more friends to sit with them as long as they eat a peanut-free lunch. This makes the situation much more tolerable.

- ✔ All students with any sort of food allergy sit at the same table — typically a table that's more frequently and thoroughly cleaned and better supervised. This provides students with a greater likelihood of sitting at a table with a classmate.

- ✔ Only students with peanut allergy sit at the table. This may be fine, but more often it results in some fourth or fifth grader getting stuck at a table with a first or second grader. This sure takes the fun out of lunch, and remember, for young kids, the favorite part of their day may just be lunch or recess.

Dealing with non-peanut allergens at lunch time

Peanut allergy is definitely the scariest allergy in the cafeteria, due to peanut's notorious reputation for triggering life-threatening reactions, but if your child is allergic to milk, egg, or some other food, you're no less concerned about protecting her safety.

Although some schools are willing to arrange for a milk-, egg-, or wheat-free table, such arrangements are more difficult to implement and increase the odds that your child will be sitting at a cozy table for one. The solution? The peanut-free table may still be the best option, simply because it's typically cleaned more thoroughly and is better supervised.

In the most extreme situations, you may be able to get an aide to supervise your child's lunch. This would usually occur only with a 504 plan, as discussed in the section later in this chapter, "Going Behind the Scenes with 504 Plans."

Being careful what you ask for

Public schools are required by law to provide a safe environment for your child, so administrators may overreact to your requests out of fear. If you request special accommodations, without specifying exactly what you want, you may be unpleasantly surprised at what you get.

If, for example, you request that your child not be exposed to a particular allergen in the cafeteria, the school may decide that your child needs to eat in the nurse's office or library. Your child may find that a quiet lunch in solitude is perfectly acceptable, or he may look at it as punishment for having an allergy. Unless you're careful about what you ask for, you may find that you've backed yourself into a corner you can't get out of. Be careful what you ask for.

Taking a few sensible precautions

For most children, a few simple precautions are sufficient for ensuring safety in the lunchroom. Consider the following precautions, and remain flexible, so you can modify the precautions based on the school's facilities, your child's age, and the nature of the food allergy:

- ✔ **Make sure your child has a clean place to sit.** This is especially a concern if your child is scheduled to eat during a later lunch shift. Your child should have a designated safe seat, where she sits every time she eats lunch. A properly trained adult should be in charge of cleaning the seat and table before your child's lunch shift. Having a fellow student clean the table is usually inadequate.

- ✔ **Create a buffer around your child.** Seating your child at the end of the table next to a classmate who's eating only safe foods is typically the best option.

- ✔ **Have your child pack a placemat.** Eating off of a placemat or plate can prevent your child's food from picking up any allergenic remnants off the table.

By high school, your child can safely leave most of these precautions back in junior high. Your child should still avoid sitting at a dirty table with messy eaters, but special seating arrangements generally are unnecessary.

The ultimate peanut-free zone . . . a horror story

I thought that I had seen the most draconian peanut-free zone policies possible, until one of my patients described how her school had demarcated its peanut-free zone.

My patient, a fifth grader at the time, was returning to school to begin a new year and was invited to take a tour of the new peanut-free arrangements. The school had placed its peanut-free table in an alcove that was separated from the other children. They painted large arrows on the floor that she was prohibited from crossing as she made her way to the table. She was further dismayed to find that the table was labeled with a large red sign banning any other children from crossing another series of lines that quarantined the table.

Her parents, who had been among those who pushed the school to create a peanut-free table when she was in first grade, were now asking me for a letter to permit her to sit elsewhere.

Packing for Lunchtime: Cafeteria or Brown Bag?

Eating the cafeteria food may be a risky proposition, even for students without food allergies, but most students enjoy buying lunch at least some of the time, so the option is worth investigating.

When deciding whether to allow your child to buy school lunch, consider your child's food allergy, the knowledge and experience of the food service staff, and the menu selections:

- ✔ If your child has an isolated allergy, such as peanut, and the school and food service staff are well indoctrinated in reading labels and following precautions to avoid cross-contamination, your child may be able to eat a variety of foods on the menu.

- ✔ If, on the other hand, your child is allergic to milk, egg, wheat, or other allergens commonly used as ingredients in many foods, then cross contamination may be too risky, particularly if the food service staff is inexperienced.

- ✔ If the menu is loaded with items that contain the allergen that your child is allergic to, brown bagging it may be the best option. Even with a well-trained and very careful food service staff, the risk may not be worth it.

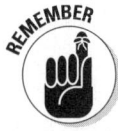

If you decide to let your child buy lunch, even part of the time, have a detailed meeting with the food service staff, from the top down, to review ingredients, policies, and procedures. This is necessary, even if the food service staff has had experience with preparing foods for students with food allergies.

After you've done your homework, if you still feel uncomfortable with the idea of your child eating the school lunch, then brown bagging may the best solution. In addition to preventing reactions, the food is likely to be much better.

Protecting Yourself without Becoming a Party Pooper

Although most people view lunchtime as the most menacing threat to children with food allergies, the risk of accidental exposure looms larger in the perilous party scene and at snack time. In fact, any eating activity that disrupts the normal routine is far more risky than the relatively well-controlled environment of the lunchroom.

Without becoming the school's party pooper mascot, your child can keep parties and snack times safe by following a few simple precautions:

✔ **No sharing food.** Instruct your child never to share, trade, or accept food from others, even if it looks safe or the giver swears that the food is completely allergen free. Follow one rule about sharing food — never do it!

✔ **Bring a safe party food alternative from home.** For scheduled parties, send in a safe party food for your child, volunteer to cater the party yourself, or have your child's teacher keep a store of safe party foods available for surprise parties.

✔ **Host the party in the cafeteria.** If possible, keep party foods out of the classroom, so students can return to an allergen-free classroom after the party.

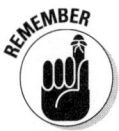

Parties often pose the most serious risks for three reasons: they break routine, often include problem foods (such as desserts with peanut, egg, milk, and wheat), and involve eating foods in the classroom, increasing the risk of exposure.

Taking Your Allergies on a Field Trip

Like parties, field trips disrupt the normal routine. One day your child is sitting in the classroom, and the next, he's off to the dairy farm to learn the fine art of homogenizing milk.

When you hear about a planned field trip, your ears should perk up, and you need to ask a few questions to find out where the class is going, what they're planning to do, where they're planning to eat, and who's responsible for making sure the medications get on the bus and providing emergency medical treatment. Consider the following issues at least a few days before the planned departure date:

- ✔ **Is the class going somewhere that could be hazardous?** A milk-allergic child may be better off skipping the field trip to the local dairy farm, and a student with wheat allergy may want to forego the bakery tour. With sufficient early warning, the teacher may be willing to work with you to choose a safer destination, but if the itinerary is already set, your child may have to remain behind.

- ✔ **Who's in charge of your child?** In most cases, the teacher takes a group of children, and other groups are assigned to parent chaperones. At this point, the teacher should be well informed of your child's allergy, so having your child in the teacher's group may be best. If that's not possible, volunteer to chaperone or at least talk to the parent who's going to be assigned to your child's group.

- ✔ **Who's responsible for packing, carrying, and administering the medicines?** The medicines need to be available at all times, not left sitting on the bus.

- ✔ **Is a cell phone going to be available at all times, if anything comes up?**

- ✔ **Can you go on the trip?** In some schools, parents are diplomatically uninvited. Others prefer you to go. Offloading the responsibility onto you sure makes the teacher's life easier.

Going Behind the Scenes with 504 Plans

Most schools do everything possible to provide students with a safe educational environment and are willing to implement necessary policies and procedures to accommodate students with even the most severe food allergies. If your school's policies and procedures are inadequate and its administrators or staff members are unwilling to provide accommodations that you and your doctor think are necessary, you have legal recourse.

Three key laws protect the rights of disabled individuals in schools and other institutions that receive federal funding. I describe these laws and show how they apply to food allergies in the following sections. Unfortunately, some schools don't know the laws or mistakenly believe that they only protect the rights of students who are physically or mentally handicapped or require educational modifications.

Section 504

Section 504 is a civil rights law with a twofold purpose: " . . . to prohibit discrimination on the basis of disability in education or employment in any program or institution receiving federal funds, and to ensure that students with handicaps or disabilities receive a free and appropriate public education." Public schools and private preschools and daycare centers that receive federal funds must comply with this law and its regulations to qualify for financial assistance.

Sometimes, students with less obvious disabilities, such as life-threatening food allergies, are not considered "disabled." However, students have been able to have their health- and learning-related concerns successfully addressed at school under Section 504. Under Section 504, a school district must consider the individual needs of a child and provide related services or necessary program modifications to enable that child to attend school. The school must provide these modifications at no cost to the parents.

The law provides that students with disabilities must be educated with non-disabled students, and students with disabilities must receive the same or equal access to educational opportunities or extracurricular activities that are provided to students without disabilities. Students cannot be excluded from going on field trips, eating in the cafeteria, or participating in class projects because of their food allergies.

Schools must comply with Section 504 as a prerequisite for receiving federal funds. Failure to provide an appropriate public education is a violation of a student's civil rights and can jeopardize the school's federal funding. If you've done everything you can and the school remains unresponsive to your requests, call the United States Health and Human Services Department at 1-800-368-1019, e-mail ocrmail@hhs.gov, or visit www.hhs.gov/ocr to file a complaint online.

For more information about 504 plans, including a Question and Answer section and links to additional useful Web sites, visit the Council for Educators for Students with Disabilities, Inc. Web site at www.504idea.org.

The Individuals with Disabilities Education Act (IDEA)

IDEA requires schools to evaluate any student suspected of having special needs and to provide for that student's educational needs in the least restrictive environment, as appropriate for the individual child. IDEA specifies that parents of children with disabilities and school personnel are equal partners in the planning process that creates the goals, program and environmental modifications, and services that are written into the Individualized Education Plan (IEP). An IEP or other written plan is not required by Section 504, but IDEA reinforces your child's rights to a fair education.

The Americans with Disabilities Act (ADA)

The Americans With Disabilities Act (ADA), further extends the rights and responsibilities provided under Section 504. ADA states "no individual shall be discriminated against on the basis of disability in the full and equal enjoyment of the goods and services . . . of any . . . public accommodation."

The ADA states that public accommodations, including any school receiving federal funding, must take such steps as may be necessary to ensure that no individual with a disability is excluded, denied services, segregated, or otherwise treated differently than other individuals because of the absence of auxiliary aids and services. Noncompliance with the ADA can result in civil and criminal penalties or even loss of federal assistance.

Citing the law to gain cooperation

When a school seems reticent to ensure the safety and full participation of your child in their curriculum, you may have no choice but to cite the laws that ensure your child's rights. Bottom line, the law requires the school to:

- ✔ Not deny a child admission based on the child's disability.
- ✔ Recognize children with life-threatening food allergies as disabled and protected under federal law.
- ✔ Work with parents to enable students to safely participate in all activities with their peers.
- ✔ Provide services and program modifications under section 504 for disabled students, even if they're not eligible for special education.
- ✔ Provide necessary accommodations, so no student is excluded from field trips, eating in the cafeteria, or class projects because of their food allergies.

✔ Provide an appropriate public education to eligible students.

✔ Provide benefits and services detailed under Section 504, regardless of whether the student is considered a special student under IDEA.

✔ Have an appeals procedure in place (required both by IDEA and Section 504) to field complaints from any parent who feels that their child is not receiving the benefits and services they need.

Chapter 14

Empowering Your Adolescent or Teenager

*B*eing a teenager is tough, even if you don't have food allergies. You're trying to figure out how to navigate a world that doesn't really understand you and perhaps doesn't really want to listen. You're young. You're naturally driven to break away from your parents and other authority figures. You have less to lose. You're invincible, unbreakable, shatterproof! So, what's up with all the worry, the rules, the restrictions?

As a parent of a teenager, you're probably fighting conflicting emotions and thoughts. You want to loosen the reins to give your child more freedom and responsibility. At the same time, you want to rein in your teen, set some healthy limitations, and provide guidance on how to make good decisions.

When you add food allergy to the mix, the situation can become even more tense and unstable. Out of fear for the health and safety of your teenager, you may try to impose additional limitations. Your teenager, already saddled with more limitations than he can bear, may tend to react against the additional restrictions — restrictions that many of his friends don't have. Couple that with normal peer pressure, and your teenager (quite understandably) may place himself in high-risk situations, sometimes just to prove to himself that he can.

This chapter explores the challenges of being a teenager with food allergies and being a parent of a teenager with food allergies and explains some ways parents and their teenage "children" can work together to cope with the realities of the situation.

Fostering an Atmosphere of Empathy

Families often become embroiled in battles due to differences in perspective. The parents' job is to protect their children. The child's job is to become independent. These two goals are often diametrically opposed, even when it comes to dealing with health issues.

The key to successfully resolving any conflict and effectively teaming up to properly manage a food allergy is empathy. Establish common ground. Work toward understanding one another's concerns, fears, and needs. Respect the challenges that each of you face. Only then can you begin to collaborate and see food allergy for what it really is — an inconvenient and sometimes dangerous reality that needs to be supervised and managed.

Whether a teenager has a newly acquired food allergy or an allergy that developed in early childhood, the food allergy is a huge burden — physically, socially, and psychologically. Studies show that food allergy has a marked effect on quality of life, and this typically peaks in adolescence when the effects of being different are always magnified.

Acknowledging the injustice

No doubt about it, food allergy sucks. As a parent, you may be tempted to soothe your teenager's angst concerning food allergy by pointing out everything in life that could be deemed as being worse — diabetes, AIDS, blindness, hearing loss, acne, and any other health issue you can think of, but the fact is that your teenager is dealing with food allergy, and for him or her, it sucks. It also sucks for you, as a parent.

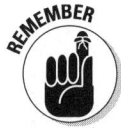

I hate to sound like some family therapist on TV, but the fact is that only by admitting how you truly feel about food allergy can you validate one another's feelings and then work through them to a more logical resolution.

Feeling the sting of teenage teasing

In the perfect world, the most effective way to prevent accidental exposure would be to inform everyone that you have a food allergy, so they wouldn't accidentally expose you to the food that makes you ill. In junior high and even in high school, telling everyone that you have a food allergy can be like hanging a sign on your back that says "Kick me!" Any exposed weakness is a vulnerability that the school bully may quickly pick up on and begin to exploit.

Teasing can range from minor verbal harassment to really dangerous stuff. I have seen hundreds of incidents in which "harmless" teasing escalated into intentional food exposure or at least an attempt to knowingly expose someone with food allergy to an allergenic food. I've seen peanuts thrown at kids and milk blown through a straw across the lunch table at school into the face of an allergic teen.

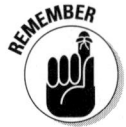

Nip it in the bud. Work to make your school a tease-free zone. "Harmless" teasing can quickly escalate into ugly scenes, and the more dangerous this becomes, the more aggressively your school needs to deal with it. Knowingly exposing someone who has a severe food allergy to an allergen is the equivalent of assault with a deadly weapon.

Some strategies that I teach my patients, and occasionally have to use myself, are listed here. (Note that I use the phrase "have to" rather than "had to." Even at this point in my life the teasing hasn't stopped. Not that long ago a well-educated colleague jokingly offered me a doughnut saying, "Would you like some peanuts?") Here are some strategies to deal with insensitive idiots:

- ✔ **Just ignore them.** Most teasers tease to get a rise out of you — that's their reward for success. When the teasing starts, just ignore them. It may not be easy but this is usually the best approach.

- ✔ **Tell them how you feel and ask them to stop.** This can be effective, especially if the teaser is generally a friend or at least a decent person. For others, however, this may be just the kind of reaction they were hoping for and may only make things worse.

- ✔ **Tell an adult.** This is essential if the teasing is affecting your life and whenever it crosses the line to the point to being dangerous. A responsible adult needs to know about this.

I always remind my patients that everyone gets teased at some point, whether they have food allergies or not. If it is potentially harmful, it must be taken seriously and reported to an adult. Appropriately, some schools have taken a very tough stand against teasing. Otherwise, shake it off — don't let it get to you. If the teasing really bothers you, bring the behavior to the attention of a parent, teacher, guidance counselor, or other trusted adult.

Dealing with restrictions and limitations

No matter how lenient you are as a parent, you're always too strict for a teenager. No matter how responsible of a teenager you are, your parents are always going to worry about you. When decisions and disagreements over food allergy are complex only one thing is certain — the parent is likely to be overly protective, and the teenager is likely to take too much of a risk.

I'm not about to tell parents how to raise their teenage children. And I certainly wouldn't try to tell a teenager how to raise her parents. All families are different, everyone's allergies are unique, and every family has the right to approach the same situation in its own way. I offer no one-size-fits-all approach. I know teens with the same food allergy who have never been permitted to ride the school bus, while others have traveled on their own to foreign countries.

If you and your teenager lock horns on a particular issue, consider taking the matter to your doctor for discussion. Your doctor is unlikely to make the decision for you, but he may be able to defuse the emotional dynamite, highlight the facts, and explain the potential risks and rewards, so you can arrive at a more reasonable consensus. Some parents are far too restrictive, and teens are far too prone to taking risks. The trick is to find a happy medium.

Sizing up the situation: Newly developed or long-standing allergy?

The way you approach food allergy may depend on whether the food allergy is something totally new or has been a family issue for some time. For newly developed allergies, the special issues may include

- The need to learn about food allergies from scratch, at a time in life when medical concerns are hardly a favorite topic.

- Potentially intense frustration and anger generated by the eternal question, "Why me?"

- A positive realization that this is a serious problem that needs to be dealt with. If the reaction was relatively recent, it could lead to less risk taking and a determination to learn about and take control of the food allergy . . . at least as long as the reaction is still fresh in mind.

With long-standing food allergies, other issues are more likely to bubble to the surface during the teenage years:

✔ Some teenagers accept their food allergy as a part of their lives. They take the necessary precautions to avoid the problem foods, and they remain prepared for emergencies.

✔ Some teenagers may become too complacent, especially if they haven't had a reaction in some time. They may doubt whether the allergy is real or still present, which may lead to more risk taking.

✔ Unexpressed frustration and smoldering anger may find expression in unpredictable ways. The teenager may not even realize that the root cause of some unacceptable behaviors lies with resentment over having a food allergy.

✔ Long-term parent-child issues may arise if parents have been overprotective and the teen suddenly finds himself in a situation in which he's expected to take on more responsibility.

Empowering Your Teen to Take on More Responsibility

The teenage years are a transitional period — a bridge from childhood to adulthood. As such, teenagers often demand more freedom, while parents encourage them to take on more responsibility in just about every aspect of their lives — homework, jobs, driving, dating, and health. With food allergy, the challenges are amplified but should certainly be manageable. Here are some suggestions that may help you weather the storm:

✔ **Avoid the blame game.** Both parties are attempting to achieve the same goal — successful management of the food allergy. As long as you keep this in mind, you may be able to avoid the blame game.

✔ **Transfer ownership of the allergy.** This can be tough, especially for parents who've been managing their child's allergy for several years. At some point, parents need to transfer ownership of the allergy, and the teenager must accept more of the burden. Agreeing to a slow, gradual transition may work. As parents see that the teen is able to handle small responsibilities, they will be more comfortable letting the teen handle the big ones.

✔ **Ask the doctor.** Teenagers can play a more active role during office visits by asking questions about medications, treatment options, whether certain situations are safe, and so on.

✔ **Transfer responsibility when dining out.** Most teenagers are perfectly capable of communicating with a restaurant server or cook. The next time you dine out, encourage your teen to ask the questions about ingredients and food preparation, or, if you're the teenager, ask your parents to let you do the talking.

✔ **Hand over control of the medications.** The key to success is the ability of the person who has the allergy to responsibly manage her own medications. Teens need to prove that they will always have their medicines with them when they leave the house. I give parents permission to nag their teens until the teens show that they've fully assumed the responsibility.

✔ **Discuss common scenarios.** Talk about the best way to handle specific events, such as a school dance, summer camp, hanging out at the mall, or going to parties. By drawing up a game plan well in advance, you may be able to avoid some risky surprises and create an experience that's less stressful and more enjoyable.

✔ **Rehearse difficult situations.** Knowing how to react in a specific situation before that situation arises is often critical in helping a teen make the right decisions and take the right actions. Role-play different scenarios — for example, say you're at a party with friends and someone offers you a cookie, what do you do? If you have a severe reaction, what would you do? If the teen might need epinephrine, have them use an expired autoinjector on an orange or grapefruit to demonstrate its use.

✔ **Analyze past mistakes.** Teens should open up to their parents about situations they've encountered and mistakes they've made without the threat of punishment hanging over them. Parents can then suggest a potentially more effective course of action for the next time a similar situation arises.

✔ **Analyze past reactions.** Discuss what happened and how you can prevent it from happening again. This proves to parents that the teen is mature enough to use past mistakes to build future successes. I tell all my patients that we all make mistakes and that reactions happen no matter how hard you try to prevent them. Success is measured not simply by the ability to prevent a reaction but also by the ability to learn how to more effectively prevent and deal with future reactions.

We all need to recognize that gaining independence is a process for both the teen and the parents. Teenagers are often ready, willing, and even able to be independent all at once. Parents may not be ready, willing, or able to accept that independence, and they're rarely willing to accept it all at once. Take it one step at a time and be patient with one another. Realize that in a way, you're both raising each other.

Getting a Little Help from Your Friends

Managing a food allergy is a team sport. Naturally, as a teenager, you may want to cut your parents from the team and take on more of the responsibility yourself. When you choose to do that, however, fill the empty slot with someone who's more capable, at this stage of the game, to assist you.

You don't have to tell everyone that you have a food allergy, but let your closest friends know about it. Describe the symptoms of an allergic reaction, review prevention strategies, and explain what they should do if you experience a reaction when you're together. Having a responsible friend keep an eye on you may calm your parents and make them more willing to let you wander a little farther from their protective embrace.

Friends can form a protective shield around you without making you feel like a little kid. I frequently see friends who are far more willing to speak up about the food allergy than the person with the allergy. I see friends who will virtually attack a restaurant waiter and even go in to inspect the kitchen while the allergic teen is too shy to ask a single question. I see friends show up at appointments to learn more about food allergy. I've even seen friends head off to college together, so the friend can keep her pal safe on campus. Ask one of your closest friends to be a pal, as explained in the following sidebar, "Be A PAL."

Be A PAL

FAAN has formalized the value of friends with its Be A PAL (Protect A Life from food allergy) program. The program encourages those with food allergies to teach their friends about what they can do to help prevent a reaction and what to do should a reaction occur. According to FAAN, your PAL should know the following:

✔ The foods you need to avoid.

✔ That foods can be hidden in unexpected places, so you need to ask questions about what's in the food and how it's prepared.

✔ The symptoms you may have when experiencing an allergic reaction.

✔ The medicine you need to take if you have a reaction and where you keep it.

✔ What to do and who to call in case you have a reaction.

Nothing is more important to teens than their friends, so make your friends an integral part of your support network and protection program. I encourage all my patients with food allergy, especially teens, to talk to their friends and teach them about food allergy. I have seen friends prevent numerous reactions and take quick action in the face of reactions. Every time I witness or hear about a friend saving a friend from an allergic reaction, I realize what a beautiful thing friendship can be.

Mastering the Art of Acceptable Risk Taking

Unrestrained joy, unfettered impulse, and a fair amount of risk taking are part of the beauty of youth. Unfortunately, risk taking often manifests itself in unacceptable and life-threatening ways, particularly with food allergies. A recent study reveals that an alarming number of teenagers with food allergies admit to purposefully ingesting problem foods, and that many teens also fail to carry their medications with them. Perhaps this is why fatal food reactions are most common among adolescents and young adults.

Now, I'm not one to throw a wet blanket on spontaneous teenage exuberance, but I do get more than a little concerned when I hear about teenagers knowingly ingesting suspect foods and not carrying their medications. In fact, I'm dumfounded when I hear such things, because in order to continue taking risks as a teenager, living another day is rather important. By figuring out how to take less life-threatening risks, you can pack a lot more acceptably risky activities into your life.

Teenagers rarely intentionally take risks with their food allergies. Few teenagers knowingly ingest problem foods to see what will happen or head out of the house without their epinephrine autoinjectors for the thrill of it. In most cases, they simply have an overwhelming and very understandable need to fit in and be "normal." The best way to achieve a sense of normalcy is to make food allergy feel more normal. Increased education and open communication between food allergic teens and their parents, friends, and doctor can increase the sense of normalcy and help teens master their independence while at the same time staying happy, relaxed, and safe.

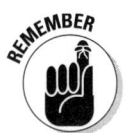

While life is never entirely risk-free, knowingly ingesting a suspect food or conveniently forgetting to carry life-saving medications is never acceptable. The key is to find out which risks are okay and which are not and then do whatever you can to limit the risks. While eating out may never be risk free, for example, carefully choosing a restaurant and asking the right questions can make eating out an acceptable risk. Eating dessert, however, no matter how tempting or how much your date pushes you to do so, may never be an acceptable risk.

Documented food allergy risk taking

Researchers from the Mount Sinai School of Medicine and FAAN used an anonymous questionnaire to survey 174 food allergy patients between the ages of 13 and 21.

The survey data revealed that more than half of the respondents admitted to knowingly consuming a potentially unsafe food. Only 61 percent always carried their epinephrine. Carrying rates varied by activities or circumstances. Activities such as traveling and going to restaurants had high carrying rates. However, the rates were much lower for certain peer-related social activities, such as going to a friend's home, participating in sports activities, wearing tight clothing, or attending a school dance.

The majority of respondents also indicated that education of their friends would make living with a food allergy easier. However, they did not want to educate their peers themselves. The researchers also concluded that patients who take the most risks by eating problem foods and not carrying epinephrine are the ones who are likely to feel "different" because of their food allergies.

Laying Down Some Safe Dating Guidelines

A food allergy can certainly cramp your style on a date. Fortunately, by agreeing to a few key dating rules up front, you can make your date safer, more enjoyable, and perhaps even make you slightly less anxious:

- ✔ **Let your date know about your allergy.** In addition to assisting you in avoiding problem foods, your date may need to know about your food allergy to save your life in the event that you experience a severe reaction. If you're nervous about what to say, practice with a friend what you should say and how to say it.

- ✔ **Keep your explanation brief.** No need for a full medical history or a dissertation on food allergy. Your date should understand, however, that an allergic reaction could be very serious.

- ✔ **Discuss the limitations up front.** Let your date know which foods you can and cannot eat and which restaurants you can eat at. Clearly explain other restrictions before the date moves too far along. You may, for example, tell your date that you are allergic to peanuts and she needs to avoid eating peanuts and to brush her teeth and wash her hands if she has eaten peanuts before the date. I know, telling your date to be sure to brush her teeth and wash her hands may take some of the romance out of the evening, but it may also keep you out of the emergency room, which is not the most romantic place, either.

Eating out

Eating out, especially on a first date, always generates some anxiety. In a public restaurant, few people like to call attention to themselves, particularly when trying to impress a date. The trick here is to follow the rules discussed in Chapter 11 in a way that's a little less obvious but just as effective. Here are some suggestions that can make your dinner out safe without making you feel as though you're eating on stage in the spotlight:

- **Steer clear of risky restaurants.** If you're allergic to fish or shellfish, and your date or your friends seem to be leaning toward seafood, steer them in a different direction before the decision process gets too far along. (This is when it really helps to have a PAL on your side.) The same goes for Asian foods and peanut allergy. If you have a milk allergy, your date needs to know up front that finding a safe restaurant may be very difficult.

- **Pick a restaurant well in advance.** Do as much legwork as possible before you even get to the restaurant. If possible, pick a place you've dealt with before and always call ahead of time and speak with the manager or chef. Preparation well in advance streamlines the ordering process.

- **Keep your date and your friends at ease.** To handle unplanned meetings at restaurants, let your friends or your date know that they should not be offended if you join them for dinner without ordering anything. You may simply order a soda or water or eat a snack you brought from home.

- **Carry a chef's card.** The first chef's card was created by a very smart teenager who had severe food allergy and hated to ask too many questions publicly. A chef's card does not replace calling ahead and asking questions but it can streamline the process of ordering your meal and may allow you to get a safe meal without calling much attention to your allergy. Chapter 11 provides a sample chef's card.

Acquiring a few safe-kissing skills

Not to be an alarmist, but when you have a severe food allergy, even a "harmless" kiss can be fatal. In 2006, a teenager in Canada died of an apparent allergic reaction that may have occurred after kissing her boyfriend who had just eaten peanut.

Before this incident occurred, I warned my patients about kissing. Now, this is often the first question that parents of teenagers ask me. The teens themselves don't ask the question. In fact, they're often mortified when their parents ask this embarrassing question, but they do listen intently to the answer.

A fatal kiss

Can a kiss actually contain enough of an allergen to cause a fatal reaction? This is the question that researchers sought to answer in a recent study. The answer they arrived at is "Yes," individuals with food allergies are at risk of experiencing a reaction when kissing someone who has recently eaten the food to which they are allergic.

The researchers measured the level of peanut allergen in an individual's saliva after eating a peanut butter sandwich — both before and after the participants brushed their teeth. The study found that despite tooth brushing, allergen levels were detectable for up to four hours after a participant ate peanut butter. The study's authors concluded that in addition to brushing their teeth, individuals who have consumed a food should wait several hours before kissing someone who's allergic to that food.

Anyone with a food allergy and everyone who's in a close relationship with someone who has a food allergy should consider the risk. While it may be an uncomfortable topic to bring up, it's definitely more comfortable to talk about it than to have a reaction. Be honest and open. If your date really cares about you, she'll understand and want to learn about what she can do to keep you safe.

When you're just getting to know someone, you may not feel quite ready to tell the person about your food allergy. That's perfectly understandable. Until you're ready to open up about your food allergy, however, stay on the safe side by following these precautions:

- ✔ **Avoid food-related activities.** For example, plan dates before or after mealtimes.

- ✔ **If you eat, make sure you both eat only safe foods.** Consider packing a picnic lunch.

- ✔ **Hold off on the kissing.** Avoid kissing until you can be honest with your date and feel that your date will respect your food restrictions.

When you do get ready to kiss, make sure your date knows how serious your food allergy is and what he or she needs to do in order to prevent you from having a reaction. Many teens tell me that their date has agreed to avoid the allergy-causing food on days when they will be hanging out together. Others say their boyfriends or girlfriends have cut the allergen out of their diets entirely.

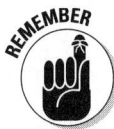

Dating is all about spending time with a person you like to learn whether you are comfortable with each other. If your date isn't understanding or is pressuring you to take chances that might harm you, he may not be right for you! On the other hand, if your new boyfriend makes an effort to learn about food allergy and is genuinely concerned, he should automatically score a few points with you (and your parents).

Chapter 15

Preventing and Outgrowing a Food Allergy

*F*ood allergies are not the most predictable of illnesses. In some families, one child becomes allergic to peanut on his first exposure to it, while a half dozen of his siblings can chow down on peanuts without the slightest hint of a reaction. A milk allergy becomes a lifelong companion to some, while other kids suffer through a few milk-sensitive years and then can chug a carton of milk without incident.

We (doctors and researchers) can't reliably predict the onset of food allergy or the course it will eventually take, but we can provide some advice on possible strategies for preventing its onset and perhaps hastening its departure.

This chapter explores the possibility of preventing food allergy in the first place. It then delves into the likelihood of someone outgrowing an existing food allergy. Here, I rank your chances of shaking a food allergy based on the food or foods you react to and your sensitivity to those foods. I reveal various techniques that may hasten the "cure." And I guide you through the process of safely introducing problem foods . . . with the approval and assistance of your doctor, of course.

Preventing Food Allergies: Hope or Hype?

The dramatic increase in the prevalence of food allergies over the past 20 years or so proves that the medical community hasn't exactly made great strides in the prevention department. But we're hard at work trying to figure out why food allergies are on the rise and what we can do to prevent the onset of these allergies.

In the following sections, I provide a brief overview of what we currently know in the areas of food allergy prevention and point out the most promising studies. Families that have a history of allergies may be able to improve the chances that their children, especially their youngest children, can avoid the onset of food allergy and perhaps other allergic conditions, including asthma, by following the recommendations offered here.

The only two prevention strategies I recommend unconditionally are breast-feeding (over bottle feeding) and the avoidance of tobacco smoke. These two strategies can't guarantee that your child will successfully dodge the food allergy bullet, but they can improve the odds.

Stressing early intervention

Food allergies typically arise in the first two years of a child's life, so prevention strategies focus on these critical years. For high-risk families (families with a history of allergic conditions, including asthma and allergic rhinitis), many doctors recommend avoiding highly allergenic foods, including milk, egg, and peanut, in the first two years of an infant's life. Sometimes, doctors also recommend that breastfeeding mothers avoid eating high-risk foods over the duration of the breastfeeding years.

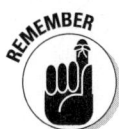

No studies have proven conclusively that strict avoidance is effective in preventing the onset of food allergies. In fact, a certain amount of exposure at the right time may be beneficial, but since we don't know how much exposure at what age is optimum, and because the ideal amount of exposure and the ideal age may vary from one person to another, we generally recommend that high-risk families avoid high-risk foods during the critical ages — up to three years of age.

Focusing on baby formulas

Because food allergy is more prevalent in developed countries, especially in children, we asked ourselves, "What's different about the way we raise children in developed countries?" One difference that immediately pops up on the radar screen is that instead of breastfeeding their children, parents in developed countries rely more heavily on baby formula, most of which is manufactured from — you guessed it — cow's milk.

Tiffani Hayes, a pediatric nutritionist, and I published an article in September of 2005, in which we reviewed the data from several studies on baby formulas. What we discovered is that alternatives to cow's milk formulas — including extensively hydrolyzed casein formulas and partially hydrolyzed whey formulas — are appropriate alternatives to breast milk for allergy prevention in infants at risk.

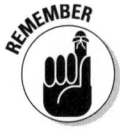

Because nobody can predict the onset of any allergy-related disease in any family, parents who cannot or choose not to breastfeed should consider the use of extensively hydrolyzed casein formulas and partially hydrolyzed whey formulas — hypoallergenic baby formulas. This becomes even more important for families who have other children with allergic diseases such as atopic dermatitis (eczema), food allergy, asthma, and allergic rhinitis. Consult your doctor prior to giving birth to discuss the pros and cons of breastfeeding and different types of baby formulas.

Clearing the smoke from the room

One of the few factors that have been proven without a doubt to contribute to the onset of all types of allergies and asthma is cigarette smoke. If any of the thousands of other good reasons to quit smoking can't convince someone to give up smoking for good, perhaps the fact that cigarette smoke has been proven to increase a child's vulnerability to allergic conditions will be sufficient.

Taking action to prevent the onset of food allergies and asthma

Parents in families that have a strong history of food allergy and asthma are often highly motivated to do whatever it takes to prevent the onset of food allergies and asthma in all their children. The problem with giving strict recommendations, however, is that we currently have very little conclusive proof on preventive strategies that work. Recommending questionable prevention strategies can lead to other problems, such as malnutrition, or simply waste your time and money on something that's not effective.

My recommendation is to study the evidence for yourself, discuss the options with your doctor, keep up on the latest breakthroughs in food allergy research, and make the choices that you think are best for your child. In the following list, I describe prevention strategies we've studied. The most effective strategies are listed first followed by more questionable options:

- ✔ **Avoid tobacco smoke.** Tobacco smoke is proven to contribute to the onset of all allergy-related conditions. Avoiding exposure to tobacco smoke, especially in the early years of life, can help stave off asthma, food allergies, and other allergy-related conditions.

- ✔ **Breastfeed exclusively.** If possible, avoid baby formula for at least the first six months of your infant's life. If you must use formula, choose a hypo-allergenic formula. Although breastfeeding has not been conclusively proven to prevent food allergies, it is far safer than cow's milk and has so many other health benefits that doctors don't hesitate to recommend it.

- ✔ **Use hypo-allergenic baby formulas.** This is a good idea for all families who cannot or choose not to breastfeed or as a supplement to breastfeeding.

- ✔ **Restrict your diet while pregnant or breastfeeding.** Some studies show that this is effective, and some don't. I recommend that all mothers consider avoiding peanut and tree nuts during the last trimester of pregnancy and while breast feeding, especially mothers in high-risk families. I do not routinely recommend restricting other common allergens, such as milk and egg, since the evidence is not strong enough to justify putting the mother or baby at nutritional risk.

- ✔ **Introduce probiotics.** Probiotics are beneficial bacteria, such as those in yogurt. Some evidence shows that probiotics may help in preventing the onset of food allergies. Refer to Chapter 9 for details on probiotics.

- ✔ **Waiting to introduce solid foods in the baby's diet.** Some studies have shown this to be effective, and others have not. I recommend that babies in high-risk families not be started on solids until 6 months of age.

Ranking the Likelihood of Outgrowing an Allergy Food by Food

A majority of children, even those with the most severe food allergies, often simply outgrow their allergy. When this occurs, what exactly happened to make the person less sensitive to the problem food? We don't know for sure. All we know is that sometimes the body makes a few internal adjustments and the immune system stops overreacting to a particular food.

What are your or your child's chances of outgrowing a food allergy? I can't say for sure on a case-by-case basis. Some food allergies are easier to outgrow, and some people's bodies seem better equipped than others to outgrow a food allergy. I can, however, reveal some factors that may increase your chances of outgrowing a food allergy, such as the type of food and the severity of the reactions. In the following sections, I explore the chances of outgrowing each of the most common food allergies.

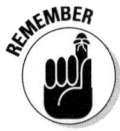

In general, the less severe your food allergy, the more likely you are to outgrow it.

Charting your chances with cow's milk

In the United States, cow's milk allergy affects about 2.5 percent of children during their first two years of life. Fortunately, most kids (approximately 80 percent) will eventually outgrow their milk allergy, most within a few years of their diagnosis.

Food allergy's growing tenacity

Based on my observations, I'm afraid that food allergies are becoming not only more common over the years but also more tenacious. I don't have any official studies or data to back me up, but I've noticed that over the past decade or so, fewer people seem to be outgrowing their food allergies.

Fortunately we now have studies underway to try to explain this trend and shed some light on why this phenomenon is occurring, assuming it really is occurring. Perhaps the answers will lead to a future cure or more effective treatments. Stay tuned.

Your chance of outgrowing milk allergy depends a great deal on whether your allergy is IgE-mediated or not:

- ✔ Non-IgE mediated cow's milk allergy is almost always a transient condition that passes with age. Non-IgE mediated milk allergy typically causes more subtle, delayed symptoms, such as allergic colitis, as discussed in Chapter 7.

- ✔ IgE-mediated cow's milk allergy is a more stubborn variety that persists in about 20 percent of children, maybe more.

If you or your child has milk allergy, ask the doctor to specify whether it is IgE-mediated or non-IgE-mediated. Outgrowing a non-IgE-mediated milk allergy is almost guaranteed. Time is on your side. If the milk allergy is IgE-mediated, then track the levels of M-IgE (milk-specific IgE) from one year to the next and look for a significant drop in M-IgE levels. Studies show that people with a higher percentage drop in the M-IgE level in a single year are more likely to develop a milk tolerance regardless of how high their M-IgE level when first diagnosed. In one study, a percentage drop of 50, 75, 90, and 99 percent correlated with a 31, 45, 66, and 99 percent chance of passing a milk challenge, respectively. Once your M-IgE level drops far enough, your doctor may want to consider performing a food challenge to determine whether you've outgrown your milk allergy.

Outgrowing an allergy to eggs

In the United States, egg allergy affects about 1 to 2 percent of children. As with milk allergy, however, a majority of kids outgrow egg allergy within a few years:

- ✔ About half of those diagnosed with egg allergy outgrow the allergy within a couple years.

- ✔ About two thirds outgrow the allergy by the time they're five.

- ✔ Even more children become less sensitive to eggs, even if they don't completely outgrow the allergy.

As with cow's milk allergy, the rate at which egg-specific IgE (E-IgE) levels drop may determine the likelihood that a child has outgrown the allergy. In a group of children who developed egg allergy before the age of four, the percentage drop in E-IgE in one year correlated with the likelihood that the child would pass a food challenge performed at that time. An E-IgE drop of 50, 75, 90, and 99 percent correlated with a 52, 65, 78, and 95 percent chance of passing the food challenge, respectively. As with milk allergy, if your E-IgE level falls sufficiently, performing a food challenge for egg may confirm a developing tolerance for egg.

Winning out against wheat and soy allergies

Although we haven't performed specific studies on the likelihood of outgrowing a wheat or soy allergy, the prognosis for outgrowing either allergy is very positive:

- 80–90 percent of those with a wheat or soy allergy outgrow the allergy by the age of five or six years.

- In a study of children with food allergy and allergy-related dermatitis, 50 percent of the children with soy allergy outgrew it in a year, and 67 percent outgrew it within two years. Only 25 percent of the children with wheat allergy outgrew their allergy within a year, and only 33 percent outgrew the wheat allergy within two years.

As with milk and egg, those who are more sensitive to soy and wheat may have a more difficult time outgrowing their allergies.

Overpowering a peanut allergy

Until recently, most food allergy specialists concurred that people rarely, if ever, outgrew a peanut allergy, and almost every study supported that belief. Relatively recently, however, new studies have shown that approximately 20 to 25 percent of people who have peanut allergy eventually outgrow it.

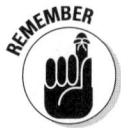

What does this mean for you or your child who's been diagnosed with peanut allergy? It means that outgrowing peanut allergy is rather unlikely, but don't give up hope, and don't let anyone convince you that outgrowing a peanut allergy is impossible. A substantial percentage of people lose their sensitivity to peanut, so I recommend asking your doctor to reevaluate you or your child at least once a year, at least up to the age of six years:

- Test PN-IgE levels annually and monitor these levels over time. Low or undetectable levels of PN-IgEa are a pretty good indication that you've outgrown a peanut allergy, but about 30 percent of those with low or even undetectable levels of PN-IgE still experience reactions.

Fighting peanut allergy with peanuts?!

The funny thing about a peanut allergy is that if you outgrow the allergy and then continue to avoid peanuts, you may actually be more likely to become allergic to peanuts again.

We performed a follow-up study in 36 patients who had a clear history of peanut allergy. Of the 36 patients, three of them (8 percent) experienced a recurrence of peanut allergy after having successfully passed a peanut challenge. A six-year-old girl was representative of the three who experienced a relapse. When she was a year old, she ate a peanut butter cracker. Within five minutes, she broke out in hives and her face swelled up. Her PN-IgE level at diagnosis was 2.79 kUA/L, and she had no history of other food allergies. At age 4.5 years, her PN-IgE level was 1.1 kUA/L, and she passed a peanut challenge. She subsequently ate only "may contain peanut" products until approximately 1.8 years after the initial challenge.

One day, she decided to eat some Butterfinger ice cream. Within 15 minutes of taking two bites of the ice cream, she developed hives, coughing, difficulty breathing, throat tightness, abdominal pain, vomiting, and diarrhea. A repeat PN-IgE level was greater than 100 kUA/L. All three patients who relapsed after successfully passing the peanut challenge consumed concentrated peanut products less than once a month. In other words, the patients who relapsed had avoided peanuts!

In contrast, none of a group of 23 patients who ate peanut more frequently after having passed their peanut challenge had recurrent peanut allergy. Thus, infrequent exposure may be a risk factor for re-sensitization. This may also be why recurrence is virtually unheard of with other common food allergies, such as milk and egg. Even if you hate milk after outgrowing your allergy, you're probably getting some form of concentrated milk on a regular basis, because it's such a common ingredient.

✔ If you haven't had a reaction in the past year or two and your PN-IgE level tests below 2 kUA/L, discuss with your doctor the possibility of an oral peanut challenge to determine if you've outgrown your peanut allergy.

✔ If you pass the peanut challenge, consult with your doctor about eating peanut regularly. Not eating peanut regularly may be a risk factor for re-sensitization, as explained in the following sidebar.

Don't try this at home. Food challenges, particularly peanut challenges, should always be performed in a controlled setting with emergency medications readily available.

Shaking a tree nut allergy

Tree nut allergy may actually be tougher to outgrow than peanut allergy, although few studies prove it. In our own study, we found that about 9 percent (9 of 101) children with tree nut allergy outgrew their allergy. The rate of resolution corresponded to the TN-IgE (tree nut specific IgE) level:

- ✔ TN-IgE level below 5 kUA/L, 58 percent resolution.
- ✔ TN-IgE level below 2 kUA/L, 63 percent resolution.
- ✔ Undetectable TN-IgE level, 75 percent resolution.

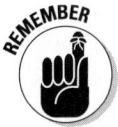

As with peanut allergy, monitor your TN-IgE level closely from one year to the next. If the TN-IgE level drops below 5 kUA/L, consult with your doctor to determine if a tree nut challenge would be advisable.

Surmounting a seed allergy

Allergies to sesame, sunflower, or other types of seeds tend to persist, although no studies provide conclusive evidence to support this. Your doctor may want to monitor your IgE levels for sesame and perform a sesame challenge if your IgE level drops, but we have no specific sesame-specific IgE levels or percentage drops to recommend for testing.

Overcoming other food allergies

Milk, egg, and peanut are the main players in childhood food allergies. Wheat, soy, and sesame play relatively minor roles. Some other foods make cameo appearances. These include certain fruits, vegetables, and cereal grains other than wheat. Fortunately, most kids outgrow allergies to fruits, veggies, and grains within a period of six to 12 months. Many of the reactions may represent intolerances or irritant reactions rather than true food allergy. Of course, in at least a few cases, children do develop severe IgE-mediated allergies to these foods that may persist.

I haven't said much about seafood (fish and shellfish) up to this point, because seafood allergies more commonly develop later in life. In any event, seafood allergies are perhaps the most tenacious of the bunch. Estimates of seafood allergy resolution range from 3.5 percent for fish to 4 percent for shellfish.

Whipping multiple food allergies

Some kids seem to be allergic to everything — milk, egg, wheat, peanut, you name it. You may think that these poor kids are just destined to remain allergic to everything. Well, that assumption holds some truth — as a general rule, multiple food allergies may slightly reduce your ability to outgrow any food allergy, but an inability to outgrow one food allergy doesn't affect your ability to outgrow a different food allergy.

We found this rather surprising. When we began our studies, we predicted that if a child could not outgrow a food allergy that was relatively easy to outgrow, such as milk or egg, the child would never outgrow a stubborn peanut allergy. Boy, were we wrong. Several children we studied had persistent milk or egg allergy but managed to lose their peanut allergy. Go figure.

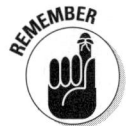

Your chances of outgrowing one food allergy has nothing to do with your ability or inability to outgrow another food allergy. Monitor all your food-specific IgE levels and treat each food allergy as a separate condition.

Accounting for other allergic conditions

Having other allergic conditions, such as asthma or eczema or hay fever, may also reduce the chance of outgrowing a food allergy. In other words, a child with just food allergy may have better odds of outgrowing his food allergy than a child with food allergy plus asthma or eczema. Most children, however, have other allergy-related conditions in addition to their food allergy, so studying food allergy in isolation is a bit difficult.

The results of our studies showed that the presence of other allergic conditions reduced the chances of outgrowing some food allergies, such as milk, but the presence of other allergic conditions did not affect the likelihood of outgrowing peanut allergy.

Speculating on the Timing

When patients and their parents hear the good news that food allergies can be outgrown, they often ask how long it'll take — a year, two years, five years? Timing is tough to predict. Some children outgrow a milk allergy before they're out of diapers. Others have to wait until they get their driver's license. A number of less fortunate food allergy sufferers never seem to shake their allergy.

Nobody can accurately predict the date and time you can expect to outgrow your food allergy or even guarantee that you'll outgrow it, but I can give you a general idea of what to expect based on IgE levels and exposure:

✔ In our studies, the best predictor of timing is the level of food-specific IgE. For example, consider three two-year-olds with milk or egg allergy who have IgE levels (RASTs) of 1, 15, and 75 (all on a scale of 0 to 100). The child with the level of 1 is likely to outgrow the food allergy very soon, if she hasn't done so already. The child with the level of 15 could still outgrow her allergy, but it'll probably take her at least three years. The child with the level of 75 is unlikely to outgrow her allergy, but if it were to happen, it would take at least five to seven years.

✔ Another predictor is how a patient responds to a food challenge or accidental exposure. If a child reacts to a tiny exposure, for example, especially if it is a significant reaction, he is likely to be at least a few years away from outgrowing the allergy, no matter what the other test results say. On the other hand, someone who tolerates more of the food before reacting is logically closer to losing the allergy.

These predictors are just that — indications of the likelihood of outgrowing a food allergy in a certain period of time. They offer no money-back guarantee. As I said earlier in this chapter, some people with undetectable levels of a food-specific IgE may continue to react to the food.

Prodding Your Allergy to Vacate Sooner

Food allergies are like uninvited guests who stay long past their welcome. So, how do you get them to leave? The best advice I can offer is based on the best information we currently have — strictly avoid the problem food.

In practice, some children rapidly outgrow their food allergies without strict avoidance, while others fail to outgrow their food allergies despite the most stringent diets. Because strict avoidance is so difficult, understanding the impact of continued exposure on the natural history of food allergy would be helpful. However, until we do, the majority of children with food allergy are more likely to benefit from strict avoidance, at least to dodge symptoms and hopefully to hasten the departure of their food allergies.

Strict avoidance has been the mainstay of food allergy management and continues to be the best treatment approach to prevent reactions, keep the condition from worsening, and hasten the process of becoming allergy-free. This advice, however, may change in the future, as we gather more data and explore other treatment options.

Monitoring and Managing Your Allergies

You and your doctor should keep an eye on your food allergies and tweak the treatment approach as your body adjusts. This is particularly important when treating food allergies in children, because children are more likely to outgrow their food allergy and because they're more dependent on certain foods for normal growth and development. To stay abreast of the changing nature of food allergies in your child, work with your doctor to:

- Ensure proper nutrition, growth, and development.

- Track accidental exposures and reactions to ensure that avoidance measures are adequate and that you're recognizing reactions promptly and treating them appropriately.

- Have sufficient supplies of fresh emergency medications, including epinephrine autoinjectors, for home and for your child's daycare, school, and wherever else she spends time.

- Ensure that all caregivers understand the allergy management plan and emergency medical treatment plan. Your doctor should provide you with an allergy management plan in writing.

- Evaluate your child regularly to determine whether she's outgrown her food allergy. In our clinic, we typically test once a year, but longer or shorter intervals may be more appropriate is some situations. A child with a reaction to fruit, for example, may be evaluated every six months, whereas an older child with persistent peanut allergy may not require annual testing after the first few years if he shows no sign of improvement.

Your child's allergist may choose any of several methods to evaluate your child for the disappearance of food allergy, including information on accidental exposures, skin-prick testing, in-vitro testing, or blood tests. No single method has proven most effective. In our clinic, we typically rely on clinical history and CAP-RAST (FEIA) testing to monitor food allergy progression in our patients. We generally do not perform repeat skin testing, because we think it doesn't change our management in the majority of cases, although other centers perform repeat skin testing on a regular basis.

If a child hasn't had a reaction in the past six to 12 months, I recommend that the child be re-evaluated in the following ways based on the problem food:

- **IgE-mediated cow's milk or egg:** About 50 percent of children who have a milk or egg allergy shake the allergy by the age of 6 years old. We recommend retesting yearly with CAP-RAST testing. The rate of decline can predict the likelihood that a challenge will be negative. We usually offer a food challenge for milk and egg when the M-IgE or E-IgE level is less than 2 kUA/L, which gives the patient an approximately 50 percent chance of passing the challenge.

✔ **Non-IgE-mediated milk or egg:** Kids tend to outgrow non-IgE-mediated milk and egg allergies more quickly. If the child has had no recent reactions from accidental exposure, a careful challenge is warranted by the age of two or three years old. Be careful, though. If your child has been diagnosed with food-protein induced enterocolitis syndrome (FPIES), reintroducing milk or egg poses a significant potential risk. Prior to reintroducing milk or egg, your doctor should perform a careful food challenge under close supervision in a hospital setting.

✔ **Peanut or tree nuts:** If you have a peanut or tree nut allergy, consult your doctor to obtain annual CAP-RAST testing. If your TN- or PN-IgE level is less than 2 kUA/L, you and your doctor may consider a supervised challenge. If the challenge confirms that you've outgrown your peanut or tree nut allergy, your doctor may advise you to eat the problem nut at least once a month to prevent re-sensitization. We don't know the optimal amount you should eat, but we generally recommend a single serving — for example, the amount of peanut in a peanut butter sandwich or a candy bar with nuts. Follow up with your doctor for at least a year to ensure that you're not experiencing recurrent symptoms. In patients with persistent peanut allergy, or if the CAP-RAST remains unchanged for several years, less frequent testing is usually sufficient.

✔ **Wheat and soy:** Children usually outgrow their wheat and soy allergies more quickly than allergies to milk or egg. If your child has a wheat or soy allergy, see your doctor yearly for reevaluation with CAP-RAST testing. When wheat- or soy-specific IgE levels are low, you and your doctor may consider attempting a supervised food challenge. "Low" levels for wheat and soy are not as well-defined as they are for other common allergenic foods.

✔ **Other foods:** If you're allergic to some other food not included in this list, we recommend annual evaluations and testing. As mentioned previously, repeat evaluation can be less frequent if the allergy is showing little sign of improvement.

Testing negative doesn't mean you've outgrown your allergy, nor does testing positive mean that you still have it. A negative test merely enables you and your doctor to gauge the likelihood that you've outgrown your food allergy and that a food challenge may be safe and useful. Only by successfully passing a food challenge can you be certain that the allergy is gone.

Never perform a food challenge on your own — proceed with caution under your doctor's supervision, and with full emergency equipment and medications on hand to treat possible reactions.

Safely Reintroducing the Problem Foods

Say you've managed to raise your child with a severe food allergy for a couple years. You've mastered the fine art of avoidance. Your kid doesn't mind not eating a particular food. In fact, he seems to dislike the food. Why would you even consider taking the risk of re-introducing the problem food? Why not leave well-enough alone? I have several good answers to offer for that question:

✔ Knowing that your child has outgrown the food allergy can reduce your family's anxiety.

✔ Your child automatically increases the variety of foods he can safely consume.

✔ By not knowing that your child has outgrown the food allergy, you may increase the risk that your child will become re-sensitized to the food.

Based on your child's history, the severity of past reactions, the most recent test results, and the problem food, your doctor may decide that your child is ready for a food challenge or for you to try to re-introduce the food at home (if the risk of a severe reaction is very low).

If your doctor recommends that you re-introduce the problem food at home and you're not comfortable doing that, request a supervised food challenge in the doctor's office. If your child passes the food challenge without incident, you're likely to be less worried about adding the food to your child's diet. I rarely recommend introducing the food at home if the child has a peanut allergy or has had acute reactions to the problem food until the child passes a food challenge.

Confronting your allergies with food challenges

Although CAP-RAST tests provide a fairly good indication of whether you've outgrown an allergy, they offer no guarantee. You can have low food-specific IgE levels and still experience an allergic reaction, or you can have relatively high food-specific IgE levels and safely consume the food. The only way to be certain that you've outgrown your food allergy is to try eating the problem food — challenge your system.

The problem with challenging your system with a food that has made you ill before is that it can be somewhat risky, particularly if you experienced severe reactions in the past. To increase safety, we normally perform a food challenge in our clinic under doctor's supervision with emergency equipment and medication on hand.

What can you expect from a food challenge? A food challenge typically proceeds as follows:

1. Your doctor or your doctor's assistant feeds you a specific amount of the problem food that you're likely to tolerate.

2. You sit in the room for a period of time under close observation for any signs of a reaction. (If you react, the doctor or assistant obviously treats you for the reaction.)

3. Pass the food challenge, and the doctor sends you home with instructions for safely re-introducing the food at home. Usually you start with the amount of food that you ate during the food challenge and then gradually ramp up the dose over the course of a week or more.

Inviting problem foods into your home

If your doctor recommends introducing the food into your child's diet at home, follow the doctor's instructions carefully and proceed slowly. Gradually increase the amount of the problem food in the diet over the course of 1 to 2 weeks. When introducing milk into the diet, I typically advise parents to start with one teaspoon on the first day or two and then double the dose every one to two days. If you get up to 4 to 6 ounces in a day with no reaction you're probably home free.

Once you can tolerate a full serving of the food over a period of several days, your doctor is likely to lift all restrictions, so you can consume all forms of the food.

Part IV
The Part of Tens

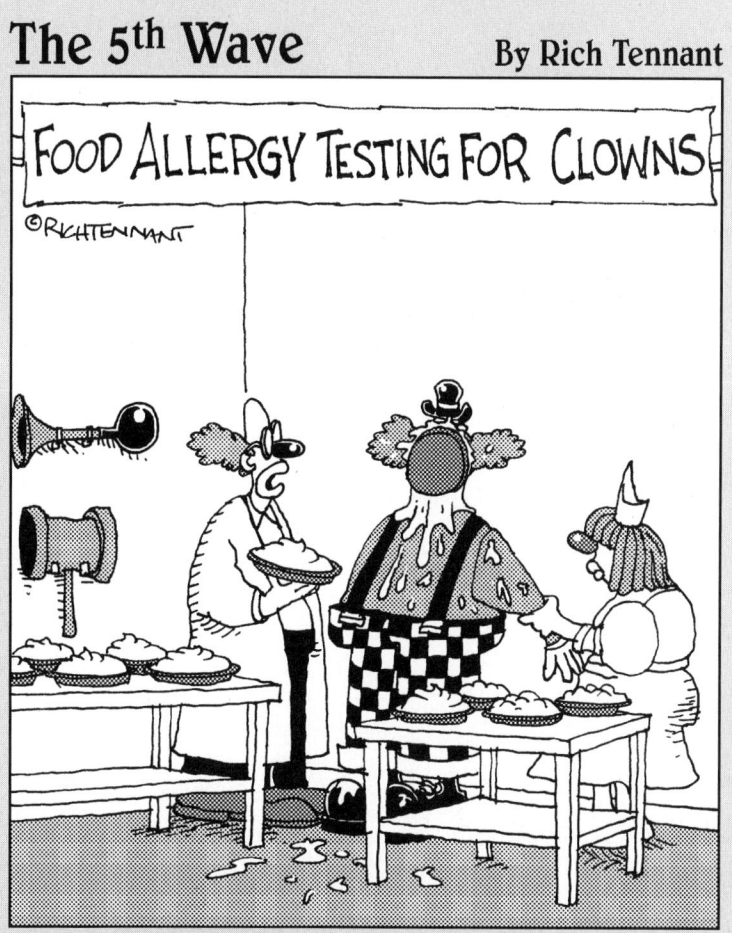

FOOD ALLERGY TESTING FOR CLOWNS

"Well, you're not allergic to banana cream..."

In this part . . .

At the end of every *For Dummies* guide is a Part of Tens — a veritable dessert tray that complements the main course and packs your belly to bursting with practical tips, tricks, and advice.

This Part of Tens is no different. Here you discover ten key food allergy lessons to pass along to your children, ten tips to enlighten your child's caregiver at daycare or preschool, ten common dietary substitutions to help out in the kitchen, and the top ten food allergy Web sites where you can gather even more advice and support.

Chapter 16

Teaching Your Child Ten Key Food Allergy Lessons

*R*aising children and teenagers who have food allergies is even more challenging than living with your own food allergy. Not only do you have to steer clear of problem foods in grocery stores and restaurants, but as a parent, you have to protect your child at school and after school and educate your child to protect herself and eventually take ownership of her food allergies. Moreover, you need to pull off this juggling act in a way that doesn't instill unnecessary fear and anxiety.

In this chapter, I reveal the top ten talking points that you, as a parent, should pass along to your allergic children to help them successfully handle their food allergies both physically and emotionally.

Finding Comfort in Numbers: Lots of People Have Food Allergies

One of the most frequently lodged childhood complaints is this: "That's not fair!" Parents, grandparents, teachers, and babysitters drill the fairness rule into kids from before the time the kids even learn the language. The rule is one of the critical lessons to learn in the socialization process. Without it, total chaos would certainly ensue. Adults would be wrestling in the streets, intentionally smashing into one another on the roads, and strangling their co-workers.

By about 5th grade, children slowly experience the epiphany that life isn't always fair. Children who have allergies often pick up on it much sooner — typically around the age of 3 or 4 years — when they realize that they can't eat everything that their friends and siblings are eating.

As a parent, the most you can do to overcome your child's frustration is to let your child realize that he's not alone. Following are some tips on how to help your child find comfort in numbers:

- ✓ **Tell your child that nearly 12 million people in the United States alone have food allergies.** That's a lot more people than she can count on her fingers and toes. Three million children in the United States have food allergies — that's about 1 in every 25 kids.

- ✓ **Connect with parents in your neighborhood who are struggling with food allergies in their families.** The more you network with other parents, the more you realize that you and your child are not the only people struggling with food allergies.

- ✓ **Join a local food allergy support group or create a mini-support group at your child's school.** In a support group your child has contact with other children in the neighborhood whom life is treating not so fairly. In the process of finding support for your child, you also gain support for yourself, along with some practical information and tips, allergist recommendations, and suggestions concerning other useful resources.

- ✓ **Encourage your child to visit FANKids (the Food Allergy & Anaphylaxis Network's Web site for kids) at** www.fankids.org **or FANTeen (Food Allergies in the Real World) at** www.faanteen.org. See Chapter 19 for more Web sites, including FAAN's main Web site.

 You can track down a local food allergy support group by asking your allergist, searching the Web, contacting FAAN, or talking with your allergist. Your county or city health agency may also be able to provide you with a list of local support groups.

Decoding Labels and Asking Questions

Children are often much more capable of taking on additional responsibility than we, as parents, give them credit for. From birth, they struggle to control their environment. As teenagers they often mutiny in an attempt to take control of your house. You can empower your children and teenagers to take more control of their food allergies by providing them with the information and tools they need to do the job:

- ✔ **As soon as your child can read, teach her how to read food labels, as I explain in Chapter 6.** Make a game out of it to see who can spot the hidden foods on a candy bar label or a box of cereal. Advise your child to read the label every time before unwrapping a food — manufacturers sometimes change the ingredients in a food, so just because a food *was* safe doesn't mean it's always safe.

- ✔ **Foster a sense of curiosity about food allergies by encouraging your child to ask questions.** By learning to ask questions, your child becomes less dependent on you for the answers. When she eventually ventures out on her own to a local eating establishment, she is better prepared to grill the cook and restaurant manager for information about what's in the food.

 Treat your child's food allergies matter-of-factly, with the detachment of a scientist. Children can quickly spot your fears, whether you express them verbally, in your tone of voice, or through your facial expressions or body language. I know that suppressing your own fears and concerns can be a monumental task, but do your best to keep them in check.

Teaching Your Friends a Thing or Two

Your child doesn't have to stand up in front of the entire second grade class and give a PowerPoint presentation on food allergies, but he may be able to gain acceptance and support by teaching classmates and friends about his food allergy. Encourage your child to engage her friends and playmates in discussions about her food allergies. Friends often prove to be great protectors, both medically and socially.

 Sometimes simply stating that you have a food allergy and that eating a particular food makes you sick is sufficient to spark a healthy dialogue with playmates.

Sitting at the Cleanest Table in the Cafeteria

As I explain in Chapter 3, allergens, including peanut protein are easily cleaned from cafeteria tables with common household cleaning solutions Not all school cafeterias, however, follow strict cleanliness guidelines, especially when they have multiple shifts of students shuffling in and out. Encourage your child to sit at the cleanest table in the cafeteria or ask one of the kitchen crew to wipe off the table before lunch.

To maximize safety without having to draw too much attention, consider packing wet wipes and a small placemat in your child's lunchbox, just in case. If your child has a peanut allergy, and the school has a peanut-free table, that may be the safest option and hopefully does not result in too much isolation. To limit the isolation factor, a friend who intentionally does not bring in peanut butter can sit with your child.

Eating Off a Plate or Napkin

Even if your child's school has a great food allergy policy in place and an immaculately clean cafeteria, encourage your child to eat off a small plate or a napkin, both at home and away from home. If a few errant scraps of food or allergen residue remains on a table, a plate or napkin can prevent them from finding their way into your child's meal. Besides, eating over a plate or napkin keeps everything a little cleaner. Packing a small placemat, as discussed in the previous section, is a great idea, but if you forget to pack it, a paper plate or napkin is usually available.

Steering Clear of Sloppy Eaters

You've been in a lunchroom, and you know that not all kids strive to achieve the same standards of lunchroom etiquette. If your child has severe reactions to peanut butter and happens to sit next to some kid who has peanut butter all over his hands and somehow can't keep his hands off other kids, a change in seating arrangements may be in order.

Advise your child to steer clear of any sloppy eaters, but if the sloppy eater happens to be your child's best friend, a little education may be in order.

Your child or a responsible adult may need to teach the friend a thing or two, as explained earlier in this chapter.

Avoiding Lunch Room Food Swaps and Food Fights

More trades occur in the average school cafeteria in an afternoon than in a day at the New York Stock Exchange. Sandwiches and snacks always look a little tastier when they're sitting on someone else's plate.

For a child who has food allergies, however, food swapping is taboo and may be dangerous. Your child has no way of knowing what's in a food that's not in its original wrapper, how that food was prepared, or what it touched between the other kid's house and the school. Make sure your child understands how important it is to eat only what he brings to the table — only foods that you, your child's parents, have approved.

Your child's school should have a no-tolerance policy concerning food fights. Some kids may think they're just having fun, but to subject a fellow student who has a severe food allergy to a food fight is borderline assault.

Stocking up on Some Healthy, Yet Yummie Snacks

Up until junior high, most schools are party schools . . . at least some of the time. Teachers celebrate birthdays, Valentine's day, Halloween, and parents send in all sorts of goodies for the class. To enable your child to participate fully in the festivities, send in some allergen-free snacks on the day of the party. Better yet, deliver a small supply of snacks for the teacher to keep on hand, or volunteer to make treats for the whole class. I know many mothers of food allergic children who have simply become the baker for all parties.

Ask the teacher to send a letter home to parents explaining that a child in the class has a particular food allergy and informing them that when their snack day rolls around to please send in a snack that's free of the problem food. Include a list of common names used for the food, as explained in Chapter 6.

Asking for Help Immediately when You Start Feeling Funny

Children are often too embarrassed to ask for help when they're feeling ill at school, but when your child has a food allergy, the sooner she gets appropriate treatment the better, especially if she experiences severe reactions.

Foster an awareness in your child of the potential early warning signs and symptoms of a reaction. Teach your child the following three important points:

- ✔ Your symptoms may differ with each reaction, so be aware of all the potential symptoms, as described in Chapter 2.

- ✔ You may start feeling funny right after eating, but symptoms can occur at any time. The most common initial symptom is itching in the mouth so warn them to be on guard for this one.

- ✔ Inform your child that she is to seek assistance immediately if she notices any of these early warning signs:

  - Itching, especially in or around the mouth.

  - A sense that something is terribly wrong. We often refer to this as "a sense of impending doom," which is incredibly common even before other symptoms start.

  - Rash.

  - Queasy feeling.

  - Tightness in the throat or any difficulty breathing.

Even if your child knows what to do, he may be too embarrassed or physically unable to ask for help. Teachers and caregivers may need to intervene. Chapters 12 and 13 provide additional suggestions on policies and procedures for daycare, preschool, and kindergarten through high school.

Carrying a Health Emergency Card

Every child should carry a health emergency card that includes her name and address, parents' work and phone numbers, family doctor's phone number, a list of any health conditions she has; and brief instructions on what to do in the event of an emergency. Figure 16-1 shows a sample card for a child who has a food allergy.

> **Jane Doe**
> 2222 North Walnut Drive
>
> **I have food allergies:**
>
> **Call 911**
>
> **I carry a Twinject. Remove the green cap (exposing the gray cap) and remove the red cap. Hold the gray cap firmly against the outside portion of my upper thigh, press down firmly, count to 10, and remove. If the needle is exposed, I received the injection. If not, re-administer the injection. Call 911.**
>
> Dad (Joe) at home: (555) 555-5555
> Mom (Mary) at work: (555) 111-1111
> Doctor Bob Wood: (555) 222-2222

Make the creation of a health emergency card a fun group project. Create a custom card for each member of the family or each student in the class. Encourage your child to personalize his card with funky (but legible) fonts, wild colors, and a cool background. Most kids love to create their own publications on the computer.

Wearing a medical ID bracelet is another option. See Chapter 11 for details.

Chapter 17

Packing Ten Key Food Allergy Tips for Camp, College, and Other Outings

- -

- -

*E*ventually, your child is going to venture out on her own, leaving the allergy safe house you call home. This may begin with something simple like a sleepover at a friend's house, but over time may include summer camp, vacation with a friend's family, travel to a foreign land as an exchange student, moving off to college, or hiking the Appalachian Trail.

Venturing out presents both a challenge for your child and an opportunity for him to experience more freedom and assume more responsibility for managing his food allergy. In this chapter, I provide ten tips to help smooth the transition, ease your mind as a parent, and make the experience a little safer.

Packing Fresh Medications

A week or two before your child (or teenager) heads out to a friend's house, camp, college, or some other venture, check the food allergy medications to ensure the following:

- Your child has sufficient supplies to last the duration of the sojourn.

- Medications are in their original prescription bottles and are clearly labeled with your child's name. (Many camps and other institutions refuse to administer medication that's not in its original prescription bottle.)

- Expiration dates indicate that the medications are not to expire until after your child returns home.

- Detailed prescription information that describes how much of the medication to take and when your child should take it.

- At least two epinephrine (EpiPen or Twinject) autoinjectors, if prescribed. Check the expiration dates on the injectors, too.

- If plane travel is needed, be sure you have a letter from your doctor permitting you to carry medicines on the plane.

When your teenager decides to study abroad for a semester or seek his fortune in college or in the more real world, arrange for a doctor's visit soon after your teenager arrives at his new destination. Most colleges have an on-campus clinic complete with doctors and nurses, but your teenager must know exactly who to contact in the event of an emergency or when he's running low on his medications. Ask your child's allergist for a recommendation. Allergists have access to board-certified allergy specialists around the country through their specialty societies. This information may be of use in identifying an appropriate provider in another part of the country if the travels are within the U.S.

Taking Your Allergy Free Diet on the Road

At home, where the kitchen is well-stocked with allergen-free foods and snacks and everyone is well-versed in proper food preparation, remaining reaction free is manageable, if not always easy. On a trip, try your best to re-create the controlled situation of your home, by taking the following actions:

- **Speak directly to the head of the food service at the camp, school, or other institution.** Ask the head honcho to explain policies regarding food allergy and how they educate the kitchen staff about food allergy.

- **Inquire about how they use the specific foods that concern you.** Some camps and schools, for example, have a self-serve peanut butter bar that can create a real mess.

✔ **Ask to see the menu before you arrive.** This may help you to identify other red flags.

✔ **Ask about food in the bunks, dorm rooms, and other areas where your child may come into contact with others.** Consider arranging for a single room, or at least obtain assurance that your child will not have to room with a peanut-snack addict.

✔ **Arrange a visit to the kitchen.** Any place you can trust should be happy to have you inspect their kitchen. Examine the foods they have on their shelves, and ask questions about food preparation and risks of cross-contamination.

✔ **Once you have sorted out the menu and the kitchen set-up, you and your child can select safe foods for her stay.** After the initial inspection, however, your child will need to remain vigilant about any changes in the menu or food preparation. For longer stays, such as spending the school year on campus, intermittent calls or meetings with the food service manager can keep you in the loop, as well.

✔ **Have your child pack enough snacks to last him for the duration of his trip plus a few extras, just in case.** On a trip, allergen-free snacks may not be as readily available as they are at home.

Most summer camps have a camp store or canteen where the campers can purchase snacks. Consider having your child's snacks stored in the camp store, so he doesn't eat them or give them all away on his first day. This can also help your child feel more like one of the gang when everyone lines up in the camp store to buy snacks. People working the camp store should know your child has a food allergy and that they need to read the label every time before dispensing any snacks to your child.

Packing Emergency Information and Instructions

Prompt, well-trained, and well-coordinated action is essential to properly deal with allergic reactions, especially severe reactions. Like CPR, if you have to teach someone what to do during the emergency, the lesson may already be too late. No matter how long your child plans to be away from home, send emergency information and instructions to your point person. (See the next section for details about selecting a point person.) You may include allergy information on a health form, application, or (preferably) as a separate document that can be copied and distributed to key personnel. Instructions should include the following:

✔ **List the foods that your child is allergic to.** Include specific foods along with common names that appear on labels. See Chapter 6 for details.

✔ **Describe the specific symptoms that your child typically experiences, along with symptoms that your child may experience, as described in Chapter 2.**

✔ **Provide step-by-step instructions on how to administer medications.** You can find instructions for using EpiPen at www.anaphylaxis.com. Instructions for using Twinject are available at www.twinject.com. Provide *trainers* (an EpiPen or Twinject look-alike that is used to familiarize people with the device) and make sure everyone who might need to is fully familiar with this device. (Trainers are typically provided along with your prescription.)

Identifying One or More Point Persons

The support network you built at home and in your community does your child little good when she hits the road. Before she sets out, create a new support network at the planned destination. Begin by identifying and contacting your *point person* — a responsible adult, preferably one who knows about food allergies, who communicates directly with you and distributes essential information to all those who need to know. In a camp situation, this may be the camp director or nurse. In college, the campus medical center and the resident assistant in the dorm may be good choices.

Educate your point person, as explained later in the section, "Training Counselors and Other Personnel," so he knows the foods that your child is allergic to, potential symptoms to watch for, and emergency procedures. Make sure that this person is comfortable with the epinephrine injector and that she completely understands your emergency action plan. Have your point person pass this information to others who are responsible for your child. In a summer camp situation, for example, the following people need to know what to look for and what to do in the event of a reaction:

✔ Counselors

✔ Camp nurse

✔ Drivers

✔ Cooks and cafeteria workers

✔ Camp store workers

✔ Lifeguards

✔ Volunteers who may visit the camp

Tweaking Your Emergency Plan

Your existing emergency plan may be foolproof at home, but when your child travels, that plan is often useless. Tweak your emergency plan to fit the situation. A solid emergency plan contains the following items:

- ✔ Immediate treatment in the form of medications, including epinephrine autoinjectors.

- ✔ Name of the person or people who are best equipped to deal with a severe reaction, including how to contact them immediately.

- ✔ Location and contact information for the nearest emergency care facility.

- ✔ Transportation to the emergency care facility. Find out whether the ambulances that service the area carry epinephrine or not, and if you can request that a unit capable of administering epinephrine be sent.

- ✔ Communication on the way to the emergency care facility — a cell phone.

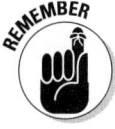

Everyone who cares for your child should know the emergency plan details well in advance of any possible reaction.

Training Counselors and Other Personnel

If the people who are caring for your child or teen are not well trained in dealing with food allergies, consider holding a brief training session. This is especially useful for summer camps that have little or no experience with food allergies. Your training presentation should include a description of food allergy, the fact that even small exposures can be deadly, and instructions on the use of all medications. Make it clear that they really do not want your child to die on their watch.

Practicing a "mock" reaction scenario can be very useful for the people who will be caring for your child or teen with food allergy.

Work with your point person to schedule your presentation, so that everyone who's going to care for your child can be present. You can find plenty of free training materials at the Food Allergy and Anaphylaxis Web site: www.food allergy.org. FAAN also has specific programs on camps and colleges to help train both you and them.

Giving Your Child a Refresher Course

Although your child's new support network may need to get up to speed on food allergies, your child shares responsibility for her own care and safety. Remind your child of the following key precautions:

✔ Never share food or drinks.

✔ Read the labels, and don't eat any unlabeled foods.

✔ Ask your counselor or the cook if you're unsure of the ingredients in a particular food.

✔ Follow the rule of thumb, "If in doubt, don't take chances with a food."

✔ Seek help if you suspect the beginning of a reaction, even if you don't have any noticeable symptoms.

In Chapter 16, I present other key lessons to teach your child that apply to all situations.

Choosing a Food Allergy–Friendly Camp

In many cases, your child chooses the camp he wants to attend based on one single criteria — where his friends are going. In other cases, you, as a family, make the choice. Whether your choice is already made for you or you're shopping for an appropriate camp, gather the following essential information:

✔ Has the camp had other campers with food allergies and how has it handled these cases? (You may be able to have the camp contact parents of children with food allergies who attended the camp and are willing to talk with you.)

✔ Who's the medical person in charge and who's second in command (for when the primary medical person is unavailable)? Ask about their credentials and their knowledge and experience in dealing with food allergies.

✔ Where will your child's epinephrine and other medications be stored and how readily available will they be? Can your child carry her own medications? How many people at the camp will be trained in giving the epinephrine shots?

✔ How far away is the nearest emergency medical treatment? Onsite emergency care may be insufficient in a case of very severe reaction.

✔ What outings may the camper be going on during her stay? How accessible are medications and emergency treatment on these outings?

✔ Does the camp have a system in place to keep all camp personnel well informed? See "Identifying One or More Point Persons," earlier in this chapter for details.

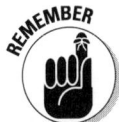

In most states, the camp cannot provide medicines or just keep epinephrine on hand. Each family must provide the medications for their child. You can never depend on others even if they are supposed to have it.

Educating Bunkmates and Roommates

Bunkmates and roommates can play a key role in intervening when a reaction begins. Oftentimes, people with food allergies are too embarrassed or confused to seek help themselves or ask if a particular food is safe. Someone with a clearer mind who can spot the early warning signs may be better at sounding the alarm.

Encourage your child to talk about his food allergies with bunkmates and roommates. If a counselor is involved, perhaps she can introduce the topic of food allergies and present a brief training session that covers prevention, common symptoms, and emergency procedures.

Buddying Up with a Food Allergy Savvy Pal

Whether a child or teenager is at camp, college, or on a field trip, she typically clicks with one peer more than others. The duo may become inseparable and do everything together. This person should know about your child's food allergy, be well-trained in spotting the early warning signs of a reaction, and know how to respond in the event of a severe reaction.

When our clinic works with a family to send a patient off to a new situation, many families bring along the best friend or future roommate to get them a special lesson on what their friend is allowed or not allowed to do. I love these visits.

Surviving and thriving with the buddy system

Last year, a long-time patient of mine with very severe food allergy was preparing to go off to college. She had multiple food allergies — milk, egg, peanut, tree nuts, and sesame, and her parents agonized over her safety. Her father, in fact, referred to college as her "death sentence" and had initially refused to let her go. To make matters worse, she had been a bit of a risk taker and had had several recent reactions. We had many hours of discussion about the approach to college and implemented all the tips described in this chapter. Most important among them, they worked with the food service manager to determine which foods she could eat and which eateries on campus would be prepared for her.

Perhaps the best move we made was to arrange a private room for my patient and her best friend from high school. The room included a microwave oven, so they could cook their own allergy-free meals, if needed. We arranged for the friends to visit campus together the spring before school started, and we went over all the precautions in detail, including safe foods, spotting reactions, administering medications, and even rules that my patient's dates had to follow. Knowing that her best friend was going to vigilantly police her activities, her parents were able to breathe a major sigh of relief. I am happy to say that my patient completed a reaction-free freshman year, and all of us feel that she has made a huge leap forward in becoming an adult with potentially deadly food allergy.

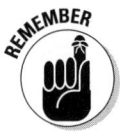

In college particularly, having a food allergy buddy to pal around with is very helpful, especially if your friend has a tendency to wander off with the first babe or hunk that saunters past. The friend can not only assist you in the event of a reaction, but also help spot dangerous situations and support you emotionally if you have to leave when the party was just starting to rock.

Chapter 18

Substituting Foods and Ingredients: Ten Common Dietary Substitutions

*C*learing the cupboards of the foods that ail you doesn't condemn you to a lifetime of rice cakes and distilled water. The world offers an abundance of tasty and nutritional substitutes for the most common troublesome foods, and the food industry is pumping out more variations each year.

In this chapter, I present you with a veritable buffet of substitutes for the most common problem foods, including milk, eggs, wheat, and peanuts. With the information in this chapter, you can restock your cupboards with healthy foods and ingredients that taste good, too.

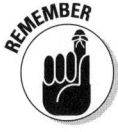

As you search for a replacement for a food, always make sure that the replacement does not contain small amounts of that food or another food that you are allergic to. Also be aware that many companies produce the substitute food on the same equipment as the food you are trying to avoid, such as the soy ice cream on the real ice cream equipment or soy nut butter on the peanut butter equipment.

Discovering Peanut and Peanut Butter Alternatives

Food manufacturers are beginning to get the message about the seriousness and rising incidence of peanut allergies. Nestlé, for example, now has an entire product line of peanut-free snacks, manufactured in a peanut-free environment, and clearly labeled as peanut free. The SoyNut Butter Company manufactures a peanut-free, tree-nut-free product, cleverly called Soynut-Butter (www.soynutbutter.com). And several companies produce tree-nut butters, including cashew and almond butter, and spreads made out of sunflower seeds.

You can satisfy your craving for peanuts with tree nuts, but people who are allergic to peanuts are commonly allergic to tree nuts, as well. You don't want to risk triggering another allergy by pursuing a substitute, so check with your allergist first to assess the risk. Some people find sunflower seeds or roasted soybeans or chick peas to be a suitable substitute, and they're less likely to cause a reaction in those with peanut allergies.

Before trying a peanut or peanut butter substitute, read the label carefully to make sure it doesn't contain peanuts or other ingredients you're sensitive to, and always check with your allergist first.

Replacing Milk, Ice Cream, and Yogurt

When you're allergic to milk, seeing celebrities and athletes with milk mustaches asking you if you "Got milk?" is probably not all that appealing, and it doesn't have to be. Although milk is packed with calcium and fortified with vitamin D, so are a host of other beverages and foods, including rice milk, soy milk, oat milk, potato milk, and calcium-fortified juices, cereals, and breads. See Chapter 6 for guidance on how to obtain sufficient calcium in your diet (and fat and protein, for infants and children). Your allergist and nutritionist can recommend other nutritional alternatives.

Ice cream and yogurt lovers rejoice! You don't have to give up these tasty treats. Health food stores and specialty markets typically carry several milk-free products to cater to customers who have milk allergy or are lactose intolerant. Try several products until you find one or more you like. Remember, however, that products manufactured solely for those who are lactose-intolerant are not safe alternatives for people with milk allergy — lactose-free products often contain the milk protein that triggers reactions. See Chapter 6 for details on how to spot milk on food labels.

To replace milk in recipes, substitute 1 cup of milk with ¾ to 1 cup water, fruit juice, soy milk, or rice milk. (Because substitutes are more watery than milk, try using less of the substitute and adding 3 tablespoons of canola oil to make up for the loss of fat.) You can pick up recipes for evaporated milk, sweetened condensed milk, buttermilk, heavy cream, light cream, sour cream, yogurt, and chocolate at the Food Allergy Kitchen (www.foodallergy kitchen.com). When you get there, click Substitutes.

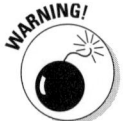

Products labeled as dairy free often contain milk. Go figure. Read the labels carefully before trying any of these products. When in doubt, scratch the item off your grocery list.

Discovering a Better Butter

Your grocery's dairy section is no doubt packed with butter substitutes, including margarine, but be careful, because many margarines contain milk solids. If you're looking for something to spread on your toast, consider using olive, sesame, or canola oil and either spreading it or spraying it on your bread. You can spice up the oil with seasonings to improve the taste. Health food stores also carry spreads made of tahini (sesame) and sunflower seed oil that may be suitable replacements, as long as you're not allergic to those seeds.

Margarines, cooking oils, and vegetable shortening are also suitable substitutes for butter in baking, assuming the products don't contain milk solids or other food items that trigger your reactions.

Checking Out Some Cheesy Substitutes

For cheese connoisseurs, soy- and rice-based cheese substitutes don't quite stack up to a slice of Swiss or a chunk of cheddar, but people who are allergic to milk often find a suitable substitute in soy- or rice-based cheese products. Kids who grow up eating cheese substitutes don't even miss the "real thing," because they've never had it, and many adults quickly acquire a taste for it. Some people love this stuff simply because they can use it to make pizzas and macaroni and cheese.

Not all cheese substitutes are created equal. Try several products to find the ones you like, and try them in different recipes. Just be sure to read the labels carefully and weed out any products that contain traces of milk.

For those who can't stomach cheese substitutes, try eating something else entirely. If you're not allergic to sesame seeds, try spreading hummus on your crackers and bread instead of cheese. Hummus is primarily made up of garbanzo beans and tahini (a sesame seed spread). Other replacements for cheese spreads include tofu; paté; and Taramasalata — a Greek sandwich filling made with fish, roe, olive oil, lemon juice, and garlic.

Taramasalata often contains bread crumbs, so if you have a wheat allergy, consider mixing up your own batch, without the bread crumbs.

Trading in Your Chocolate

True chocolate allergies are rare. If you react to chocolate, you're more likely intolerant of it or something else (like milk or egg) in the product may be triggering the reaction. In such cases, eating a product that has pure chocolate or cocoa, as long as it doesn't have milk or eggs, is safe.

Baking (also called cooking) chocolate is typically pure chocolate. Almost all grocery stores also carry cocoa powder for baking. Cocoa is chocolate with most of the cocoa fat removed.

If you have a chocolate intolerance, you can substitute cocoa in most recipes with carob or carob powder. Use 1½ to 2 times as much carob as cocoa. You can also purchase carob chips to use in place of chocolate chips in cookies and muffins.

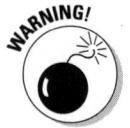

If you have a peanut or tree nut allergy, always read the fine print on the package to make sure the chocolate or chocolate substitute is safe — meaning it doesn't contain peanuts or tree nuts.

Whipping up a Fake Egg Mixture

When you're allergic to eggs, you have to scrape sunny-side up and over-easy off your breakfast menu. Commercial egg substitutes, which are usually designed to lower cholesterol, often include egg whites, so be careful. I recommend a product called Egg Replacer from Ener-G Foods. You can learn more about it by visiting ener-g.com or calling (800) 331-5222.

When you're baking, eggs are fairly easy to replace. Try the following substitutions:

✔ Substitute ½ mashed banana for 1 egg in cake recipes. Bananas are a pretty good binding agent; that is, they help the other ingredients stick together.

✔ Replace each egg in the recipe with ¼ cup of applesauce. Applesauce is another good binding agent.

✔ Mix 1 tablespoon of gelatin or fruit pectin with 3 tablespoons of water. (Use immediately before the mixture congeals.)

✔ Use 1 tablespoon of corn starch or arrowroot powder per egg along with 3 tablespoons of water to dissolve the powder. This works well for recipes that need a little leavening.

✔ Mix ¼ teaspoon xanthan gum with ¼ cup of water and let stand for about five minutes. You can then whip this like an egg.

When shopping for dairy-free and egg-free products, look for products labeled "Vegan," and check the label to confirm the absence of milk and eggs. Vegans are strict vegetarians who avoid not only meat but also any animal products, including milk, cheese, and eggs.

Finding a New Staple: Wheat-Free Breads

Bread is the staple of many a western diet, but for those who are allergic or intolerant of wheat products, most breads spell misery. Fortunately, wheat doesn't have a monopoly on the bread industry. Several companies bake breads out of rice, quinoa (pronounced "keen-wa"), amaranth, buckwheat, potato, and other grainy, starchy stuff. Common products include the following:

✔ **Rye bread or rye crackers:** Some rye breads and crackers contain wheat flour, so you may need to check with the manufacturer to make sure the product is 100 percent rye. (Many people who have wheat allergies are also allergic to rye, so rye may not be an option.)

✔ **Gluten-free breads:** Most gluten-free breads are made with a combination of rice, soy, and other types of non-wheat flours.

✔ **Oat cakes:** Delicatessens, health food stores, and upscale grocery stores often carry oat cakes, but if you're allergic to milk, make sure the oat cakes are entirely milk-free, as well.

✔ **Rice cakes:** Most grocery stores carry rice cakes and typically shelve them in the cereal aisle. They're a little on the dry and crunchy side, but a little jam or other spread can make them quite tasty.

Grocery stores often shelve their wheat-free breads and other healthy stuff in a separate section, which is great for those of us with food allergies. If your local grocery isn't in tune with the times, you may have to visit a specialty market or health food store.

Breakfasting with Wheat-Free Cereals

Wheat-based cereals rule the cereal aisle, but plenty of alternatives are also available, including corn flakes, puffed rice or rice flakes, kasha (buckwheat), porridge oats, rolled oats, millet flakes, or quinoa flakes. For hot cereals, try oatmeal or brown rice cereals, grits (basically corn meal), or millet.

Some of these cereals can be a little on the dry side. Try letting the milk (or soy or rice milk) soak in a little longer, or add more liquid or raisins, chopped apples, or bananas to moisten it.

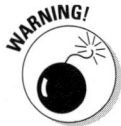

Before eating any cereal advertised as being made from a grain other than wheat, check the label for any trace amounts of wheat and if you have any lingering doubts, contact the manufacturer.

Baking Your Goodies with Wheat-Free Flour

Because so many bakery products contain wheat, many people with wheat allergies choose to bake their own breads. You can find a host of wheat-free and gluten-free flours and flour mixtures at just about any health food or specialty food store, or you can make your own mixture. Here are a couple suggestions:

✔ Mix 2 parts brown rice flour 1 part soy flour and 1 part tapioca flour. Substitute 1 cup mixture for 1 cup wheat flour. (You may need to add more liquid to your recipe, because rice flour tends to soak up more moisture than does wheat flour.)

> ✔ Mix 6 parts white rice flour with 2 parts potato starch and 1 part tapioca flour. Substitute 1 cup mixture for 1 cup wheat flour. (You may need to add more liquid to your recipe, because rice flour tends to soak up more moisture than does wheat flour.)
>
> ✔ Substitute 1⅓ cup ground rolled oats or 1⅛ cups oat flour for a cup of wheat flour.

Many wheat- and gluten-free flours and mixtures include their own recipes and instructions for using the flour as a substitute in your other recipes.

Baking powders also contain trace amounts of wheat. To make your own substitute, blend ⅓ cup baking soda with ⅔ cup cream of tartar and ⅔ cup potato or arrowroot starch and store it in an airtight container.

Discovering Safer Thickening Agents

When most chefs want to thicken their gravies, soups, and stews, they reach for wheat flour or corn starch, but if you have a wheat or corn allergy, these options end up on the chopping block. Fortunately several thickening agents work nearly as well, including the following:

> ✔ Sago flour
>
> ✔ Tapioca
>
> ✔ Arrowroot
>
> ✔ Rice flour
>
> ✔ Potato flour or starch

To thicken stews, soups, and gumbos, try using okra. Okra works better as a thickening agent if you grind it up or cook it thoroughly before adding it to the pot.

Chapter 19

Exploring Ten Outstanding Food Allergy Web Sites

*I*n my humble opinion, *Food Allergies For Dummies* is the ultimate resource for information and advice about food allergies. I have to admit, however, that various Web sites provide resources I couldn't possibly offer in this book, including late-breaking research results made available after printing, the ability to network with other food allergy sufferers, an opportunity to post direct questions to specialists, and assistance in advocating for policy changes locally and nationally.

In this chapter, I steer you toward what I consider to be the top ten food allergy Web sites and describe the most valuable tools and features you can expect to discover at each site.

Tapping Online Resources at FAAN: Food Allergy & Anaphylaxis Network

When you're not sure where to turn for help with food allergies, few sites are better than FAAN's (www.foodallergy.org), where a panel of the world's leading experts in food allergy carefully scrutinize every piece of information before it's posted. Here you find plenty of information and resources presented in easily recognizable categories, including the following: Common

Food Allergens, Anaphylaxis, School & Childcare, Advocacy, Research, Recipes, and the Daily Tip.

This site also provides links to areas specifically for teenagers and children and to an area where teachers and school administrators can find information on how to implement a food allergy program. The site is bilingual in English and Spanish.

If you're having trouble convincing your child (or an unmotivated family member) to read this book, refer them to this Web site. It offers something for everyone in an engaging and easily accessible format.

Communing with the Allergy & Asthma Network Mothers of Asthmatics

When you want some practical information on how to care for your child, ask a mom. This site (www.aanma.org), created and maintained by moms and other committed individuals, lets you do just that. Once you land on the home page, click Breatherville USA to jump to the main content area or click En Español for the Spanish version. If you click the Breatherville USA link, the site presents you with an interactive map you can click to visit the desired content area.

Click once anywhere on the interactive map to activate it. Then you can mouse over different buildings on the map to display a pop-up box that contains a description of the building. Click the building to access its offerings.

Since you're interested in food allergies, click the Farmer's Market to jump to the food allergy page. Here you'll find an online library packed with information that covers the top food allergy topics, including the following:

- Detecting food allergies
- Symptoms of food allergy
- Follow the food allergy clues
- Adverse reactions to food
- Symptoms of anaphylaxis
- Using epinephrine
- Living with allergies
- Reading food labels

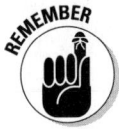

Don't limit yourself to the Farmer's Market just because it focuses on food allergies. Visit the other buildings in Breatherville, including America's College of Allergy & Asthma (where you can take an online course), the Childcare Center (for parents and care givers), City Hall (for advocacy tips), the Pharmacy (for information on available medications), the School House (for tips on keeping your child safe and healthy at school), and the News Room (where you can find information on the latest breakthroughs). The site also features a Play Time playroom for kids.

Investigating the Food Allergy Initiative

The Food Allergy Initiative (FAI; www.foodallergyinitiative.org) is a non-profit group that raises funds to fuel research into effective treatments and cures for food allergies. This site is one of the easiest sites of the bunch to navigate, because it offers three ways to skip to the desired content:

- ✓ Use the navigation bar that runs across the top of the page to access the main content areas, including Food Allergy Information, Living with Food Allergies, Restaurant Training, Research, Public Policy, and Downloads.

- ✓ Scroll down for links that match those in the navigation bar but offer descriptions of each content area. By scrolling down, you can preview areas before visiting them.

- ✓ Click the links that run across the center of the opening page for quick access to information on how to deal with the eight most common food allergies: Peanuts, Eggs, Milk, Shellfish, Wheat, Tree Nuts, Soy, and Fish.

Don't leave this site without clicking the Download link to see what it has to offer. Here you find a collection of PDF documents and Microsoft Word files that include an Authorization for Emergency Medical Treatment, an Emergency Medical Plan (in several languages), and Restaurant Cards (also in several languages).

Poking Around in the Food Allergy Kitchen

The Food Allergy Kitchen (www.foodallergykitchen.com) is an online repository for food allergy recipes, dietary substitutions, menu planning strategies and tips, cooking questions and answers, and tips for managing food allergies. This site also features a Links link that recommends additional food allergy Web sites, many of which are included in this chapter.

From the home page, you can click a link to order the FoodAllergyKitchen Cookbook online or subscribe to the bi-monthly newsletter that features articles, cooking tips, seasonal ideas, recipes, safety alerts, tips for reducing stress, and recipes for those with multiple food allergies.

Visiting AAFA: Asthma and Allergy Foundation of America

The Asthma and Allergy Foundation of America (www.aafa.org) created and maintains this site to provide the latest available information and advice to allergy sufferers, family members, and other concerned individuals and to assist in advocacy.

The opening page makes the site look like a stodgy billboard intended merely to convey the group's vision statement and promote the many useful programs it offers for sale, but if you dig a little deeper, you find an outstanding collection of free materials.

Rest your mouse pointer on the **Allergies** tab and then click **Food and Drug** to call up an alphabetical list of a couple dozen links, that cover the most common food allergies, allergy testing for children, and various treatment options and therapies. Each link takes you to a one-page information sheet that provides an excellent overview of the topic along with links to additional resources on the Web.

Click the Ask the Allergist link on the opening page to e-mail a specific question to an allergy specialist. You can also register to participate in live online chat room discussions.

Accessing Anaphylaxis Canada

If you or your child has a life-threatening food allergy, head to Anaphylaxis Canada (www.anaphylaxis.org) for information and advice. This site features a navigation bar that provides quick access to a definition of anaphylaxis and a page that reveals practical strategies and tips for living with anaphylaxis.

Children and teenagers can click the Safe4Kids link to head to a special activities and games area where they can learn more about their allergies and how to manage them while having fun.

Dropping in on the American Academy of Allergy Asthma & Immunology

The American Academy of Allergy Asthma & Immunology Web site (www.aaaai.org) opens with a page that caters more to allergy professionals than to patients, so upon arrival, click the **Patients & Consumers** tab to skip to the good stuff. Here you find links to the Topic of the Month, a Find an Allergist/ Immunologist searchable directory, and several useful tools, including a Patient Gallery, Medication Guide, an A to Z index of conditions, printable brochures, and allergy and asthma headline news.

The Patient Gallery isn't a collection of photographs of allergy patients. Clicking this link calls up a page with eight buttons for various allergy and asthma topics. Click the Food Allergy button for a list of clickable food allergy topics in several categories that include General Information, Signs and Symptoms, Diagnosis and Management, Medications, For Kids, and Additional Resources.

This site offers content in both English and Spanish and has special areas just for kids and for seniors. Click the Patients & Consumers Contact link to communicate directly with AAAAI via e-mail.

Attending the American College of Allergy, Asthma, & Immunology

The ACAAI (www.aaaai.org) is a professional organization for allergy specialists that's committed to improving patient care and educating patients. As soon as you arrive at the home page, click the **Patient Education** graphic — it's really big, you can't miss it. Clicking Patient Education pulls up a page with a navigation bar that runs down the left side of the page.

For food allergies, try the following links in the navigation bar: A-Z Allergy Topics, Find an Allergist (searchable directory), Glossary, Healthcare Plans (a checklist for evaluating healthcare plans for coverage of allergy care medications), Interactive Quizzes, Patient Support, and Questions.

Joining the Anaphylaxis Campaign

The Anaphylaxis Campaign (`www.anaphylaxis.org.uk`) is a charity organization directed by the top allergists in the UK. Although the site is careful to explain that professional care is essential in properly treating allergies, it offers a great collection of information and resources to empower patients and caregivers. Here you can find general information about anaphylaxis, food alerts for new popular food products that contain known allergens, guidance for schools and pre-schools, information for young adults, and information and advice for healthcare professionals and companies in the food industry.

Gathering Additional Information at AllAllergy.net

If you haven't yet found the information and resources you're looking for on the Internet, turn to AllAllergy.net (`allallergy.net`) for additional leads. This site acts as a gateway to other Web sites that focus on all types of allergies. Links to sites are organized by category, including Articles, Organizations, Publications, Events, Products, Databases, and Contents. The site also features a handy search tool.

Chapter 20

Responding to a Severe Reaction:
Ten Do's and Don'ts

*T*aking the necessary precautions to prevent allergic reactions is no guar-antee that a reaction won't occur. Hidden ingredients, unlabeled foods, and cross contamination are always possible, so remain prepared at all times, carry your medications with you, and remain at the ready to respond in a hurry.

If you or a loved one experiences a reaction, despite your best efforts at avoidance, what should you do? In this chapter, I provide ten do's and don'ts to assist you in successfully responding to a severe reaction and preventing future recurrences.

Identify the Symptoms

Severe reactions can escalate in a hurry but may begin with more subtle symptoms, such as an itchy mouth, panic, or an impending sense of doom. The earlier you respond to a reaction, the better the outcome, so make sure that you, your friends, and your family can recognize the signs and symptoms:

✔ **Mouth:** Itching or swelling of the lips, tongue, or mouth

✔ **Throat:** Itching or a sense of tightness in the throat, hoarseness, or a hacking cough

- ✔ **Skin:** Hives, itching, or swelling of the face or extremities
- ✔ **Gut:** Nausea, abdominal cramps, vomiting, or diarrhea
- ✔ **Lungs:** Shortness of breath, repetitive coughing, or wheezing
- ✔ **Heart:** Lightheadedness, fainting
- ✔ **Anxiety:** Panic or sense of impending doom

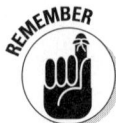

Each reaction can present different symptoms. If your symptoms typically consist of breaking out in hives, you have no guarantee that your next reaction will begin with hives. You may experience anxiety, nausea, a tightening of the throat, or any of the other symptoms described above.

Tell Someone Immediately

Whether you experience a reaction alone or when accompanied by others, always tell someone else immediately. A common mistake people make, especially in social situations, is to wander off from the crowd and try to attend to the reaction themselves. They follow their natural impulse to avoid becoming party poopers, or in the case of teens, just look different.

The problem with this approach is that a reaction can progress from relatively subtle symptoms to a life-threatening situation in a matter of minutes. You can faint. Your airway can become restricted to the point at which you can't talk.

At the first sign of a reaction, tell someone. If you're alone, call 911, a nearby family member, or a neighbor. If you're on a date, tell your date. If you're with friends or family members, tell them. Make sure someone stays with you until the crisis is resolved.

Remain As Calm As Possible

Feeling anxious and nervous in the midst of a severe reaction is certainly understandable, and I'm not about to tell you Don't Panic! I do recommend, however, that you remain as calm as possible. When people panic, they generally make mistakes and often forget the emergency action plan they carefully reviewed with their doctor.

You know what you need to do at this point — take your medications, call 911, and wait for help to arrive. Sometimes taking decisive action can reduce some of the anxiety.

Consider rehearsing your emergency action plan in preparation for a possible future reaction. I know this may sound a little corny, but sometimes if you act it out on your own, your body will "remember" what you need to do, even when your brain is in panic mode.

Respond Immediately

Patients often let a reaction escalate unnecessarily because they question their instincts. They think that some relatively minor symptoms will just go away on their own or that calling 911 is a sign that they've officially become drama queens. Because a severe reaction has the potential to become a life-threatening reaction, however, an immediate response is critical. The faster you can reverse the overreaction of your immune system, the better the outcome and the faster you'll start feeling better.

If a friend or loved one is experiencing a reaction, don't let the person talk you out of administering medication or calling 911. Act immediately. Err on the side of overreacting. You can apologize later . . . if you think you need to.

Administer Medications

Medication is key to successfully thwarting a reaction, and an epinephrine autoinjection is best. If you have an autoinjector, give yourself an injection immediately. If an autoinjector is unavailable and you can swallow, Benadryl is the next best option, and liquid or Fastmelt Benadryl is preferable. How much Benadryl should you take? Consult your doctor prior to experiencing a reaction to determine an effective, safe dose.

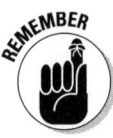

Antihistamines have no life-saving properties. If you throat is swelling closed, it will do nothing and is never a substitute for epinephrine.

Call 911

Whenever you or a loved one experiences a severe reaction, call 911 immediately after administering medication. If you don't have medication, calling 911 immediately is even more important. When you call, be sure to provide the dispatcher the following information:

- ✔ You're experiencing anaphylaxis.
- ✔ You need epinephrine.
- ✔ Your current location.

 If you're the one experiencing the reaction, have someone else place the call for you. Some doctors recommend that anyone experiencing anaphylaxis lie down to help alleviate symptoms with low blood pressure. I don't recommend it for everyone, but if you feel faint or lightheaded, lie down.

Don't Drive Yourself

Calling 911 and waiting for the EMTs to arrive with epinephrine and additional medical supplies and equipment is usually the best option, but if an emergency room is nearby, having someone drive you to the emergency room is another good option.

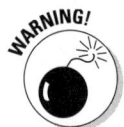 Whatever you do, don't try to drive yourself. If symptoms escalate on your way to the hospital or emergency room, you could have a serious accident or even a minor fender bender that could delay treatment. Ask a friend, family member, or neighbor to drive you.

Call Your Doctor

Your doctor is not the person to call when you're in the midst of a severe reaction, but after you've obtained emergency treatment, call your doctor or allergist and report in. Your doctor may want to see you for a follow-up, provide you with prescriptions for medication refills or new medications, and offer advice on follow-up treatment in the hours after your initial reaction.

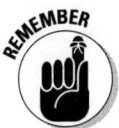 As soon as possible after receiving emergency treatment, call your doctor or allergist or have someone call for you. Your doctor should be aware that you've experienced a severe reaction.

Call Family or Friends

In some cases, a complete stranger may come to your assistance during a severe reaction, in which case you end up in the emergency room with no way home and nobody to watch over you. Call a friend or family member or have the hospital place a call to let them know what happened and ask them to drive you home and stay with you.

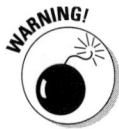 In the hours after a severe reaction, symptoms may recur. You face the greatest risk in the four hours immediately after receiving emergency treatment, during which time, you should remain in the emergency room under observation. Ask a responsible adult to watch over you until the risk of recurring symptoms passes.

Review What Happened

Figuratively speaking, you want to do a post mortem after any reaction, particularly a severe reaction, while that reaction is fresh in your mind. Jot down the following details:

- ✔ Where you were when the reaction occurred
- ✔ What you were doing when you first experienced symptoms
- ✔ What you had eaten just prior to experiencing symptoms
- ✔ The amount of time that passed between when you ate the suspect food and when symptoms appeared

 Take your notes to your next doctor's appointment, describe what happened, and discuss possible adjustments to your food avoidance strategies to avoid similar situations in the future.

Part V

Appendixes: Allergy-Friendly Recipes and Other Treats

The 5th Wave   By Rich Tennant

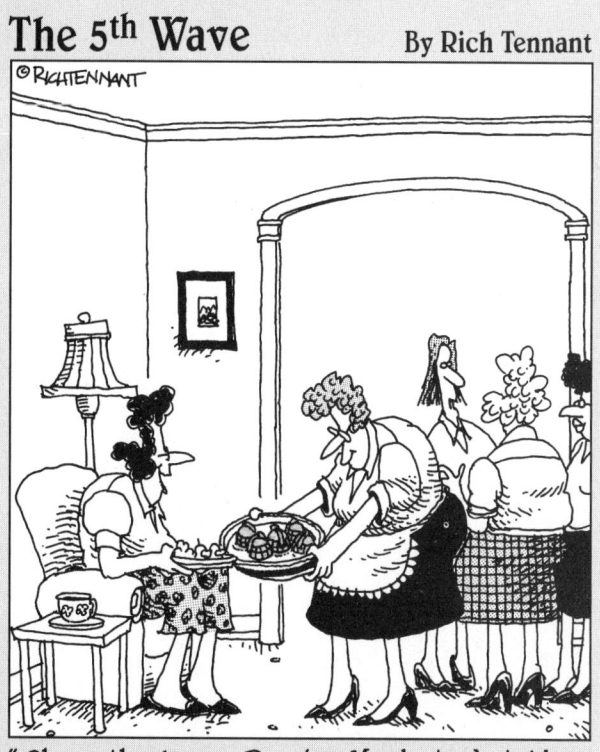

"Oh, no thank you, Bernice. My doctor's told me to avoid foods containing too much lactose, gluten, or hand grenades."

In this part . . .

*O*n your journey through this book, you probably worked up quite an appetite, and you may be wondering, "If this is all the stuff I *can't* eat, then what *can* I eat?"

In this part, I answer that question with a collection of 28 recipes plucked from the pages of a couple of FAAN (Food Allergy and Anaphylaxis Network) cookbooks. I grouped the recipes in separate appendixes so you could quickly skip to a specific meal. Appendix A covers breakfast items, B is for main courses, C is for snacks and cookies, and D is for the desserts.

In Appendix E, I serve up a collection of food-allergy-related terms and their definitions, so you can quickly look up a definition as you're reading the book or doing extra research on your own.

Bon appetite!

Appendix A

Breads & Breakfasts

*O*ften referred to as the most important meal of the day, breakfast provides the fuel to get us through the day . . . at least until lunchtime rolls around. In this section of the recipe box, I serve up six of the most popular recipes ranging from on-the-go coffee cakes and muffins to hearty pancakes.

Use the following key to know if the recipe works with your specific allergy or allergies:

- ✔ **EF:** Egg free
- ✔ **MF:** Milk free
- ✔ **NF:** Nut free
- ✔ **PF:** Peanut free
- ✔ **SF:** Soy free
- ✔ **WF:** Wheat free

Recipes in This Chapter

▶ Potato Pancakes
▶ Banana Pancakes
▶ Cinnamon Syrup
▶ Corn Muffins
▶ Cinnamon Raisin Coffee Cake
▶ Vanilla Icing
▶ Blueberry Muffins
▶ Pumpkin Bread

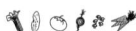

Potato Pancakes

(EF, MF, NF, PF, SF, WF)

1 cup cooked potatoes, mashed

1 cup uncooked potatoes, finely grated

½ teaspoon salt

½ teaspoon baking powder

2 tablespoons milk-free, soy-free margarine

In large bowl, combine all ingredients except margarine. Set aside. In large skillet, melt margarine over medium heat. Spoon potato mixture into skillet, forming pancakes; cook until golden brown on bottom; flip and continue cooking. Serve plain or with maple syrup.

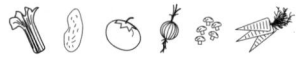

Banana Pancakes

(EF, MF, NF, PF, SF, WF)

1 ½ cups oat flour

1 tablespoon sugar

1 teaspoon baking powder

½ teaspoon baking soda

¼ teaspoon salt

1¼ cups orange juice

1 tablespoon oil

1 teaspoon vanilla extract

1½ tablespoons water, 1½ tablespoons oil, 1 teaspoon baking powder; mixed together

1 ½ cups banana, chopped

Heat nonstick griddle or skillet over medium heat. In medium bowl, combine all ingredients, except banana. Stir well. Fold in banana. Spoon ⅓ cup batter for each pancake onto griddle or skillet. Cook until top bubbles and edges are browned. Flip and cook until done. Top with Cinnamon Syrup (see next recipe).

Cinnamon Syrup

(EF, MF, NF, PF, SF, WF)

¾ cup light corn syrup

1 teaspoon ground cinnamon

1 teaspoon vanilla extract

1 teaspoon lemon juice

In small saucepan over low heat, cook corn syrup until thoroughly heated. Add remaining ingredients. Mix well. Pour warm syrup over pancakes or waffles.

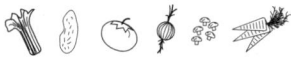

Corn Muffins

(EF, MF, NF, PF, SF, WF)

⅓ cup shortening

¼ cup sugar

1 cup Cream of Rice cereal

1 tablespoon baking powder

⅔ cup warm water

¼ teaspoon salt

1 teaspoon vanilla extract

1 teaspoon grated lemon rind

⅔ cup cornmeal

¼ cup raisins, optional

Preheat oven to 375 degrees. Line muffin tin with paper liners. Cream shortening and sugar. Mix rice cereal and baking powder in warm water. Combine with sugar and shortening mixture. Mix in remaining ingredients (and raisins, if used). Spoon into muffin cups (small muffins have a better texture). Bake 25 minutes. Makes 8 muffins.

These muffins hold together better if you let them cool a few hours or overnight.

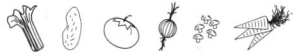

Cinnamon Raisin Coffee Cake

(EF, MF, NF, PF, SF)

1 cup plus 2 tablespoons water

2 cups raisins

1 cup brown sugar

⅓ cup milk-free, soy-free margarine

½ teaspoon cinnamon

½ teaspoon allspice

½ teaspoon salt

⅛ teaspoon nutmeg

2 cups sifted flour

1 teaspoon baking powder

1 teaspoon baking soda

Vanilla Icing (see next recipe)

1 Preheat oven to 325 degrees. Grease a 7-inch tube pan. In a medium saucepan, combine water, raisins, brown sugar, margarine, cinnamon, allspice, salt, and nutmeg; bring to a boil and cook for 3 minutes. Cool.

2 Sift flour before measuring, then sift again with baking powder and soda. Stir dry ingredients gradually into cooled mixture; beat with electric mixer until smooth. Turn into prepared tube pan and bake 35 minutes or until a cake tester comes out clean. Drizzle with Vanilla Icing (see next recipe).

Vanilla Icing

(EF, MF, NF, PF, SF, WF)

1 cup confectioners sugar

1½ tablespoons warm water

¼ teaspoon vanilla extract

Combine all ingredients and mix until smooth.

Blueberry Muffins

(EF, MF, NF, PF, SF, WF)

½ cup milk-free, soy-free margarine at room temperature

1 cup plus 2 tablespoons sugar

3 tablespoons water, 3 tablespoons oil, 2 teaspoons baking powder mixed together

1 teaspoon vanilla extract

2 teaspoons baking powder

¼ teaspoon salt

2 cups flour

½ cup water

2½ cups blueberries

1 tablespoon sugar mixed with ¼ teaspoon ground nutmeg

1 Preheat oven to 375 degrees. Line muffin tin with paper liners. In a medium-size bowl, beat margarine until creamy. Beat in the sugar until pale and fluffy. Beat in water, oil, and baking powder. Add vanilla, remaining baking powder, and salt.

2 Fold in half the flour and half the water with a spatula. Add remaining flour and water. Fold in blueberries. Scoop batter into muffin cups. Sprinkle with nutmeg-sugar. Bake 25 to 30 minutes or until golden brown. Let muffins cool slightly before serving.

Pumpkin Bread

(EF, MF, NF, PF, SF, WF)

½ cup milk-free, soy-free margarine

1 cup sugar

½ teaspoon cinnamon

½ teaspoon nutmeg

¼ teaspoon ginger

1¾ cups barley flour

1 teaspoon baking soda

½ teaspoon salt

2 teaspoons baking powder

½ cup water

1 teaspoon vanilla extract

1 cup canned pumpkin

Preheat oven to 350 degrees. Cream margarine and add sugar. Set aside. Sift together cinnamon, nutmeg, ginger, flour, baking soda, and salt; set aside. Dissolve baking powder in ¼ cup water; add to margarine mixture. Mix remaining ¼ cup water and vanilla extract together; add pumpkin. Stir well. Add to margarine mixture. Combine dry ingredients and wet ingredients. Blend together well. Pour into a loaf pan. Bake 1 hour.

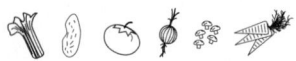

Appendix B

Main Courses

*T*o prepare an allergy-free main course, consider sticking with the basics — meat and potatoes with a vegetable on the side. For more variety, allergy-free substitutes enable you to prepare many of your favorite dishes without the problem foods and ingredients. In this section, I present the top three main courses generously provided by FAAN.

Recipes in This Chapter

▶ Turkey Soup
▶ Chicken and Rice
▶ Mexican Casserole

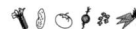

Use the following key to know if the recipe works with your specific allergy or allergies:

- ✔ **EF:** Egg free
- ✔ **MF:** Milk free
- ✔ **NF:** Nut free
- ✔ **PF:** Peanut free
- ✔ **SF:** Soy free
- ✔ **WF:** Wheat free

Turkey Soup

_(EF, MF, NF, PF, SF, WF)_

1½ pounds ground turkey

4 ribs celery, sliced

1 tablespoon olive oil

4 cups water

4 carrots, sliced

¼ cup uncooked rice

1 small bay leaf

½ teaspoon thyme

½ teaspoon sweet basil

4 teaspoons chili powder

¼ teaspoon onion powder

¼ teaspoon dillweed

4 drops red pepper sauce

2 medium potatoes, diced

1 teaspoon salt (or to taste)

¼ teaspoon pepper

3½ cups tomatoes or tomato juice

1 can green beans

1 can black-eyed peas (or other beans)

Brown turkey and celery in 1 tablespoon olive oil. Add water, carrots, rice, bay leaf, thyme, basil, chili powder, onion powder, dillweed, red pepper sauce, potatoes, salt, and pepper. Bring to a boil and simmer until vegetables are tender. Add remaining ingredients and heat through. Remove bay leaf and serve hot.

Tip: _Chicken may be substituted for turkey._

Chicken and Rice

_(EF, MF, NF, PF, SF, WF)_

1 teaspoon oregano

2 peppercorns

1 clove garlic, peeled

2 teaspoons salt

2 teaspoons olive oil

1 teaspoon vinegar

2½ pounds chicken, cut into serving pieces

1 tablespoon olive oil

2 ounces cured ham, diced

1 strip bacon, diced

1 onion, peeled

1 green pepper, seeded

1 celery stalk

1 cup water

6-ounce can tomato paste

6 green olives

1 teaspoon capers

1 tomato, chopped

2 tablespoons olive oil

2¼ cups rice

1 can pinto beans, kidney beans, or green peas, drained

3 cups water

1 Mash together the oregano, peppercorns, garlic, salt, 2 teaspoons olive oil, and vinegar.

2 Rub chicken with mashed ingredients. Place 1 tablespoon olive oil in a large deep kettle. Add diced ham and bacon and brown over high heat. Add chicken. and brown lightly. Reduce heat to moderate.

3 In blender, grind onion, pepper, celery, 1 cup water, and tomato paste. Add onion mixture to kettle. Add olives, capers, and chopped tomato, and cook for 10 minutes. Add 2 tablespoons olive oil, rice, and beans. Cook for 5 minutes.

4 Heat water to boiling and add to kettle. (Water level should just cover ingredients.) Mix well and cook rapidly; uncovered, until food begins to boil. With a large spoon, turn rice from bottom to top. Cover and cook slowly for 2 minutes.

5 Turn rice once more, cover, and cook for 10 minutes longer or until rice is cooked. Serve at once.

Tip: *1 chopped and seeded sweet chili pepper may be added when adding onion and green pepper.*

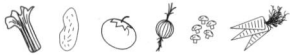

Mexican Casserole

(EF, MF, NF, PF, SF, WF)

1 pound ground turkey

2 (15- to 16-oz.) cans

kidney beans, rinsed
and drained

1 (8-oz.) can tomato sauce

½ cup mild chunky salsa

1 teaspoon chili powder

½ teaspoon salt

6 corn tortillas

Preheat oven to 375 degrees. In large skillet over medium heat, brown turkey, stirring frequently to separate; drain. Stir in beans, tomato sauce, salsa, chili powder, and salt. Line bottom of 8-inch square casserole dish with 2 tortillas. Cut 1 of the tortillas into pieces to fill in empty areas. Cover with 1/3 of meat mixture (approximately 2 cups). Repeat layers twice. Cover with aluminum foil and bake 45 minutes. Let cool 5 minutes before serving.

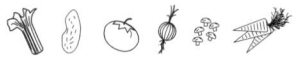

Appendix C

Snacks and Cookies

Snack time and party time often isolate those with food allergies, particularly young children. To keep these important social events festive while providing a nutritional energy boost between meals, I offer eight great cookie and snack recipes.

Use the following key to know if the recipe works with your specific allergy or allergies:

- ✔ **EF:** Egg free
- ✔ **MF:** Milk free
- ✔ **NF:** Nut free
- ✔ **PF:** Peanut free
- ✔ **SF:** Soy free
- ✔ **WF:** Wheat free

> **Recipes in This Chapter**
> - ▶ Caramel Popcorn
> - ▶ Chocolate Melt Away Cookies
> - ▶ Minty Cream Filling
> - ▶ Cinnamon Crunch Cookies
> - ▶ Molasses Cookies
> - ▶ Oatmeal Cookies
> - ▶ Rice Krispie Treats
> - ▶ Sugar Cookies
> - ▶ Traditional Holiday Sugar Cookies
>
>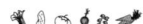

Caramel Popcorn

(EF, MF, NF, PF, SF,WF)

½ cup popping corn

1¾ cups honey

¼ cup milk-free, soy-free margarine

⅓ cup water

¼ teaspoon salt

1 Pop the popping corn. Set aside. Grease cookie sheets.

2 Combine the remaining ingredients in a saucepan and bring to a boil over medium heat, stirring continuously. Continue stirring occasionally until mixture reaches 280 degrees (use a candy thermometer).

3 Pour caramel mixture over popcorn, and stir well until coated. Spread on greased cookie sheets to cool.

Tip: *To make caramel popcorn balls, grease your hands and form mixture into balls while warm. Wrap in waxed paper to cool.*

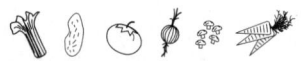

Chocolate Melt Away Cookies

(EF, MF, NF, PF, SF)

1½ cups flour

¼ cup cornstarch

⅓ cup unsweetened cocoa
powder

¼ teaspoon salt

½ cup milk-free, soy-free
margarine, softened

¾ cup sugar

3 tablespoons water, 3 tablespoons oil, 2
teaspoons
baking powder; mixed together

2 teaspoons vanilla extract

3 tablespoons water

1 In medium bowl, whisk together flour, cornstarch, unsweetened cocoa powder, and salt. Set aside.

2 In large bowl, beat margarine and sugar with electric mixer on medium speed until light and fluffy. Add remaining ingredients. Blend well.

3 Beat in flour mixture. Dough will be slightly crumbly.

4 Knead well with hands. Divide dough in half. Shape each half into log and cover with plastic wrap. Freeze 20 minutes.

5 Preheat oven to 350 degrees. Lightly grease cookie sheet. Set aside.

6 Unwrap dough and slice cookies ¼-inch thick. Bake 12 minutes. Cool completely.

7 Spread 1 teaspoon Minty Cream Filling (see next recipe) onto the bottoms of half of cookies. Top with remaining cookies, placing flat sides together. Press gently to sandwich together.

Minty Cream Filling

(EF, MF, NF, PF, SF, WF)

2 cups confectioners sugar

¼ cup shortening

1 tablespoon light corn syrup

¼ cup water

½ teaspoon vanilla extract

½ teaspoon mint extract

2 drops green food coloring

In large bowl, blend all ingredients together with electric mixer on medium speed until smooth and creamy.

Cinnamon Crunch Cookies

(EF, MF, NF, PF, SF)

1⅓ cups flour

1 teaspoon cream of tartar

½ teaspoon baking soda

⅛ teaspoon salt

½ cup milk-free, soy-free margarine, softened

¾ cup sugar

½ teaspoon vanilla extract

1½ tablespoons water, 1½ tablespoons oil, 1 teaspoon baking powder; mixed together

2 teaspoons ground cinnamon mixed with ¼ cup sugar

1 Preheat oven to 400 degrees. Grease cookie sheets.

2 Stir together flour, cream of tartar, baking soda, and salt; set aside.

3 In mixer bowl, combine margarine and sugar; beat until fluffy. Blend in vanilla. Beat in water, oil, and baking powder mixture. Gradually add to flour mixture, beating until just combined.

4 Drop by rounded teaspoons into the cinnamon-sugar mixture. Roll cookies to coat well, shaping them into balls as you roll. Arrange the balls about 1½ inches apart on greased baking sheets. Bake 8 to 10 minutes or until edges are golden brown. Transfer to wire racks to cool. Makes about 3 dozen cookies.

Tip: *This cookie mixture can go from freezer to oven.*

Molasses Cookies

(EF, MF, NF, PF, SF, WF)

¾ cup shortening

1 cup brown sugar, firmly packed

1½ tablespoons water, 1½ tablespoons oil, 1 teaspoon baking powder; mixed together

¼ cup molasses

2¼ cups barley flour

2 teaspoons baking soda

⅛ teaspoon salt

1 teaspoon ground cinnamon

1 teaspoon ground ginger

½ teaspoon ground cloves

½ cup sugar

1 Beat together shortening and brown sugar until soft and creamy. Add water, oil, and baking powder mixture and molasses. Mix well and set aside.

2 Combine flour, baking soda, salt, cinnamon, ginger, and cloves. Add to shortening mixture. Mix well. Cover and chill 2 hours.

3 Preheat oven to 350 degrees. Grease two cookie sheets; set aside. Shape dough into 1-inch balls; roll balls in remaining sugar. Place on cookie sheets. Bake 12 minutes. Move to wire racks to cool.

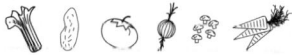

Oatmeal Cookies

(EF, MF, NF, PF, SF, WF)

½ cup shortening

½ cup dark brown sugar, firmly packed

½ cup sugar

¾ teaspoon vanilla extract

½ cup rice flour

½ teaspoon salt

2 teaspoons baking powder

6 tablespoons water

2 cups quick oats

1 Preheat oven to 350 degrees. Grease cookie sheet. Set aside.

2 In large bowl, cream shortening, sugars, and vanilla extract. Set aside.

3 In separate bowl, sift together rice flour, salt, and baking powder. Add to creamed mixture. Stir well. Add water and oatmeal; mix well.

4 Drop by teaspoonfuls onto cookie sheet. Bake 10 minutes.

Tip: Instead of washing your sifter every time you use it, hold it upside down over a garbage can and tap the bottom to get out crumbs and excess powder. If lumps are caught in it, soak it in hot, soapy water.

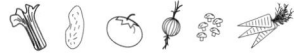

Rice Krispie Treats

(EF, MF, NF, PF, SF, WF)

¼ cup milk-free, soy-free margarine

1 package regular size milk-free, egg-free marshmallows

6 cups Kellogg's Rice Krispies cereal

1 Grease an 11-by-17-inch baking dish.

2 Melt the margarine in a large pot over low heat. Add marshmallows and stir until completely melted.

3 Remove from the heat and add Rice Krispies. Stir until the mixture is well coated.

4 Pour into baking dish and flatten with the back of a spoon. Let cool before cutting into bars.

Tip: To make an Easter bunny; shape approximately 3 cups of the mixture into a ball to form the body: Make a smaller ball for the head; using approximately 2 cups. Form the remaining cup of mixture into a ball to make the tail. Roll the tail in shredded coconut to give your Easter bunny a "cotton tail." Attach the head and tail to the body with toothpicks. Cut ears from pink construction paper and gently push them into the head. Cut whiskers from black construction paper, dip the end in honey; and attach them to the face.

WARNING: Be sure to remove the toothpicks before eating the bunny.

Tip: Shape the mixture into an Easter basket or birthday basket to fill with treats.

Sugar Cookies

(EF, MF, NF, PF, SF)

3 tablespoons milk-free, soy-free margarine, softened

⅔ cup sugar

1½ tablespoons water, 1½ tablespoons oil, 1 teaspoon baking powder; mixed together

1 tablespoon lemon juice

1½ cups flour

½ teaspoon baking soda

¼ teaspoon nutmeg

2 tablespoons sugar

1 Preheat oven to 375 degrees. Beat margarine and sugar with electric mixer on medium speed until creamy. Add water, oil, and baking powder mixture; stir well. Add lemon juice. Set aside.

2 In separate bowl, combine flour, baking soda, and nutmeg. Combine with wet mixture and stir until well blended.

3 Shape into balls and roll in remaining sugar. Place balls on ungreased cookie sheets, flatten into circle. Bake 9 minutes. Transfer to wire racks and cool completely.

Traditional Holiday Sugar Cookies

(EF, MF, NF, PF, SF)

1½ cups confectioners sugar

1 cup milk-free, soy-free margarine, softened

1½ teaspoons vanilla extract

1½ tablespoons water, 1½ tablespoons oil, 1 teaspoon baking powder; mixed together

2½ cups flour

1 teaspoon baking soda

1 teaspoon cream of tartar

1 In large bowl, combine confectioners sugar; margarine; vanilla extract; and water, oil, and baking powder mixture. Mix well. Stir in flour, baking soda, and cream of tartar. Cover and refrigerate 2 hours.

2 Preheat oven to 375 degrees. Lightly grease cookie sheet. Set aside. Divide dough in half. Place each half between two sheets of wax paper. Cut into desired shapes using holiday cookie cutters. Transfer cookies from wax paper to prepared cookie sheet. Bake 7 to 8 minutes or until edges are light brown. Transfer to wire rack. Cool. Frost if desired.

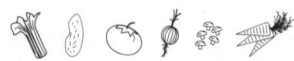

Appendix D

Cakes and Desserts

*W*hen most people bake a cake or pie or prepare some other dessert, they rely on the three staples of dessert dishes — wheat flour, eggs, and milk. Those are three of the top eight allergenic foods. If you're a dessert lover, passing on dessert is not an option, and it doesn't have to be. With these ten recipes on hand, you'll always have something to top off after the main course.

Use the following key to know if the recipe works with your specific allergy or allergies:

✔ **EF:** Egg free

✔ **MF:** Milk free

✔ **NF:** Nut free

✔ **PF:** Peanut free

✔ **SF:** Soy free

✔ **WF:** Wheat free

> **Recipes in This Chapter**
> - ▶ Fruit Crisp
> - ▶ Blondie Cake
> - ▶ Chocolate Pudding
> - ▶ Cream Filled Cupcakes
> - ▶ Hot Fudge Sauce
> - ▶ Pumpkin Pie
> - ▶ Raisin and Spice Cupcakes
> - ▶ Vanilla Frosting
> - ▶ Sweet Potato Pie
> - ▶ Wacky Chocolate Cake
>
>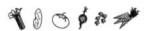

Fruit Crisp

(EF, MF, NF, PF, SF, WF)

16-ounce can sliced peaches

¼ cup cornstarch

2 tablespoons brown sugar

2 tablespoons milk-free, soy-free margarine

¼ cup quick oats

1 Preheat oven to 450 degrees. Grease a 1-quart casserole dish. Drain peaches and place in casserole dish. Set aside.

2 Blend together cornstarch, brown sugar, and margarine. Mix in oats. (Mixture will be lumpy.) Pour over peaches. Bake 20 minutes or until lightly browned.

Blondie Cake

(EF, MF, NF, PF, SF, WF)

1½ cups flour

1½ teaspoons baking powder

½ teaspoon salt

1 cup dark brown sugar, firmly packed

½ cup sugar

½ cup milk-free, soy-free margarine, softened

3 tablespoons water, 3 tablespoons oil, 2 teaspoons baking powder; mixed together

1 teaspoon vanilla extract

Preheat oven to 350 degrees. Grease 9-inch pan. Set aside. In medium bowl, combine flour, baking powder, and salt. Mix well. Set aside. In large bowl, mix brown sugar, sugar, and margarine. Beat until well combined. Add water, oil, and baking powder mixture; and vanilla extract. Beat until light and creamy. Add flour mixture and beat until well blended. Pour batter into prepared pan. Bake 30 minutes, or until light golden brown, and toothpick inserted in center comes out clean. Cool completely. Frost and decorate as desired.

Chocolate Pudding

(EF, MF, NF, PF, SF, WF)

1 cup sugar

⅓ cup unsweetened cocoa powder

5 tablespoons cornstarch

¼ teaspoon salt

3 cups water

1 tablespoon milk-free, soy-free margarine

1 teaspoon vanilla extract

1 Combine sugar, cocoa, cornstarch, and salt in a saucepan; mix well. Add water, stirring with a wire whisk until well blended. Bring to a boil over medium heat. Boil 1 minute, stirring constantly. Remove from heat. Stir in margarine and vanilla extract.

2 Pour into individual cups. Let cool to room temperature. Chill completely in refrigerator before serving.

Tip: For a less sweet taste, reduce sugar by ⅓ cup. This recipe can be used as a pie filling.

Cream Filled Cupcakes

(EF, MF, NF, PF, SF)

1½ cups flour	1 cup water
¾ cup sugar	¼ cup oil
¼ cup unsweetened cocoa powder	1 tablespoon vinegar
1 teaspoon baking soda	2 teaspoons vanilla extract
½ teaspoon salt	coarse orange sugar (optional)

1 Preheat oven to 375 degrees. Line muffin tins with paper liners. Set aside.

2 In large bowl, add all ingredients except colored sugar and mix well. Pour batter into prepared muffin tins. Bake 18 to 20 minutes or until toothpick inserted in center comes out clean. Cool 10 minutes. Move to wire rack. Cool completely. Remove paper liners from cupcakes.

3 Prepare Cream Filling (see next recipe). Pour filling into pastry bag fitted with small pastry tip. Insert pastry tip into bottom of cupcake. Squeeze filling into cupcake until cupcake starts to expand. Turn cupcake over and use filling to make a swirl design on top. Sprinkle with colored sugar if desired.

Cream Filling

(EF, MF, NF, PF, SF)

1¼ cups flour, divided	1 cup sugar
1 cup vanilla rice beverage	1½ teaspoons vanilla extract
1 cup milk-free, soy-free margarine, softened	dash of salt

In medium saucepan, combine ¼ cup flour and rice beverage. Cook over medium heat until thick, stirring constantly. Set aside and allow to cool completely. In medium bowl, whip margarine and sugar until fluffy. Add remaining flour, rice beverage mixture, vanilla extract, and salt; beat 5 minutes.

Tip: *To make a Thanksgiving cupcake, add a few drops of yellow or orange food coloring to the filling mixture. Use decorator gel to outline Pilgrim hats on the tops of cupcakes.*

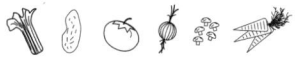

Hot Fudge Sauce

(EF, MF, NF, PF, SF, WF)

6 tablespoons milk-free, soy-free margarine

⅓ cup water

4 ounces unsweetened baking chocolate

1 cup sugar

3 tablespoons light corn syrup

⅛ teaspoon salt

2 teaspoons vanilla extract

1 In a small saucepan, combine margarine and water. Bring to a boil over medium heat, stirring continuously.

2 Add chocolate; stir occasionally until it melts. Chocolate mixture may be lumpy.

3 Add sugar, corn syrup, and salt. Boil 5 minutes. Remove from heat and add vanilla. Serve hot. Makes about 2 cups.

Pumpkin Pie

(EF, MF, NF, PF, SF, WF)

2 cups canned pumpkin

¾ cup brown sugar, firmly packed

1½ cups water

6½ tablespoons cornstarch

1 teaspoon cinnamon

½ teaspoon salt

¼ teaspoon ground cloves

½ teaspoon ginger

wheat-free pie crust (coconut pie crust works well; ¼ cup shortening, 2 cups coconut flakes, bake for 35 minutes or until light brown)

Preheat oven to 375 degrees. In a medium saucepan, combine all ingredients. Cook over medium heat until mixture begins to thicken, stirring constantly. Pour into pie crust. Bake 30 minutes or until firm. Remove pie from oven, sprinkle Coconut Topping (see next recipe) on top. Bake 5 more minutes.

Coconut Topping (optional)

¼ cup brown sugar

¼ cup coconut

Mix brown sugar and coconut. Sprinkle on top of pie.

Raisin and Spice Cupcakes

(EF, MF, NF, PF, SF, WF)

1½ cups sugar

1 cup milk-free, soy-free margarine, softened

3 tablespoons water, 3 tablespoons oil, 2 teaspoons baking powder; mixed together

2½ cups flour

2 teaspoons baking soda

2 teaspoons ground cinnamon

1 teaspoon ground cloves

½ teaspoon salt

¼ teaspoon ground nutmeg

2 cups applesauce

1 cup raisins

2 tablespoons confectioners sugar

Preheat oven to 350 degrees. Line muffin tins with paper liners. Set aside. In large bowl, beat sugar and margarine with electric mixer on medium speed until fluffy. Add water, oil, and baking powder mixture. Beat well. Stir in flour, baking soda, cinnamon, cloves, salt, nutmeg, applesauce, and raisins. Spoon batter into muffin tins, ⅔ full. Bake 30 minutes or until toothpick inserted in center comes out clean. Cool in pan 10 minutes. Transfer to wire racks and sprinkle confectioners sugar on tops of cupcakes. Cool completely before serving.

Tip: These cupcakes stay moist for days. They hold together better and are easily removed from the paper liners if made a day or two in advance. Can also be made as a cake using an 8x8-inch greased and floured pan. Bake 50 to 55 minutes at 350 degrees.

Vanilla Frosting

(EF, MF, NF, PF, SF, WF)

⅔ cup solid vegetable shortening

1-pound box confectioners sugar

3 tablespoons water

1 teaspoon vanilla extract

Cream shortening and sugar until well blended. Add water. Beat until smooth. Chill at least one hour. Beat again and add vanilla.

Tip: This frosting works well for making flowers and other decorations. It can be made with lemon or orange extract instead of vanilla.

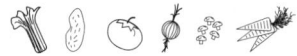

Sweet Potato Pie

(EF, MF, NF, PF, SF, WF)

1 (40-ounce) can sweet potatoes, drained

1 teaspoon ground cinnamon

dash of ground nutmeg

1 cup sugar

2 tablespoons milk-free, soy-free margarine, softened

½ teaspoon salt

1 cup apple juice

2 packets unflavored gelatin

4 tablespoons warm water

1 wheat-free pie crust, unbaked

1 Preheat oven to 350 degrees. In large bowl, mash sweet potatoes. Add cinnamon, nutmeg, and sugar. Mix well. Stir in margarine, salt, and apple juice. Set aside.

2 In small bowl, combine gelatin and warm water, stirring until gelatin dissolves. Add to sweet potato mixture. Mix well. Pour into pie crust. Bake 1 hour. Allow pie to set overnight before serving.

Tip: *This recipe was tested using a glass pie dish. Increase the oven temperature by 25 degrees if you use an aluminum pie pan.*

Wacky Chocolate Cake

(EF, MF, NF, PF, SF)

1½ cups flour

1 cup sugar

½ teaspoon salt

3 tablespoons unsweetened cocoa powder

1 teaspoon baking soda

1 teaspoon vanilla extract

1 tablespoon vinegar

5 tablespoons oil

1 cup cold water

confectioners sugar

Preheat oven to 350 degrees. Sift dry ingredients into mixing bowl. Add vanilla, vinegar, oil, and water. Blend well; pour into ungreased 9-inch square pan. Bake for 25 to 30 minutes. When cool, frost or sprinkle confectioners sugar on top.

Tip: *Omit cocoa powder, and add one mashed banana after adding water.*

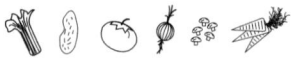

Appendix E

Glossary

• •

Adrenaline: See Epinephrine.

Allergen: Anything that triggers an allergic reaction. See also *food allergen* and *environmental allergen*.

Allergenic: A food that has the properties to trigger an allergic reaction.

Allergist: A doctor who specializes in the diagnosis and treatment of allergies. Some allergists have more knowledge of and experience with treating food allergies than others.

Amino acid: A basic building block for protein molecules.

Anaphylaxis: An immediate, severe, and sometimes fatal allergic reaction that can cause respiratory failure or shock due to a severe drop in blood pressure.

Angioedema: Swelling that typically accompanies hives and may result in welts (particularly on the face and around the eyes), stomachache (if the selling is in the intestines), or restricted or obstructed breathing (due to swelling in the airway).

Antibody: A good-guy protein that your body releases to attack what your immune system perceives as a threatening intruder. Unfortunately, when you have a food allergy, your body produces antibodies to perfectly harmless foods.

Antihistamine: Medication that prevents the body's release of histamine during an allergic reaction from affecting the tissues. Antihistamines do not stop the reaction but prevent the reaction from triggering some symptoms.

Anti-IgE antibody therapy: An allergy treatment that consists of IgG antibodies that bind with the IgE antibodies. IgG renders the IgE powerless and unable to trigger the massive release of histamines, which cause most symptoms. This therapy is still in the testing phase.

Atopic: Of or relating to allergies or asthma. Atopic conditions include asthma, hay fever, and some types of eczema.

Atopic dermatitis: Eczema that's triggered by or made worse by an allergic condition. See also Eczema.

Autoimmune disease: Any condition caused by the failure of the body's immune system to function normally. In some cases, the autoimmune system overreacts, and in other cases, it under-reacts.

Autoinjector: A device that enables patients to inject themselves with a pre-measured dose of medication, such as epinephrine. The two most common autoinjectors are the EpiPen and Twinject.

Avoidance diet: A food regimen designed to assist patients in steering clear of the foods that trigger reactions. The avoidance diet is the primary treatment approach for food allergies.

Basophils: White blood cells that protect the body from invading bacteria and viruses but that are also involved in the immune system's response to allergens. See also Mast cell.

Benadryl (Diphendydramine): An antihistamine that's one of the more effective medications in treating food allergy reactions. In the event of a severe reaction, however, Benadryl may not be effective, and epinephrine is required.

CAP-RAST: See RAST.

Complementary treatments: Any therapy that contributes to relieving symptoms but is not sufficient, in and of itself, to effectively treat a condition.

Corticosteroids: A steroid-based medication, such as prednisone, that can help prevent a recurrence of symptoms in the hours following a severe reaction and prevent late reactions, but that don't work rapidly enough to provide immediate relief.

Cross contamination: A situation in which a safe food is tainted with allergens from an unsafe food. Cross contamination can occur when a safe food is manufactured on the same equipment as an unsafe food, when safe food is prepared or served with tainted utensils, or when an unsafe food drops, splashes, or splatters into a safe food.

Cytotoxic testing: Any of several unproven methods of diagnosing allergies by exposing blood cells to suspected allergens and then examining the changes in those cells under a microscope.

Double-blind test: A treatment study in which neither the researchers nor the patients know who's receiving treatment and who's not until after the study is completed. See also Open test and Single-blind test.

Eczema: A persistent rash that is characterized by extreme dryness and itching of the skin and may or may not be caused by a food allergy. When food allergy is involved, the condition is commonly referred to as *atopic dermatitis*.

Entercolitis: Inflammation of the small and large intestine, commonly producing symptoms of fever, abdominal swelling, diarrhea, food malabsorption, constipation, and abdominal pain.

Environmental allergen: Airborne particles, including dust, molds, and pollens that trigger allergic reactions in some individuals.

Enzyme: A catalyst (speeder-upper) for the body's chemical reactions. In cases of food intolerance, you may be lacking an enzyme necessary for digesting a particular food.

Eosinophilic esophagitis: Inflammation of the esophagus often accompanied by pain, reflux, poor appetite, and difficulty swallowing.

Eosinophilic gastroenteritis: A chronic inflammation in the GI tract, sometimes localized and sometimes involving the entire GI tract. Eosinophilic gastroenteritis may or may not be related to food allergy and when it is, it's usually not IgE-mediated. See also Eosinophilic esophagitis and IgE-mediated food allergy.

Epinephrine: Another name for adrenaline, epinephrine is often administered via a shot during a severe allergic reaction to quickly alleviate symptoms.

FAHF-1: An ancient Chinese herbal formula that has proven somewhat effective in virtually curing peanut allergy in mice.

FAHF-2: A variant of this FAHF-1 that has proven as effective in treating peanut allergy in mice but is considered safer.

False negative: A test result that mistakenly shows that you're not allergic to something you really are allergic to.

False positive: A test result that mistakenly shows that you're allergic to something you're really not allergic to. False positives often convince some doctors to overly restrict a patient's diet.

Food allergen: A substance in a food, typically a protein, that triggers the immune system to overreact.

Food allergy: A condition that results when the body's immune system mistakenly identifies a particular food as an evil invader. Not to be confused with *food intolerance*.

Food challenge: An allergy test that consists of the patient consuming the food that the patient is suspected of being allergic to. Food challenges should be performed only under a qualified doctor's supervision and with emergency medications and equipment readily available.

Food intolerance: An inability of the body to digest a particular food or component of that food, typically due to the lack of an enzyme required to break down the food.

Food poisoning. The introduction of a poisonous substance, bacteria, virus, parasite, or other toxin into the body, often causing flu-like symptoms, including nausea, vomiting, and diarrhea.

Gastroesophageal reflux disease (GERD). Irritation or inflammation of the esophagus often caused by stomach acid backing up on the esophagus. Food allergy plays a role in up to one-third of cases of GERD in infants and may be the sole cause of the reflux in these cases.

Genetically engineered immunization shots: A treatment still in the testing phase that's designed to re-train the immune system to function properly by ramping up its response to disease-causing organisms and cranking down its response to food allergens.

Gluten: The protein in wheat and other grains that commonly triggers reactions in those with Celiac disease.

H2 blockers: A class of antihistamines, including Zantac (ranitidine) and Tagament (cimetidine), that are often effective when combined with antihistamines in the H1 class, such as Benedryl.

Histamine: A substance that your body produces during an allergic reaction that triggers the most symptoms, including runny nose, swelling, hives, and rashes. Histamine swells the blood vessels and makes them highly permeable.

Histamine poisoning: A condition in which enough histamine is ingested to produce symptoms very similar to those that appear during an allergic reaction. Several foods, including strawberries, chocolate, wine, and beer, may contain enough histamines to cause allergy-like symptoms.

Hives: See Urticaria.

Hygiene hypothesis: A theory that attributes the increasing incidence of food allergies in more developed countries over the past 20 years to the fact that people in developed countries are more obsessed with proper hygiene. The theory proposes that the less the immune system is exposed to germs and bacterial by-products the more energy it has to unleash on allergens.

Hypoallergenic: A product that's been produced to contain as few allergens as possible and is less likely to trigger an allergic reaction.

IgE-mediated food allergy: A food allergy in which the immune system produces IgE antibodies that trigger symptoms. Doctors can test the levels of IgE in your system to determine the likelihood that you're actually allergic to a specific food. See also Non-IgE-mediated food allergy.

Immune system: The body's defense system against bacteria, viruses, and anything else it identifies as an enemy invader. Unfortunately for those with food allergies, the immune system identifies one or more foods as harmful.

Immunoglobulin E (IgE): One of your body's antibodies that the immune system commonly releases during its overreaction to an allergenic food. Allergists often test for the presence of IgE in order to diagnose or rule out an allergy to a particular substance.

Immunotherapy: Any of various treatments designed to make the immune system more tolerant of allergens. Immunotherapy often consists of exposing the immune system to gradually increasing doses of the allergen over time.

Lactase: The enzyme required to break down lactose (milk sugar).

Lactose intolerance: An inability to digest milk sugar that triggers symptoms often mistakenly attributed to food allergy.

Leaky gut syndrome: A condition in which the walls of the intestines enable undigested food particles to pass through. Leaky gut syndrome is often mistakenly identified as a potential cause of food allergies.

Lymphocytes: White blood cells that that are the key to the immune system's response to defend the body against whatever the immune system identifies as a threat.

Mast cell: An immune system cell that releases histamine when an allergen enters the body, resulting in the most common allergy symptoms.

Non-IgE-mediated food allergy: A food allergy in which symptoms are not triggered by the presence of higher than normal concentrations of IgE antibodies. Non-IgE-mediated food allergies typically produce symptoms that appear more gradually and last longer, such as gastro-intestinal problems.

Open test: A treatment study in which researchers and patients know who's receiving treatment and who's not. Because everyone is aware of what's going on, results may be influenced by the placebo effect. See also Double-blind test and Single-blind test.

Oral allergy syndrome: A reaction restricted to the lips and mouth and is characterized by itching (sometimes severe) and swelling (usually mild). Oral allergy syndrome is most often caused by allergies to fresh fruits and vegetables in people with severe pollen allergies.

Probiotics: Beneficial bacteria, such as those found in yogurt, that may optimize the functioning of the immune system, improving its ability to defend the body against harmful bacteria and viruses while decreasing its tendency to overreact to food allergens.

Proctitis: Inflammation, itching, or soreness around the rectum which may or may not be related to food allergy. When it is related to food allergy, it's called allergic proctitis.

Protein: An assemblage of amino acid chains that's present in foods and throughout the body. Foods that cause allergic reactions commonly contain proteins that the immune system mistakenly identifies as dangerous.

RAST: Short for radioallergosorbent test, RAST is a blood test that helps diagnose the presence of IgE antibodies to specific foods. RASTs can help your doctor identify or rule out particular food allergies, but RAST results are not always conclusive. (Sometimes referred to as called the CAP-RAST or ImmunoCap test, which are the RASTs that have been best tested for the diagnosis of food allergy.)

Rotation diet: A treatment approach that consists of avoiding certain foods or food groups on a temporary basis. Rotation diets are not considered a primary treatment for people with food allergies, especially those who experience severe reactions.

Sensitization: The process by which a genetic susceptibility to an allergy develops into an actual allergy through one or more exposures to an allergen.

Single-blind test: A treatment study in which researchers know who's receiving treatment and who's not, but the patients don't. Because the researcher may unknowingly communicate, through body language, who's getting treatment and who's not, single-blind testing may also be influenced by the placebo effect. See also Double-blind test and Open test.

Skin test: An allergy test in which suspected allergens are placed below the top layer of skin to determine whether the body reacts to the substance.

Sulfite: A substance found in relatively high concentrations in some wines and food additives, including MSG (monosodium glutamate), that can cause chemical reactions in the body that produce symptoms very similar to those that appear in allergic reactions.

Urticaria: Fancy name for hives — reddish raised itchy areas that form on the skin often as the result of an allergic reaction, or a variety of other causes.

Index

• *Alphabetical* •

• Recipes by Allergy •

• *Recipes by Course* •

• *General Index* •

• *Numerics* •

• *A* •

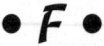

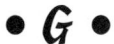

● **G** ●

• *M* •

BUSINESS, CAREERS & PERSONAL FINANCE

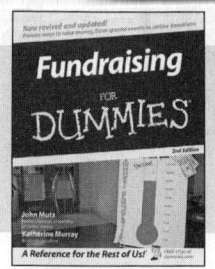

0-7645-9847-3   0-7645-2431-3

Also available:

Business Plans Kit For Dummies
0-7645-9794-9

Economics For Dummies
0-7645-5726-2

Grant Writing For Dummies
0-7645-8416-2

Home Buying For Dummies
0-7645-5331-3

Managing For Dummies
0-7645-1771-6

Marketing For Dummies
0-7645-5600-2

Personal Finance For Dummies
0-7645-2590-5*

Resumes For Dummies
0-7645-5471-9

Selling For Dummies
0-7645-5363-1

Six Sigma For Dummies
0-7645-6798-5

Small Business Kit For Dummies
0-7645-5984-2

Starting an eBay Business For Dummies
0-7645-6924-4

Your Dream Career For Dummies
0-7645-9795-7

HOME & BUSINESS COMPUTER BASICS

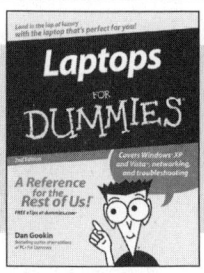
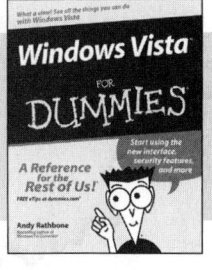

0-470-05432-8   0-471-75421-8

Also available:

Cleaning Windows Vista For Dummies
0-471-78293-9

Excel 2007 For Dummies
0-470-03737-7

Mac OS X Tiger For Dummies
0-7645-7675-5

MacBook For Dummies
0-470-04859-X

Macs For Dummies
0-470-04849-2

Office 2007 For Dummies
0-470-00923-3

Outlook 2007 For Dummies
0-470-03830-6

PCs For Dummies
0-7645-8958-X

Salesforce.com For Dummies
0-470-04893-X

Upgrading & Fixing Laptops For Dummies
0-7645-8959-8

Word 2007 For Dummies
0-470-03658-3

Quicken 2007 For Dummies
0-470-04600-7

FOOD, HOME, GARDEN, HOBBIES, MUSIC & PETS

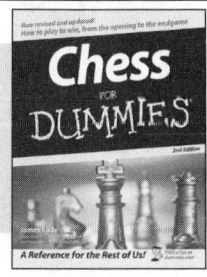
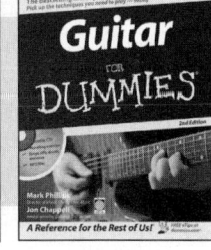

0-7645-8404-9   0-7645-9904-6

Also available:

Candy Making For Dummies
0-7645-9734-5

Card Games For Dummies
0-7645-9910-0

Crocheting For Dummies
0-7645-4151-X

Dog Training For Dummies
0-7645-8418-9

Healthy Carb Cookbook For Dummies
0-7645-8476-6

Home Maintenance For Dummies
0-7645-5215-5

Horses For Dummies
0-7645-9797-3

Jewelry Making & Beading For Dummies
0-7645-2571-9

Orchids For Dummies
0-7645-6759-4

Puppies For Dummies
0-7645-5255-4

Rock Guitar For Dummies
0-7645-5356-9

Sewing For Dummies
0-7645-6847-7

Singing For Dummies
0-7645-2475-5

INTERNET & DIGITAL MEDIA

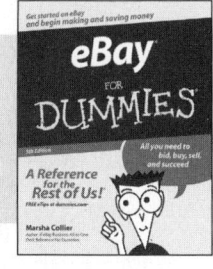
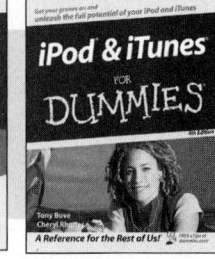

0-470-04529-9   0-470-04894-8

Also available:

Blogging For Dummies
0-471-77084-1

Digital Photography For Dummies
0-7645-9802-3

Digital Photography All-in-One Desk Reference For Dummies
0-470-03743-1

Digital SLR Cameras and Photography For Dummies
0-7645-9803-1

eBay Business All-in-One Desk Reference For Dummies
0-7645-8438-3

HDTV For Dummies
0-470-09673-X

Home Entertainment PCs For Dummies
0-470-05523-5

MySpace For Dummies
0-470-09529-6

Search Engine Optimization For Dummies
0-471-97998-8

Skype For Dummies
0-470-04891-3

The Internet For Dummies
0-7645-8996-2

Wiring Your Digital Home For Dummies
0-471-91830-X

* Separate Canadian edition also available
† Separate U.K. edition also available

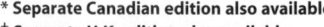

Available wherever books are sold. For more information or to order direct: U.S. customers visit www.dummies.com or call 1-877-762-2974. U.K. customers visit www.wileyeurope.com or call 0800 243407. Canadian customers visit www.wiley.ca or call 1-800-567-4797.

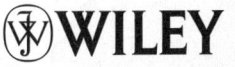

SPORTS, FITNESS, PARENTING, RELIGION & SPIRITUALITY

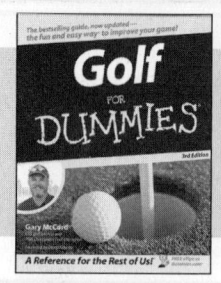

0-471-76871-5

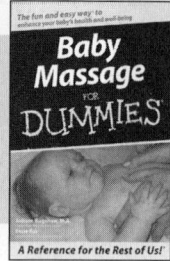

0-7645-7841-3

Also available:
- Catholicism For Dummies
  0-7645-5391-7
- Exercise Balls For Dummies
  0-7645-5623-1
- Fitness For Dummies
  0-7645-7851-0
- Football For Dummies
  0-7645-3936-1
- Judaism For Dummies
  0-7645-5299-6
- Potty Training For Dummies
  0-7645-5417-4
- Buddhism For Dummies
  0-7645-5359-3

- Pregnancy For Dummies
  0-7645-4483-7 †
- Ten Minute Tone-Ups For Dummies
  0-7645-7207-5
- NASCAR For Dummies
  0-7645-7681-X
- Religion For Dummies
  0-7645-5264-3
- Soccer For Dummies
  0-7645-5229-5
- Women in the Bible For Dummies
  0-7645-8475-8

TRAVEL

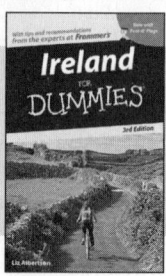

0-7645-7749-2

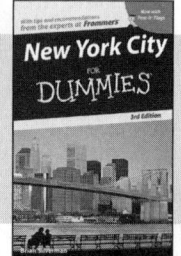

0-7645-6945-7

Also available:
- Alaska For Dummies
  0-7645-7746-8
- Cruise Vacations For Dummies
  0-7645-6941-4
- England For Dummies
  0-7645-4276-1
- Europe For Dummies
  0-7645-7529-5
- Germany For Dummies
  0-7645-7823-5
- Hawaii For Dummies
  0-7645-7402-7

- Italy For Dummies
  0-7645-7386-1
- Las Vegas For Dummies
  0-7645-7382-9
- London For Dummies
  0-7645-4277-X
- Paris For Dummies
  0-7645-7630-5
- RV Vacations For Dummies
  0-7645-4442-X
- Walt Disney World & Orlando
  For Dummies
  0-7645-9660-8

GRAPHICS, DESIGN & WEB DEVELOPMENT

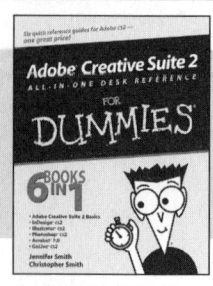

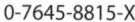

0-7645-8815-X

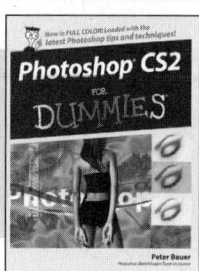

0-7645-9571-7

Also available:
- 3D Game Animation For Dummies
  0-7645-8789-7
- AutoCAD 2006 For Dummies
  0-7645-8925-3
- Building a Web Site For Dummies
  0-7645-7144-3
- Creating Web Pages For Dummies
  0-470-08030-2
- Creating Web Pages All-in-One Desk
  Reference For Dummies
  0-7645-4345-8
- Dreamweaver 8 For Dummies
  0-7645-9649-7

- InDesign CS2 For Dummies
  0-7645-9572-5
- Macromedia Flash 8 For Dummies
  0-7645-9691-8
- Photoshop CS2 and Digital
  Photography For Dummies
  0-7645-9580-6
- Photoshop Elements 4 For Dummies
  0-471-77483-9
- Syndicating Web Sites with RSS Feeds
  For Dummies
  0-7645-8848-6
- Yahoo! SiteBuilder For Dummies
  0-7645-9800-7

NETWORKING, SECURITY, PROGRAMMING & DATABASES

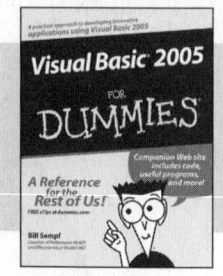

0-7645-7728-X

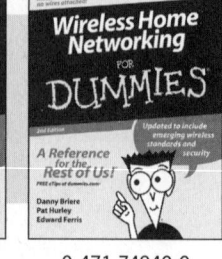

0-471-74940-0

Also available:
- Access 2007 For Dummies
  0-470-04612-0
- ASP.NET 2 For Dummies
  0-7645-7907-X
- C# 2005 For Dummies
  0-7645-9704-3
- Hacking For Dummies
  0-470-05235-X
- Hacking Wireless Networks
  For Dummies
  0-7645-9730-2
- Java For Dummies
  0-470-08716-1

- Microsoft SQL Server 2005 For Dummies
  0-7645-7755-7
- Networking All-in-One Desk Reference
  For Dummies
  0-7645-9939-9
- Preventing Identity Theft For Dummies
  0-7645-7336-5
- Telecom For Dummies
  0-471-77085-X
- Visual Studio 2005 All-in-One Desk
  Reference For Dummies
  0-7645-9775-2
- XML For Dummies
  0-7645-8845-1

HEALTH & SELF-HELP

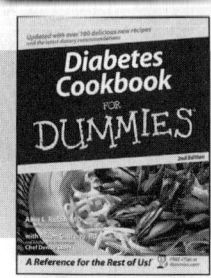

0-7645-8450-2

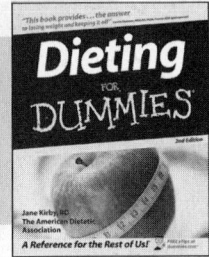

0-7645-4149-8

Also available:
- Bipolar Disorder For Dummies
  0-7645-8451-0
- Chemotherapy and Radiation
  For Dummies
  0-7645-7832-4
- Controlling Cholesterol For Dummies
  0-7645-5440-9
- Diabetes For Dummies
  0-7645-6820-5* †
- Divorce For Dummies
  0-7645-8417-0 †

- Fibromyalgia For Dummies
  0-7645-5441-7
- Low-Calorie Dieting For Dummies
  0-7645-9905-4
- Meditation For Dummies
  0-471-77774-9
- Osteoporosis For Dummies
  0-7645-7621-6
- Overcoming Anxiety For Dummies
  0-7645-5447-6
- Reiki For Dummies
  0-7645-9907-0
- Stress Management For Dummies
  0-7645-5144-2

EDUCATION, HISTORY, REFERENCE & TEST PREPARATION

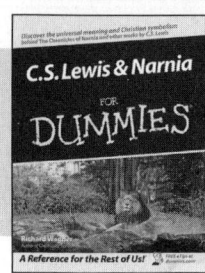

0-7645-8381-6

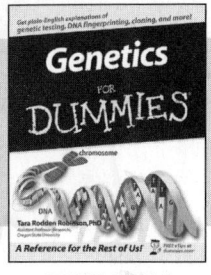

0-7645-9554-7

Also available:
- The ACT For Dummies
  0-7645-9652-7
- Algebra For Dummies
  0-7645-5325-9
- Algebra Workbook For Dummies
  0-7645-8467-7
- Astronomy For Dummies
  0-7645-8465-0
- Calculus For Dummies
  0-7645-2498-4
- Chemistry For Dummies
  0-7645-5430-1
- Forensics For Dummies
  0-7645-5580-4

- Freemasons For Dummies
  0-7645-9796-5
- French For Dummies
  0-7645-5193-0
- Geometry For Dummies
  0-7645-5324-0
- Organic Chemistry I For Dummies
  0-7645-6902-3
- The SAT I For Dummies
  0-7645-7193-1
- Spanish For Dummies
  0-7645-5194-9
- Statistics For Dummies
  0-7645-5423-9

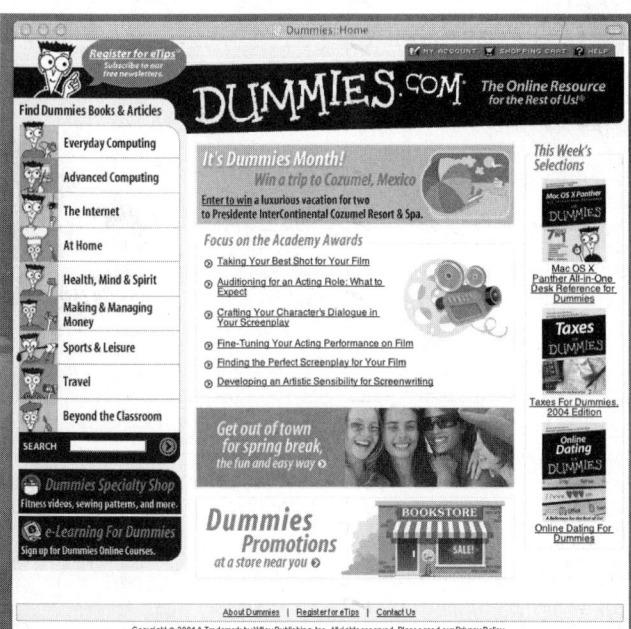

Get smart @ dummies.com®
- **Find a full list of Dummies titles**
- **Look into loads of FREE on-site articles**
- **Sign up for FREE eTips e-mailed to you weekly**
- **See what other products carry the Dummies name**
- **Shop directly from the Dummies bookstore**
- **Enter to win new prizes every month!**

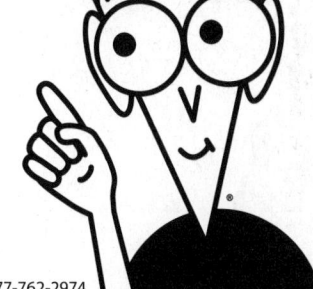

* Separate Canadian edition also available
† Separate U.K. edition also available

Available wherever books are sold. For more information or to order direct: U.S. customers visit www.dummies.com or call 1-877-762-2974.
U.K. customers visit www.wileyeurope.com or call 0800 243407. Canadian customers visit www.wiley.ca or call 1-800-567-4797.

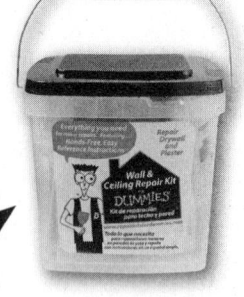
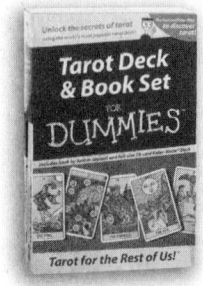
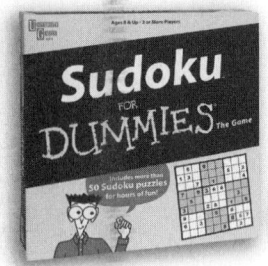
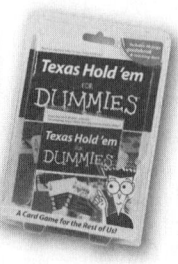
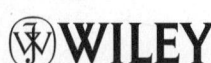